X-RAY DIFFERENTIAL DIAGNOSIS IN SMALL BOWEL DISEASE

SERIES IN RADIOLOGY

J. Odo Op den Orth, The Standard Biphasic-Contrast Examination of the Stomach and Duodenum: Method, Results and Radiological Atlas.
1979. ISBN 90 247 2159 8

J.L. Sellink and R.E. Miller, Radiology of the Small Bowel. Modern Enteroclysis Technique and Atlas.
1981. ISBN 90 247 2460 0

R.E. Miller and J. Skucas, The Radiological Examination of the Colon. Practical Diagnosis.
1983. ISBN 90 247 2666 2

S. Forgács, Bones and Joints in Diabetes Melitus.
1982. ISBN 90 247 2395 7

G. Németh and H. Kuttig, Isodose Atlas. For Use in Radiotherapy.
1981. ISBN 90 247 2476 7

J. Chermet, Atlas of Phlebography of the Lower Limbs, including the Iliac Veins.
1982. ISBN 90 247 2525 9

B. Janevski, Angiography of the Upper Extremity.
1982. ISBN 90 247 2684 0

M.A.M. Feldberg, Computed Tomography of the Retroperitoneum. An Anatomical and Pathological Atlas with Emphasis on the Fascial Planes.
1983. ISBN 0 89838 573 3

L.E.H. Lampmann, S.A. Duursma and J.H.J. Ruys, CT Densitometry in Osteoporosis. The Impact on Management of the Patient.
1984. ISBN 0 89838 633 0

J.J. Broerse and T.J. MacVittie, Response of Different Species to Total Body Irradiation.
1984. ISBN 0 89838 678 0

C. L'Herminé, Radiology of Liver Circulation.
1985. ISBN 0 89838 715 9

G. Maatman, High-resolution Computed Tomography of the Paranasal Sinuses, Pharynx and Related Regions.
1986. ISBN 0 89838 802 3

C. Plets, A.L. Baert, G.L. Nijs and G. Wilms, Computer Tomographic Imaging and Anatomic Correlation of the Human Brain.
1986. ISBN 0 89838 811 2

J. Valk, MRI of the Brain, Head, Neck and Spine. A Teaching Atlas of Clinical Applications.
1987. ISBN 0 89838 957 7

J.L. Selllink, X-Ray Differential Diagnosis in Small Bowel Disease. A Practical Approach.
1988. ISBN 0 89838 351 X

T.H.M. Falke, ed., Essentials of Clinical MRI.
1988. ISBN 0 89838 353 6

X-RAY DIFFERENTIAL DIAGNOSIS IN DIAGNOSIS IN SMALL BOWEL DISEASE

A Practical Approach

J. L. SELLINK, M.D.

Kluwer Academic Publishers
Dordrecht / Boston / London

Library of Congress Cataloging in Publication Data

Sellink, J. L.
   X-ray differential diagnosis in small bowel disease.

   (Series in radiology)
   1. Intestine, Small--Diseases--Diagnosis.
2. Intestine, Small--Radiography. 3. Diagnosis,
Differential. I. Title. II. Series. [DNLM:
1. Diagnosis, Differential--handbooks. 2. Intestine,
Small--radiography--handbooks. WI 39 S467x]
RC804.R6S455   1988   616.3'40757   87-28241
ISBN-13:978-94-010-7080-5   e-ISBN-13:978-94-009-1305-9
DOI: 10.1007/978-94-009-1305-9   87-28241

Published by Kluwer Academic Publishers
P.O. Box 17, 3300 AA Dordrecht, The Netherlands

Kluwer Academic Publishers incorporates the publishing programmes of
D. Reidel, Martinus Nijhoff, Dr W. Junk and MTP Press

Sold and distributed in the U.S.A. and Canada
by Kluwer Academic Publishers,
101 Philip Drive, Norwell, MA 02061, U.S.A.

In all other countries, sold and distributed
by Kluwer Academic Publishers Group,
P.O. Box 322, 3300 AH Dordrecht, The Netherlands

Translation: R.D.R. Birtwhistle, M.B.Ch.B.

Contents

I. Introduction

Publication of this book has been stimulated by 15 years experience with contrast fluid irrigation techniques of the small intestine and in particular by examinations performed and evaluated by colleagues.

The classification of the X-ray pathology has been arranged to give a more effective application in practice than is usually found in current handbooks. Normally this classification is adapted to that of formal anatomic pathology and internal medicine. In this book the classification is based on the radiological symptomatology. Thus, often completely unassociated conditions are found listed as a possible cause for each observed sign. When, as a result of the examination a number of pathological signs are found, a choice based on clinical probability must be made of the responsible condition.

On the X-ray's received from collegues I have frequently found abnormalities which, though clearly demonstrable, were not recognized as pathological because of insufficient knowledge of the normal picture and its variations. In other cases the abnormalities were indeed recognized but, and this after much time-wasting search through various books, attributed to an irrelevant group of diseases. Consideration of clinical data can be of assistance in reaching a good diagnosis but on the other hand can lead to faulty conclusions. It is well to remember that radiological diagnosis has its own peculiar signs with appropriate diagnostic possibilities and that these must be very seriously considered even when the result differs from that clinically expected.

It was also noticeable that abnormalities were incompletely demonstrated or completely missed because the examination was not performed adequately. Negligence in outlining the duodenum, where the filling had not been or could not be performed and duodenal abnormalities thus not visualised, occurred frequently.

All too frequently failure to maintain the proper infusion rate, by many erroneously totally under-evaluated, had the result that disturbances in motility were missed.

Additional and often too early administration of water, a measure that is seldom indicated and tends to produce more bad results than good, is quite frequently performed as a sort of panic reaction. The few indications for this procedure ought to be known and strictly followed, superfluous application costs more time and causes unnecessary discomfort for the patient.

The intention of this book with its deviant, practice dictated arrangement, should assist in enabling the radiologist, in accordance with this era of efficiency, to reach a probability diagnosis rapidly and effectively. Should he wish to make a deeper study of the conditions that he expects to encounter then he is advised to consult the known manuals and further professional literature.

A more or less thorough description of the whole scala of pathological conditions would completely miss the goal at which this book aims.

A list of references has been deliberately omitted for the sake of efficiency, a keyword index is also absent as the list of contents is for this end sufficient. No book is perfect, including this, but even so all the conditions that the author has encountered in the last 15 years and over 10.000 enteroclysis examinations are, according to their radiological signs, mentioned in one of more contexts, which is sufficient in daily practice.

Groenloseweg 49   J.L. SELLINK
7101 AC Winterswijk   *Spring 1988*
The Netherlands
Telephone 05430-19296

II. Examination technique

A. General

The objection to administration of the contrast medium by drinking is that the degree of small bowel filling is largely dependant on the emptying rate of the stomach and the amount imbibed.

In general, poor filling of the intestine means a slow transit with inconvenient thickening of the contrast medium in the ileum and an enhanced tendency to flocculation, usually beginning as high as the jejunum. Inadequate filling makes visualisation of the mucosa difficult and this is aggravated by dehydration of the barium suspension while flocculation renders any examination of the mucosa impossible. The technique of enteroclysis, also called 'Small Bowel Enema', introduced in 1970, where the contrast fluid is delivered directly into the duodenum by a tube, completely eliminates all these disadvantages.

The enteroclysis technique possesses the following advantages:

1. The administration of the contrast medium is more rapid than by drinking and is further adjustable to requirements. Even very large amounts of contrast medium can be administered.
2. Supplementary administration of transit accelerators, water or air is extremely easy through the tube.
3. The examination is fully under control and the time required very short, about 20-25 min, including the time necessary for intubation.
4. By rapid administration of a large amount of contrast medium flocculation of the barium suspension can be avoided even under the most unfavorable circumstances. Should it be desired to record this trivial phenomenon, one or two exposures can be made at e.g. 10 and 20 min after the examination.
5. The good degree of filling makes a diagnosis of celiac disease in many cases certain or highly probable which is seldom the case with a conventional follow-through examination (fig. II.1).
6. Small mucosal lesions, crossing bands, prestenotic dilatations and fistula canals are so strikingly illustrated that they are much more easily diagnosed than by the conventional method.
7. In a case of mechanical ileus the cause can usually be traced within an hour while the diagnosis 'paralytic ileus' can be confirmed in a few minutes, thus often making further examination superfluous.
8. Last but not least insight into intestinal motility and its disturbances is gained as a result of the standardised administration rate. Confirmation of both, hyper- and hypomotility of the intestine has proved to be of great importance as these signs are significant in several conditions.

B. Preparation of patients

Both for the preparation of the patient and for the adequate conducting of the examination some knowledge of the physiology of the digestive tract is essential. Some of the more important points are mentioned below:

Slow peristaltic movement is enhanced by:
    A raised fat and glucose blood level.
    Contrast media with calorific value.
    Medication with sedatives, antispasmodics and similar agents.
    Factors causing delayed gastric emptying.
Rapid gastric emptying is enhanced by:
    The patient lying on his right side.
    Isotonic stomach contents.

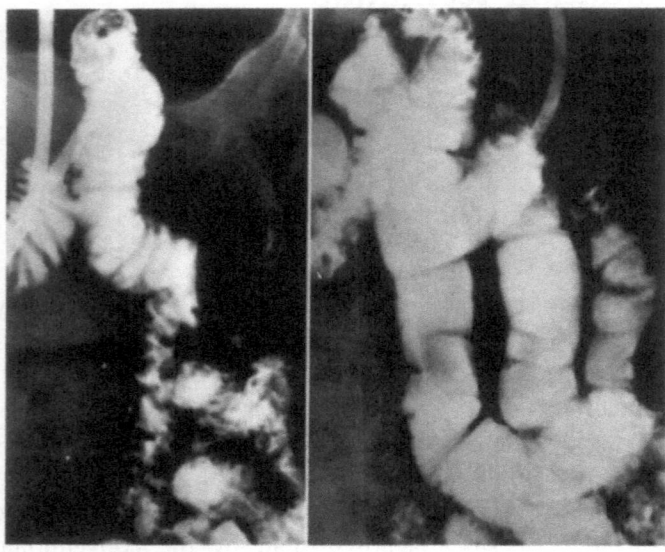

Fig. II.1. Patient with celiac disease with only slight atrophy of the mucosa in the jejunum. The presence of this disease was discovered by means of röntgenological examination (the celiac disease provocative test). The abnormalities are only visible when the intestine is well filled. The slight atrophy of the folds is similar to that seen in amyloidosis. Localization in the most proximal part of the jejunum made celiac disease the diagnosis of choice.

Stomach contents of about Ph.7.

Administration of metoclopramide.

Delayed transit in the distal ileum can be caused by:

An obstruction in this area.

Inflammation in this area.

A contaminated cecum (poor cleansing).

Remnants of food in the distal ileum.

Insufficiency of Bauhin's valve.

In the small intestine the intensity of all reflexes, including that of peristaltic movement arising from stretching of the bowel wall, diminishes gradually from the proximal to the distal end.

For small intestine examination the patient ought to appear in the department fully fasted, thus without any stomach contents. In the presence of stomach contents the stomach attempts to convey these into the duodenum, the pylorus cannot close and reflux of contrast medium from the duodenum occurs.

Further, the cecum and therefore the entire colon should be absolutely empty. A poor laxative result causes a serious delay of transit in the ileum, a markedly higher dose of contrast medium, longer examination time and poor quality of the compression details in the lower abdomen. A good method of cleansing the colon is a combination of magnesium sulphate and abundant water intake, preferably for two successive days.

Use of a rectal enema for cleansing the colon is most strictly contraindicated as reflux of enema fluid into the ileum frequently occurs and many patients are unable to rid themselves of this fluid within a reasonable time. Pre-examination diet seems to be of little significance if this method of thorough colon irrigation by oral intake is employed, but it is advisable that the last meal on the day before the examination should not be taken late or be too heavy.

C. Duodenal intubation

After some practice this procedure usually takes a few minutes in most patients and an average fluoroscopy time of 10×1 sec.

The tube should be about 135 cm long and the sightly flexible guide wire some 6 cm shorter. The so-called Sellink modification of the Bilbao-Dotter tube is specially suited for enteroclysis. Introduction of the tube through the mouth is generally the most rapid method but is so often accompanied by gagging that many patients prefer the nasal route. A minor disadvantage is the increased difficulty in manipulation of the guide wire through the fixed curve in the nasopharyngeal area. Moreover the tube must be lubricated and the nasal mucous membranes anaesthetised. Some bleeding from these membranes is sometimes unavoidable.

To avoid troublesome curling of the tube in the gastric fundus further insertion of the tube must be performed with the patient in the standing position. This is generally successful. The sitting and certainly the lying position is contraindicated. When the tube is thought to have reached the stomach cavity this can be confirmed by one or two seconds of fluoroscopy. If this is the case, the patient can lie down and proceed further with insertion of the tube himself, following the instructions of the operator. Passage of the pylorus sometimes demands a bit of patience as too much haste may be punished by curling of the tube and consequent withdrawal and starting again. The operator must take care that the guide wire does not pass the pyloric canal as its withdrawal may cause difficulties. When the tip of the tube has reached the duodenal-jejunal flexure the guide

wire can be completely withdrawn. A more proximal position for this tip enhances reflux of contrast medium into the stomach and certainly with too high an infusion rate or a reduced peristalsis, conditions which unfortunately both frequently occur.

If curling of the tube in the stomach has occurred the straight wire must be replaced by one in which the terminal 4 to 5 cm is bent at a right angle. The operator must then manipulate the guide wire with the aid of fluoroscopy until the tube assumes the proper direction. This procedure which can be performed with the patient standing or lying sometimes demands several minutes fluoroscopy. As soon as the loop has been removed the bent guide wire is replaced by a straight one and the patient can continue with insertion of the tube (fig: II.A). In thin subjects

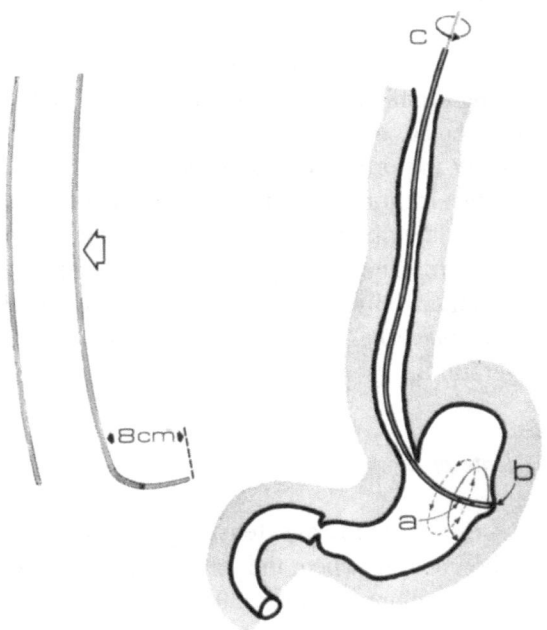

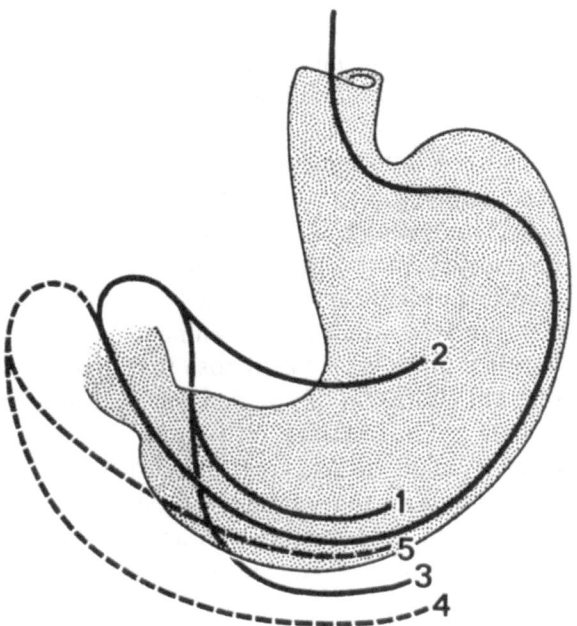

Fig. II.2A. Procedure in the event of coiling in the cardia: Insert the bent guide wire (arrows) until the tube slightly nudges the wall of the stomach (b) and then rotate at (c) until the end of the guide wire points in the direction of the antrum. Now replace the curved guide wire with a straight one. Note: if the end of the tube with the bent guide wire does not touch the wall of the stomach, it will keep springing back into the incorrect position (a). Slow rotation of the guide wire and tube together will usually avoid this problem. An upright position for this procedure is recommended.

Fig. II.2B. Possible positions of the tube when the patient is in supine position. (1) The tube is usually not correctly positioned because it passes through the pylorus in the medial direction and turns back along the side of the greater curvature in the stomach. (2) The tube is probably correctly positioned because it turns back in a plane above the level of the side of the greater curvature of the stomach. (3) The tube is almost certainly correctly positioned because it crosses the side of the greater curvature and then turns back at a lower level. (4/5) The tube passes through the pylorus in the lateral direction; the tube is then correctly positioned even if it turns back at the same level as the side of the greater curvature.

who are under medication with sedatives or anti-spasmodics the duodenum can be so dilated and lacking in peristaltic activity that the tube cannot pass the space between the aorta and the superior mesenteric artery. In this case it is better to accept this situation than to persist in an attempt to reach the ligament of Treitz, as there is considerable risk that such an attempt will be punished by retro-flexion of the tube in the duodenum. The tip then comes to lie in or near the duodenal bulb and contrast medium refluxes into the stomach (fig: IV.81). Curling of the tube in the duodenum can be corrected only by withdrawal completely into the stomach. Similarly, curling of the tube within the stomach forms a most undesirable situation as a single regurgitory movement is enough to pull the tip of the tube out of the duodenum into the stomach. A short but very hard tug on the tube often succeeds in removing the loop without causing the tip to fall back into the stomach. Passage of the pylorus can be verified by turning the patient on to his right side. Just before the vertebral column, with which it forms a right angle, the tip of the tube nearly always turns downwards into the duodenum. If the patient is very immobile in a recumbent position the sketch in fig: II.2B can be of considerable assistance in determining the position of the tube. Very con-siderable benefit can be obtained by tilting of the X-ray tube by means of telecommand equipment.

It is a grave error to suppose that there is no sense in intubation of resection stomachs due to lack of pylorus closure. A Bilroth II resection empties after drinking of contrast fluid less quickly than by the standard infusion rate of an enteroclysis. In a resection stomach, provided peristalsis is normal, no contrast medium appears proximal to the tip of the tube. Some increase of infusion rate is often desirable with resection stomachs as these occasionally show a very brisk peristaltic activity and an increased tendency to flocculation of the barium suspension.

In the presence of efficient peristalsis and nor-mal anatomy the duodenum does not always fill, so that it may be necessary to withdraw the tube a little at the end of the examination and thus complete the filling. It is selfevident that this must happen before any contrast medium has reached the transverse colon.

D. Contrast fluid and films

1. Properties

The optimal specific gravity for the contrast fluid has been determined in a series of tests on a range of subjects. The values were found to lie within the following limits; for normal patients between 1.25 and 1.30, for slender or juvenile patients 1.20 and for babies 1.15. Translated into working terms this gives values of 40% wt/vol for normal patients, 30% wt/vol for thin patients or juveniles and 20% wt/vol for babies.

Foaming of the barium suspension must be scrupulously avoided as the minute gas bubbles so produced can be very difficult to differentiate from swollen villi or lymphfollicles.

Addition of sorbitol or other hyperosmotic sub-stances to the suspension is to be avoided since they dilute the contrast medium by absorption of fluid and tend thus to give rise to flocculation. When a standard infusion system is used for daily recurring examinations the maintenance of a con-stant viscosity of the contrast medium, which is extremely important for achieving reproducable flow rates, is more easy. To this end the contrast fluid should not be cooled but stored at room temperature. The best system is to prepare the contrast fluid daily, sufficient for the examinations on the *following* day, and store it without refrigeration.

2. Rate of flow and dose

A comparative study of extensive patient material has shown that when the rate of flow of the contrast medium averages 50, 75, 100 and 125 ml/min, the amount of contrast fluid required to reach the cecum is 655, 695, 745 and 835 ml, respectively (M. Oudkerk, PhD dissertation, 'Infusion rate in enteroclysis examination', Leiden University, 1981).

Furthermore it appeared that:

1) When the rate of flow is 50 ml/min or less, filling of the intestine is so inadequate that the evaluation potential is as limited as that with a conventional transit examination. Disturbed motility, moderate obstructions, mucosal atro-

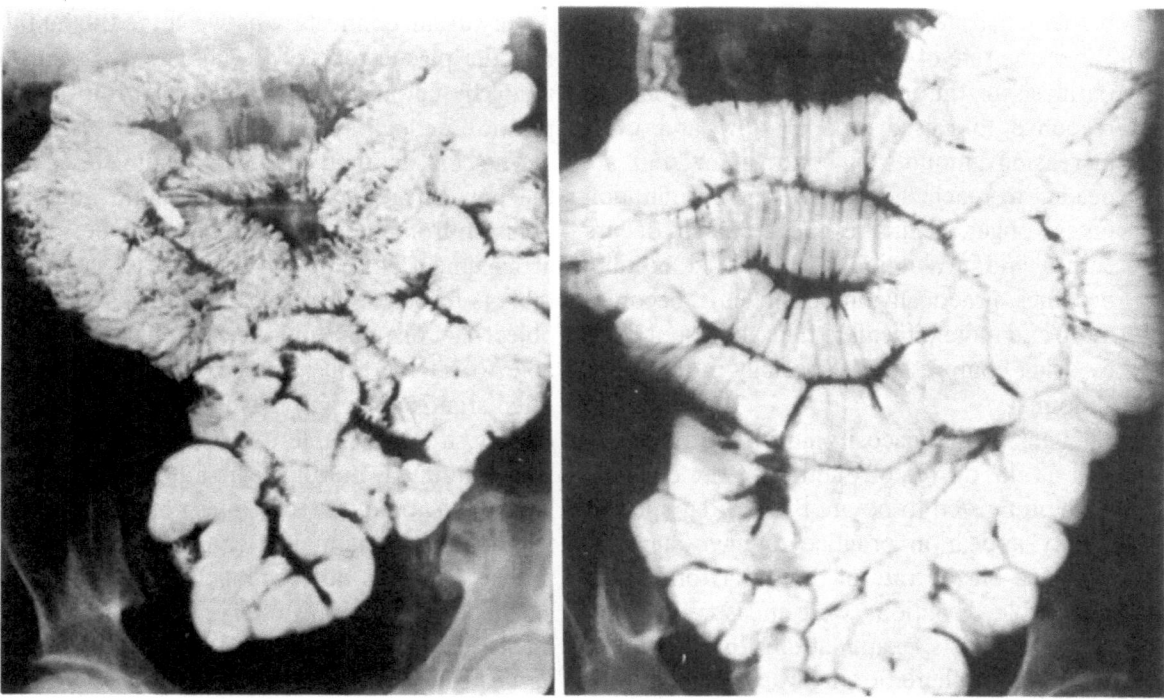

Fig. II.3A. The rate of flow of the contrast medium for the examination of this patient was 50 ml/min (left side) and 100 ml/min (right side), respectively. The hypotonia and reduced peristalsis due to the excessive use of sedatives are not apparent on the left hand film: they are however clearly visible on the right.

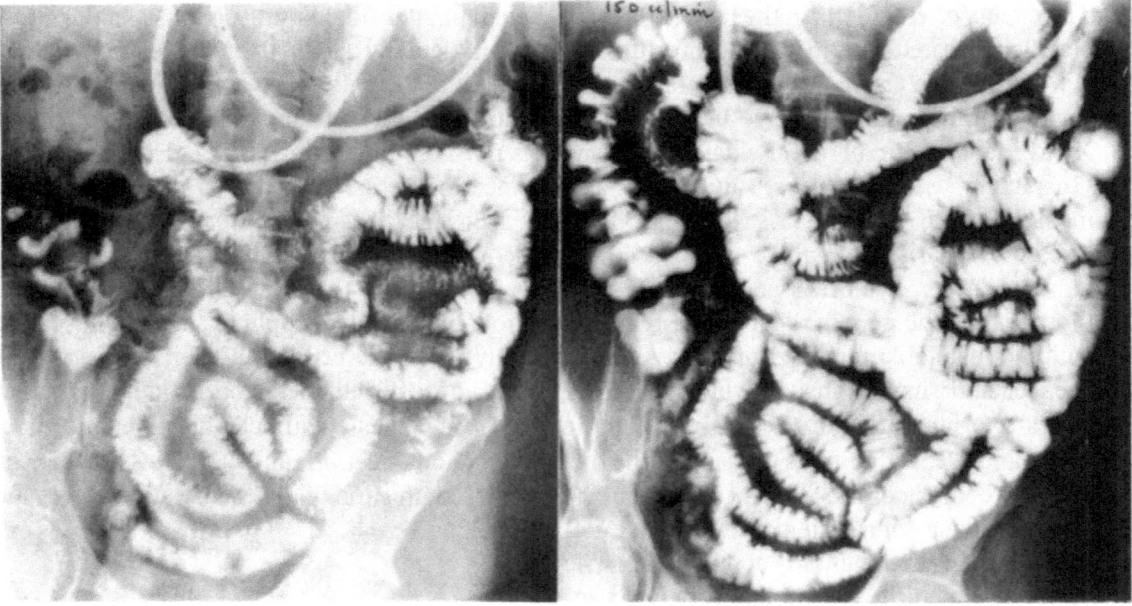

Fig. II.3B. Patient with hypermotility as a result of collagenosis. This is clearly visible on the left-hand X-ray; only 200 ml of contrast medium administered at a rate of 75 ml/min were required to reach the cecum. Because the intestinal loops were not sufficiently full for anatomical evaluation, the rate of flow was subsequently increased to 150 ml/min and additional films were taken (right side).

phy and small mucosal lesions can no longer be demonstrated

2) When the rate of flow is 100 ml/min or more, paralysis of the intestine develops sooner in response to raised rate of flow and ever-increasing amounts of contrast medium are needed to reach the cecum. The examination takes longer, reflux to the stomach occurs earlier and evaluation of disturbed motility becomes practically impossible. It becomes more and more difficult to take good spot films by using compression, especially in the lower abdomen.

3) Changes in the viscosity and temperature as well as the degree of dilution of the contrast medium needed to obtain the desired specific gravity appear in practice to have such an influence on the rate of flow that totally unacceptable deviations were measured during the enteroclysis examination. In Oudkerk's experiments therefore it was necessary to administer the contrast medium via a specially designed high-precision pump.

4) Oudkerk was able to establish with certainty that 75 ml/min is the most favourable rate of flow for enteroclysis examination and that a deviation of more than 15% is not permissible. The effects of variations in the rate of flow are clearly illustrated in fig: II.3AB. Unfortunately it would be too expensive to manufacture the very accurate pump used by Oudkerk in the X-ray department of the Leiden University Hospital in series. The most suitable and also most accurate substitute is the reasonably priced and easily obtainable pump used for kidney dialysis. The Black and Decker pump, though very cheap, is so inaccurate that it is entirely unsuitable for this purpose. An even cheaper and simpler answer which moreover appears to function more accurately than the Black and Decker pump is infusion of the day before prepared contrast fluid at room temperature, by means of a system always constructed from the same standard components. The height at which the plastic bag (originally intended for colon enema examination) containing contrast fluid must be placed to achieve the desired infusion rate for small intestine examination, can be experimentally determined

for each department and now and again checked. A very useful connection between the Bilbao tube and the plastic tube of the infusion bag can be made by cutting the proximal end from a 3 ml plastic Luerlock syringe.

The contrast fluid can best be administered with the patient prone as in this position autocompression from abdominal fat gives the best visual arrangement of the bowel loops. A telecommand table is to be prefered because of the favourable object-film distance and the convenience of being able to tilt the röntgen tube. Since the pylorus often stands open and has a latent period before closing, it is advisable to raise the speed of infusion gradually during the first 20 sec, particularly when the tip of the tube does not lie far enough within the duodenum. If after an initial dose of 600 ml the cecum is not yet reached, a second but smaller dose is administered immediately or at the most several minutes later. If the cecum has almost been reached or a confusing clump of ileal loops has developed in the minor pelvis, it is better to give only 600 ml. If the contrast medium is still far from the cecum and overprojection of intestinal loops is not too pronounced, then the second dose should be 600 ml.

If during the first infusion of 600 ml contrast medium, it is noted that peristalsis in the intestine is particularly slow, then, depending upon the weight of the patient, 20 or 30 ml metoclopramide should be added to the second dose of 600 ml. It is not wise to administer this drug intravenously since the period of action is then much shorter. Furthermore, there can be a subsequent long period, lasting 30-60 min, of greatly reduced peristalsis due to fatigue of the overloaded and probably already atrophied smooth musculature. Only when the cecum has almost been reached can a dose of 2 ml metoclopramide be administered intravenously without objection. In this case the period of action (about 10 min) is sufficient to allow completion of the examination before atony develops.

3. Number of films

The entire examination is carried out under intermittent fluoroscopy and spot films are taken using compression. If a telecommand apparatus is not available and the Bucky table is used, it is better to wait until the cecum has been reached, as seen on the survey exposures, before making spot films – not only of the distal ileum but of course of all the other loops of the small intestine.

For a standard examination of the small intestine without conspicuious abnormalities, the routine procedure is to take the following films:
$2 \times 24/30$ of the proximal jejunum after 300ml;
$2 \times 35/35$ ot the entire abdomen after 600 ml;
$2 \times 35/35$ of the entire abdomen after the cecum has been reached;
8-12 films (2-$3 \times 24/30$).

If the case is without complications, the total length of the examination is 15-30 min including duodenal intubation; the total fluoroscopy time is 3-5 min.

E. Administration of water after the barium suspension

It is often very difficult to identify small abnormalities of the mucosa in intestinal loops that coincide or have contracted. Better filling of the intestine causes a greater degree of stretching of the folds; as a result they lie in a more or less circular configuration and abnormalities are easier to identify. Each examination should, if possible, include at least a few röntgenograms of the intestinal loops in a wellfilled state. However, a high degree of filling of the intestinal loops also means that it is more difficult to project them freely by means of compression. To avoid problems in evaluation a more intensive filling should be carried out towards the end of the examination and after a number of films of the partially filled loops have already been made. In the proximal part of the small intestine, the degree of filling of the loops can be regulated fairly well by adjusting the infusion rate of the contrast fluid. In the distal part of the ileum however, this no longer applies. Instead, the degree of filling is determined by the ease with which the contrast fluid passes through Bauhin's valve to the cecum. In most cases a very reasonable degree of filling of the important terminal part of the small intestine can still be obtained by exerting pressure on the regio of Bauhin's valve with a blunt compressor.

The best way to force the contrast column onward is to administer 600 ml or more of water through the tube. Since water has a very low viscosity, a rate of flow of 150 – 200 ml/min can easily be achieved by hanging the infusion bag 40-50 cm above the level of the table. It is however possible that the patient, not being able to tolerate this rate of flow, will become nauseated. This can happen very quickly if the tip of the tube is not placed far enough into the duodenum and if the temperature of the water, which should be 30°-37°C, is too low. As soon as nausea develops, the infusion bag should be lowered so that the rate of flow will again decrease or even stop. Water infusion will not only give better X-rays of the well-filled distal small intestinal loops, but will also produce excellent double-contrast films of the jejunum (fig. II.4). The troublesome marked differences in density seen when double-contrast exposures are taken with air do not occur when water is used.

The water infusion flushes the barium suspension quite rapidly from the intestinal wall but this fails to happen if the water has been rendered viscous by addition of methylcellulose, as propagated by Herlinger.

Supplementing of the examination with water infusion is more often applied than is necessary; it provides useful additional information in 1 of 5 to 10 examinations. The indications for this procedure are summarised below. Numbers 5, 6, 7, 8 and 9 can be regarded as essential and the others left more or less to the choice of the radiologist.

1. After administration of 600 ml barium suspension the cecum is nearly reached. Alternatives are: a small supplementary amount of contrastfluid, i.v. metoclopramide or a little patience.
2. To obtain a better degree of ileal filling.
3. Patients with diminished intestinal motility, mostly as result of sedative or antispasmodic medication, and those who habitually sleep on their left side, sometimes have food residue in the ileum and cecum. More than a litre of water and additional i.v. metoclopramide is often required to wash the distal ileum completely clean.

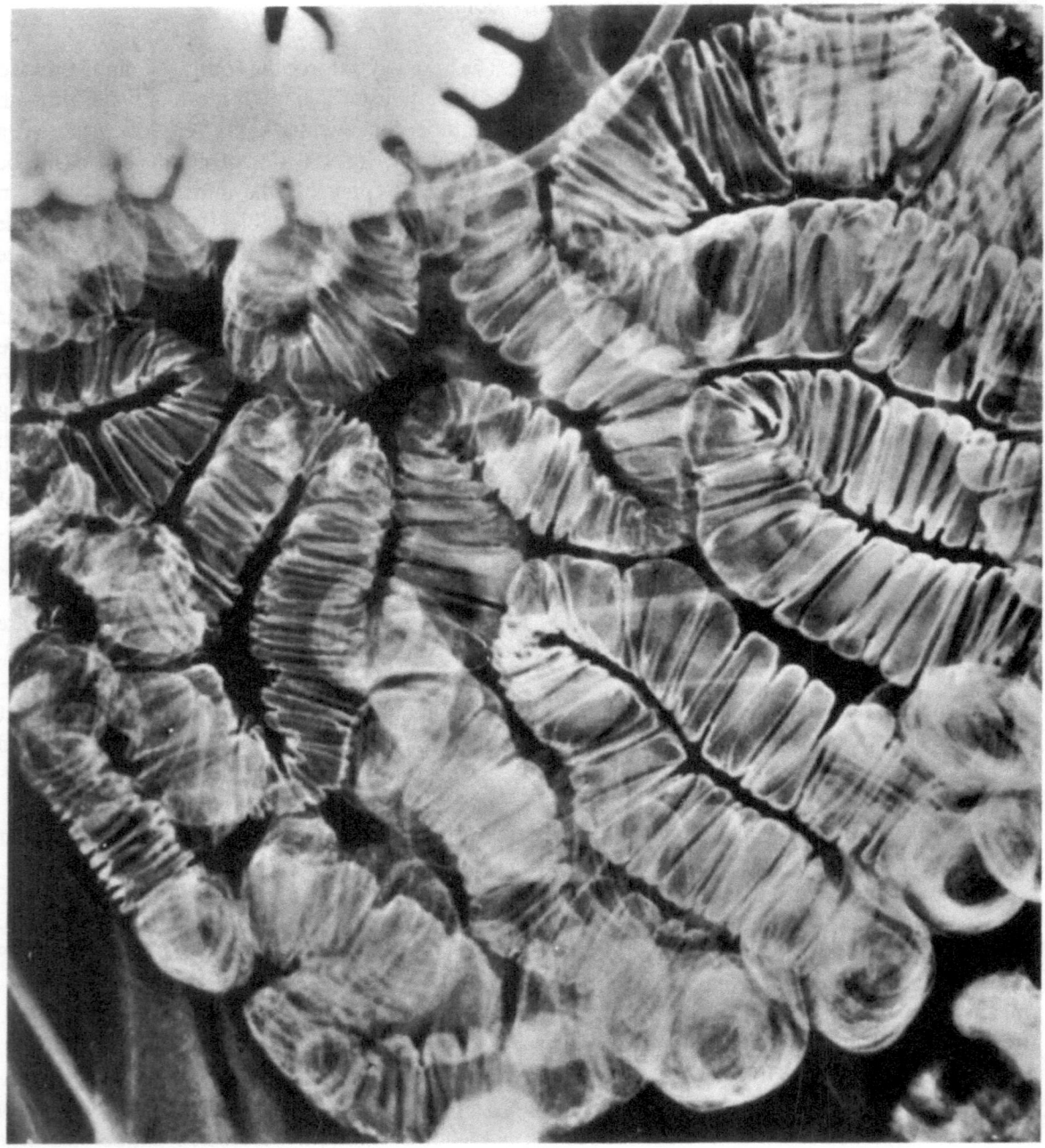

Fig. II.4.   Double-contrast exposure of jejunum after administration of plain water. A thin film of contrast fluid remains on the mucosa for 15-30 sec.

Food residues in the ileum are also seen in the presence of an incompetent Valve of Bauhini, resulting from inflammatory processes in the ascending colon or the cecum. Contrary to expectation obstructive pro-cesses are seldom conducive to prestenotic accumulation of food residues.

4. The cecum has not yet been reached even after administration of 1200 ml barium sus-pension, due to a mechanical obstruction or

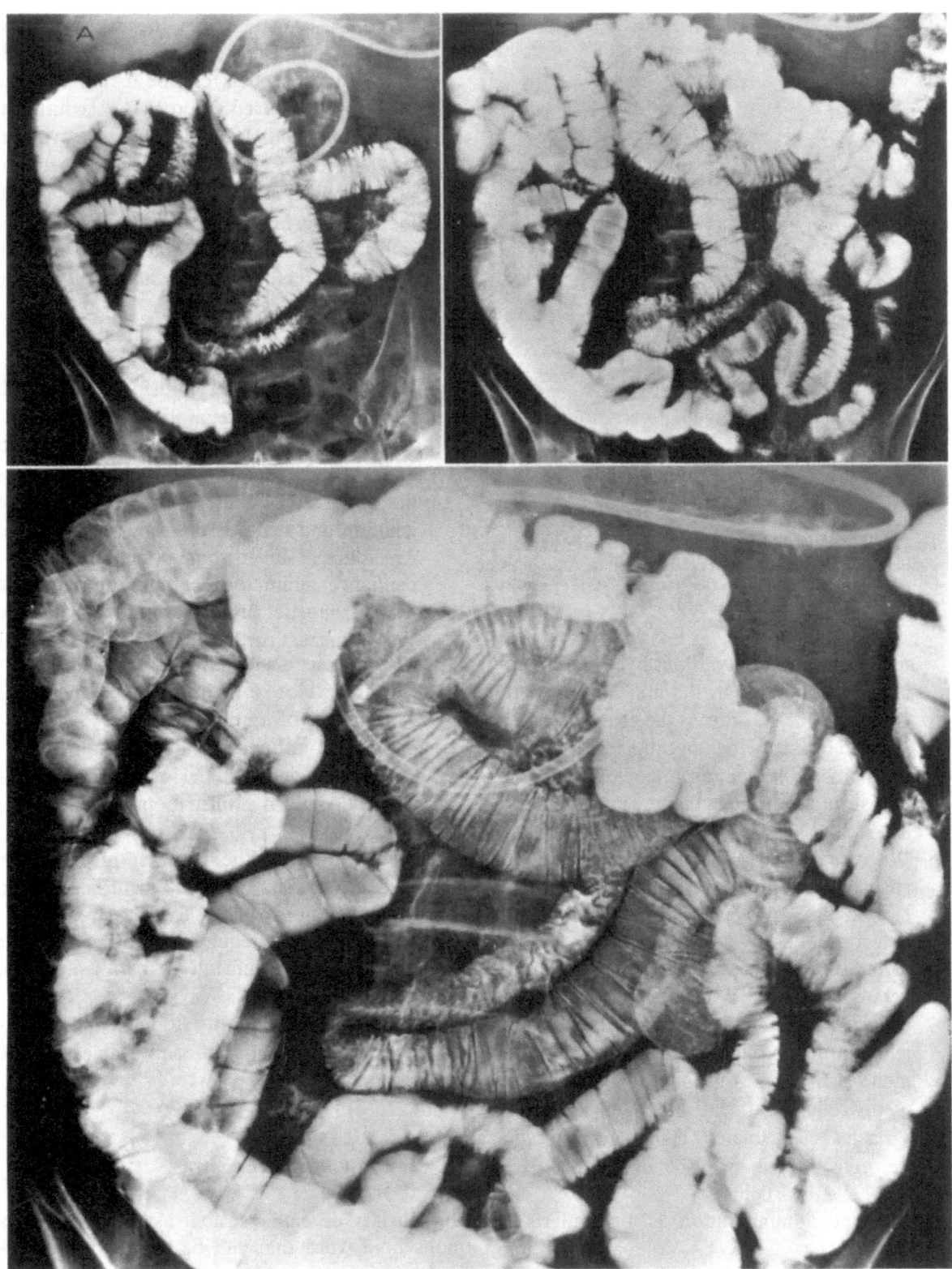

Fig. II.5. Positional anomaly of the small intestine: the ascending colon is difficult to find. Filling of the jejunal loops in the right half of the abdomen (top left). Now the ileal loops are also filled and parts of the colon are visible in the upper left quadrant. The cecum, usually located either in the lower right quadrant or high up under the liver, is not visible here (top right). After the jejunum is filled with water, the cecum and the ascending colon are visualized clearly on the right side (under).

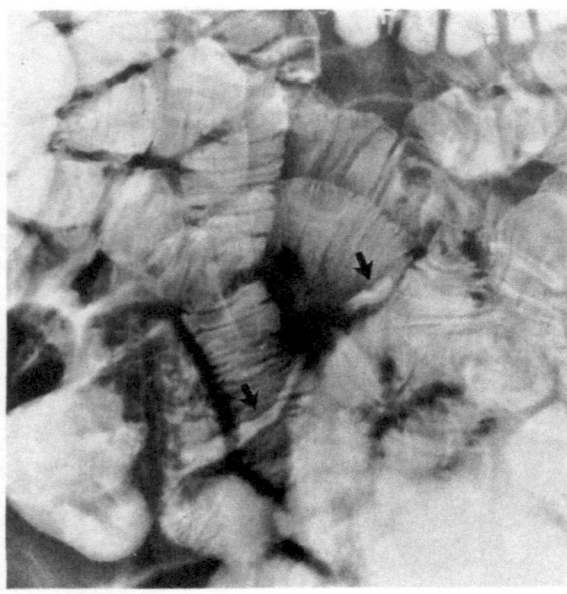

Fig. II.6. On the filling exposure the appendix was scarcely visible and free projection not readily feasible. After infusion of water an appreciably better image of the appendix is obtained.

marked hypomotility. If this hypomotility was already noticeable in the first minute of the examination, the latter is the case and can be relieved by i.v. metoclopramide. In the case of mechanical obstruction metoclopramide administration through the tube can be considered.

5. Where stenosis from tumor or ulceration is suspected but not found, rapid water infusion (150-200 ml/min) can be of assistence in the detection of relative stenosis.

6. Where the ileocecal region or an ileo-transversostomy is not visible, a spectacular clear up can be attained when the superimposed jejunum and proximal ileal loops have been made transparent by water filling (strictly *no* methylcellulose) (fig. II.5.).

7. To achieve satisfactory filling and facilitating the detection of an appendix (fig. II.6) or Meckel's diverticula.

   Water administration is particularly of value in cases where a comparatively long omphalo-enteric duct exists, as just in this condition a Meckel's diverticulum, especially if small, is difficult to find.

8. In certain rare cases the colon can for diverse reasons only be filled by oral administration of contrast medium. In these cases, after 600-1200 ml barium suspension has been administered, this bulk can be driven into the previously cleansed colon by water infusion (strictly *no* methylcellulose), with or without the help of i.v. administration of metoclopramide. The superimposed small intestinal loops are washed out at the same time. Exploratory colon radiograms are also possible using this method as adjunct to a routine enteroclysis. (fig. II.7)

9. When an operation is to be anticipated shortly after examination of the small bowel washing out with a water infusion is a useful, almost necessary preparation.

10. A supplementary water infusion, here with methylcellulose, can be considered if a splendid filling with double-contrast effect of the jejunum and ileum is desired. This method, which has assumed some popularity as independant examination technique, does not give any diagnostic profit compared with the single contrast method, but has a number of very serious disadvantages; such as:

a) it is impossible to form an adequate opinion on disturbances of motility.

b) not feasible in babies and small children.

c) compression details of the lower abdomen are, as a result of the overfilled loops, of rather poor quality.

d) disintegration of the contrast medium can occur if there is a markedly disturbed transit, whether or not resulting from obstruction.

e) the examination requires more time and is somewhat more difficult to perform than a standard enteroclysis.

f) with more reflux into the stomach and contingent vomiting it is uncomfortable for the patient.

F. Indications for aircontrast

In the last decennia aircontrast has become a household word that can be regarded as synonymous with 'Better than the Best', omission or disregard of which bears the stamp of third rate radiology. It is as though a worldwide infection has broken out under radiologists that could aptly be named 'Double contrast disease'.

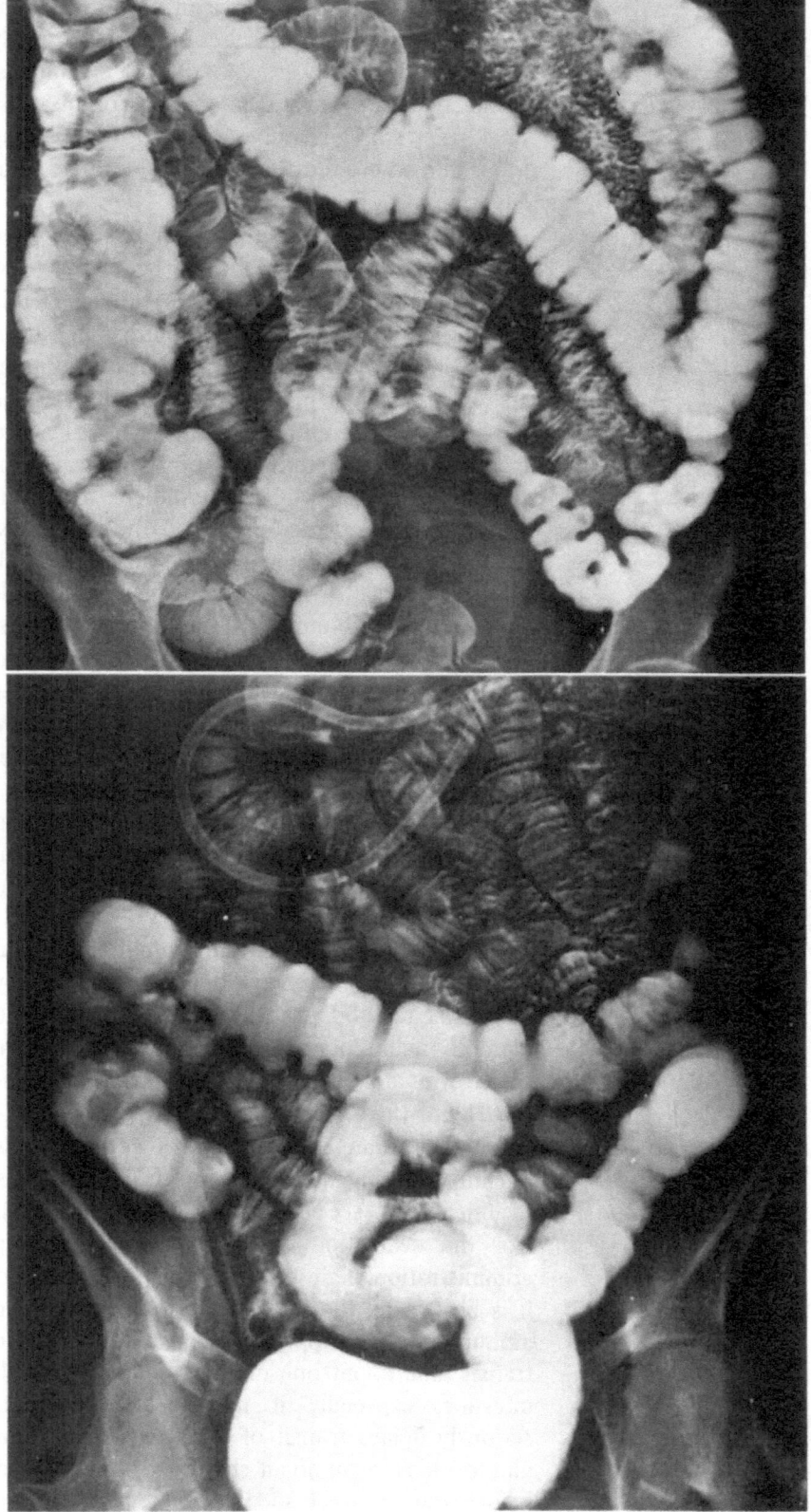

Fig. II.7. Examples of survey exposures of the colon after flushing the jejunum clean with water. Useful reproduction of the mucosa in the colon is then generally no problem.

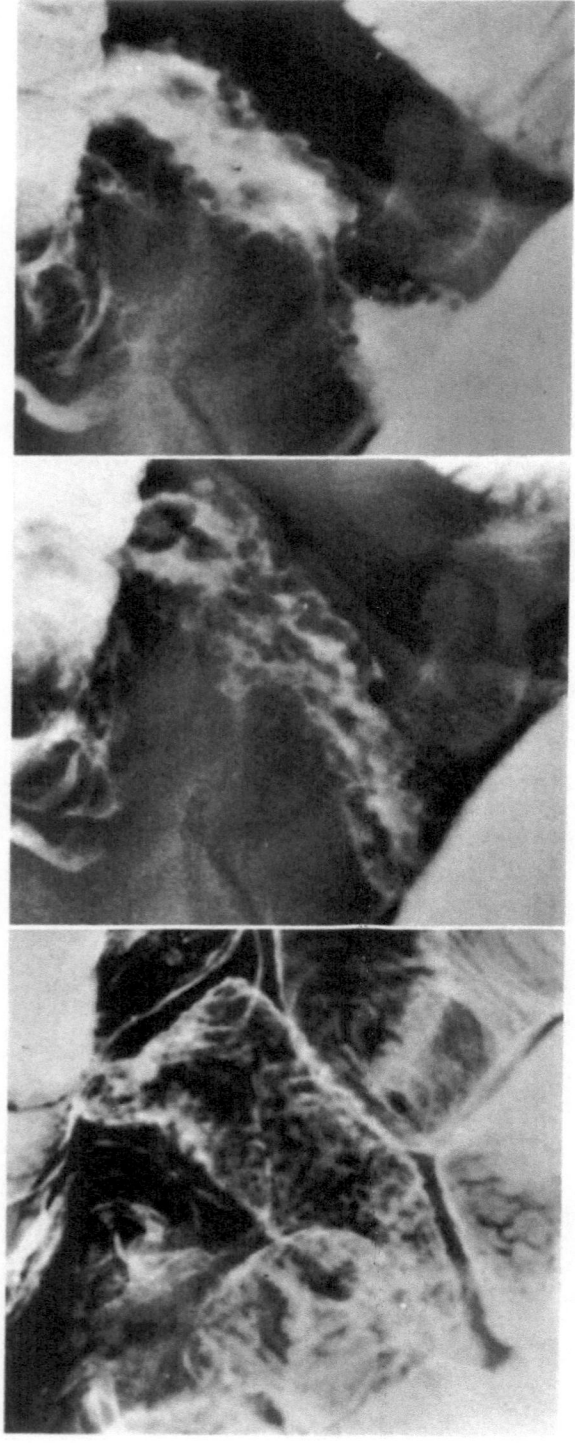

Fig. II.8. Lymphfollicles in the distal ileum, clearly visible on the double-contrast exposures but hardly or not at all when the loop was filled with barium only.

It is obvious that a standard aircontrast technique rapidly arose and that this variation of enteroclysis soon began to lead an independant existence. In my opinion aircontrast is extremely important for X-ray examination of esophagus, stomach, duodenum and colon, parts of the intestinal tract that are tubes without overlapping loops and where there is thus no hindrance from superimposition.

In the small intestine and sometimes in the sigmoid hindrance can indeed be experienced from superimposed bowel loops and it is in this situation that the value of aircontrast has been overestimated in comparison to the results obtained with full filling pictures. Meantime even the most fanatic adherents of aircontrast have learned from experience that tumors and stenoses are impossible or considerably more difficult to find in the confusion of lines produced by aircontrast than in the homogeneous white fields of a full filling. Meckel's diverticula and fistulas are seldom or never found with standard aircontrast technique and for these reasons it is being abandoned. Just as with water infusion techniques adequate evaluation of changes in motility is here not possible, but due to ignorance of these phenomena that is not felt to be a disadvantage.

Nevertheless aircontrast really has a few good indications and can be used every now and again, but exclusively as supplement to an already completed standard enteroclysis.

Small mucosal lesions and lymphfollicles can be visualised much better with aircontrast than by any other method (fig. II.8) and a troublesome clump of ileum loops in the minor pelvis is more easily evaluated and often smaller than by complete filling (fig. II.9). Let it be mentioned emphatically that administration of extra water in cases of clump forming in the minor pelvis is a first class technical error (see chapter II.H2.7 and fig. II.10). For the evaluation of small mucosal lesions administration of air via the tube is preferable and it is best to let the patient do this himself. The amount given is approximately a litre and the transit time about one minute. Air in the small intestine, especially if administered to fast, seriously delays transit of the contrast medium and for this reason no air should be administered before the contrast medium has reached the

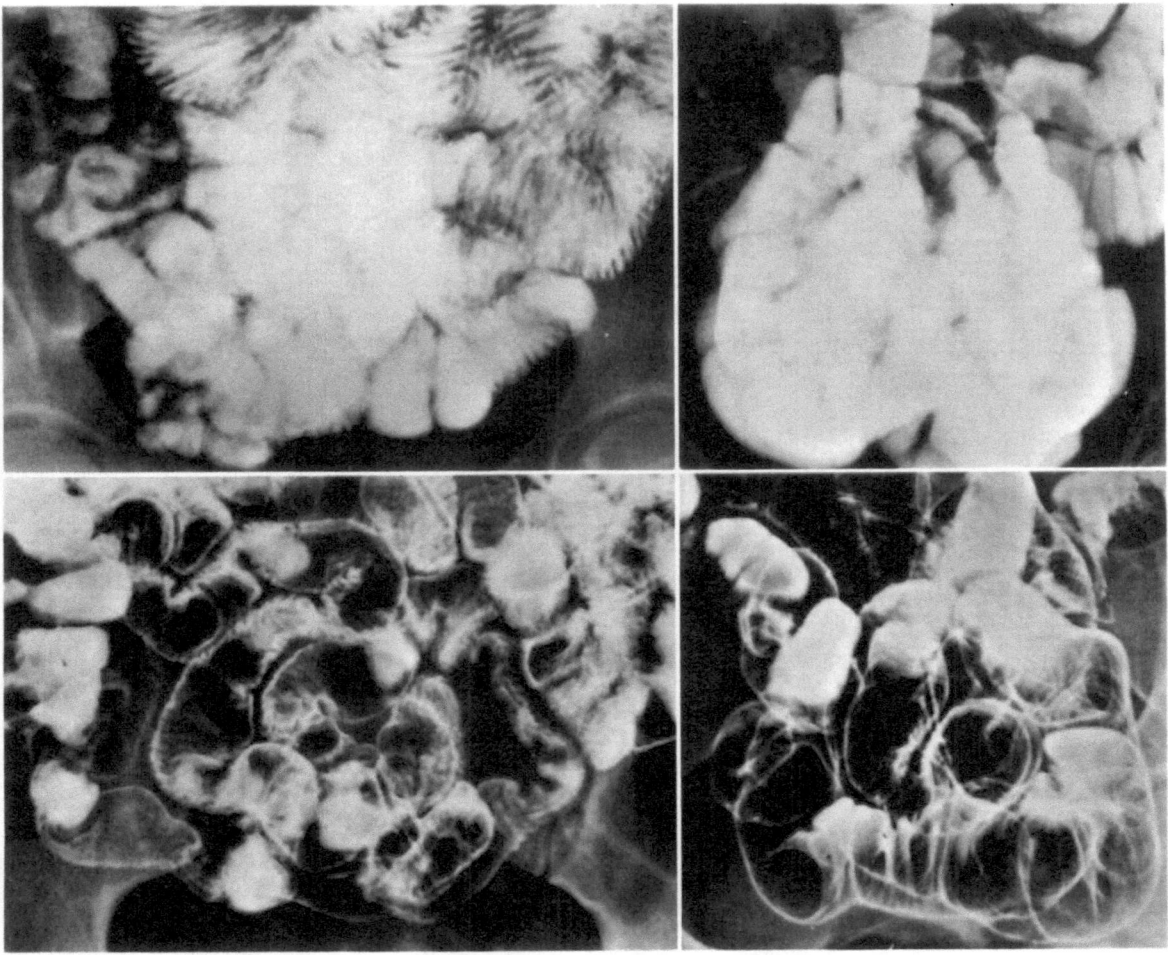

Fig. II.9. Two examples of free projection of the ileal loops in the lower abdomen and the minor pelvis by using air insufflation through the duodenal tube. The patient is in the prone position.

cecum. In the case of clump forming in the minor pelvis air can be more quickly given via a rectal cannula, this is usually sufficient and oral administration thus no longer necessary.

Where hypomotility has been observed during standard enteroclysis, oral air administration would cost too much time and the air filling of the small intestine should preferably always occur per rectum.

The indications and routes of administration for aircontrast are her shortly summarised:

lymph follicles ⎫
adhesions   ⎬ oral air administration
'minor lesions' ⎭

clump forming in ⎫ ⎧ first rectal and if necessary
  minor pelvis ⎬ ⎨ also oral air insufflation
                ⎭ ⎩

Low position of ⎫ ⎧ filling of the entire colon
  voluminous   ⎬ ⎨ per rectum
  cecum   ⎭ ⎩

The compression technique with its sequence of manipulations can best be illustrated schematically as shown in fig. II.11.

G. Special examination techniques

1. In case of ileus and subileus

An incomprehensible misconception, chiefly un-

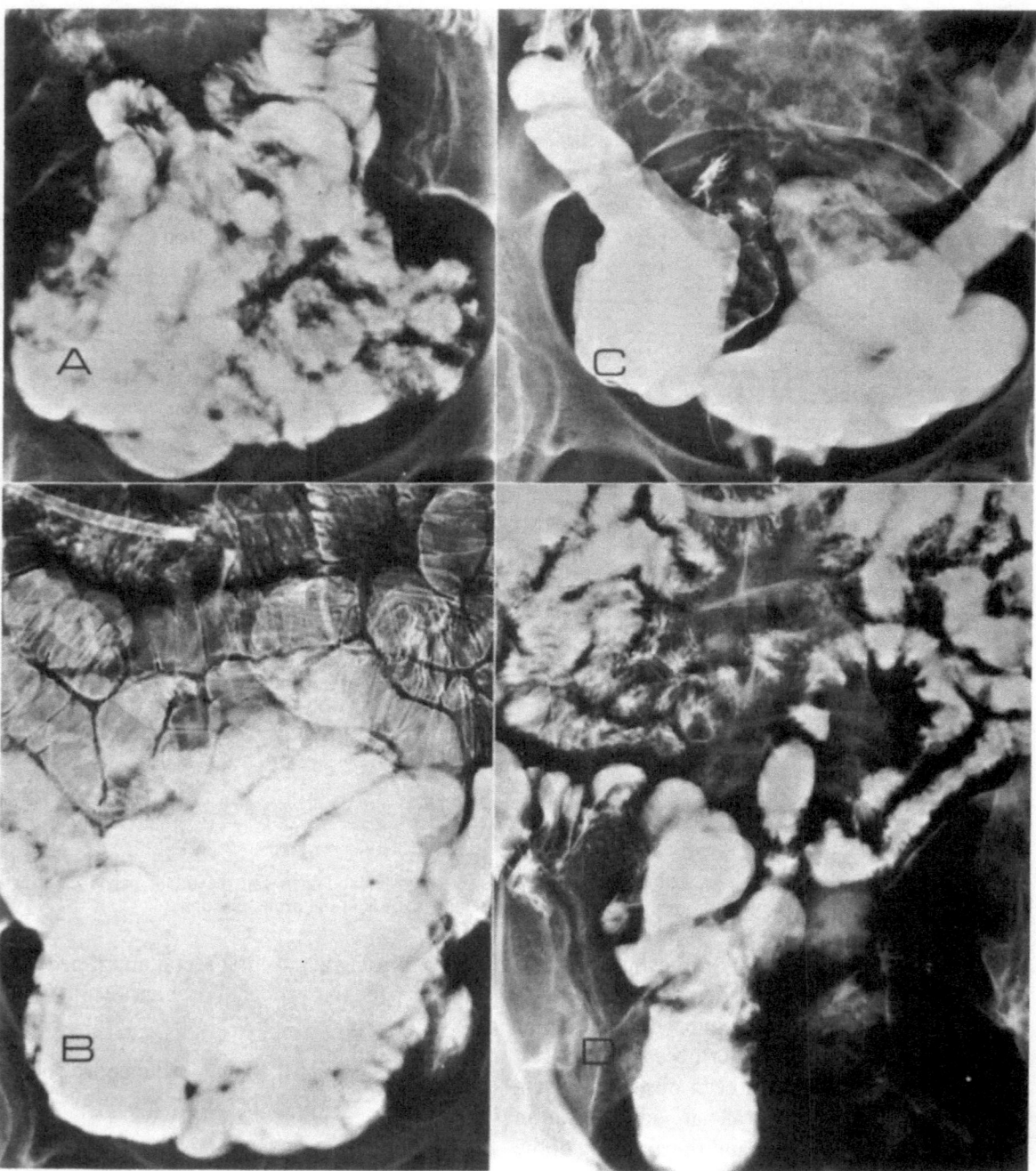

Fig. II.10. The results of an incorrect decision as to procedure during the course of the examination. There is a mass of ileal loops in the minor pelvis. (A): Because the cecum had not yet been reached, water was administered. (B): The results of this decision. Although the reasoning was in principle correct, this step was apparently taken without consideration of the problems that could be expected during free projection of the distal ileum since a previous colon examination (C) had already indicated that the ileocecal segment was deepseated. (D): The survey exposures obtained after intravenous administration of 2 ml metoclopramide, on the basis of the original situation seen in A, and air was insufflated rectally. Air insufflation via the duodenal tube would serve no purpose.

HOW TO SEPARATE ILEUM LOOPS
IN SMALL PELVIS

USE AIR AND COMPRESSION

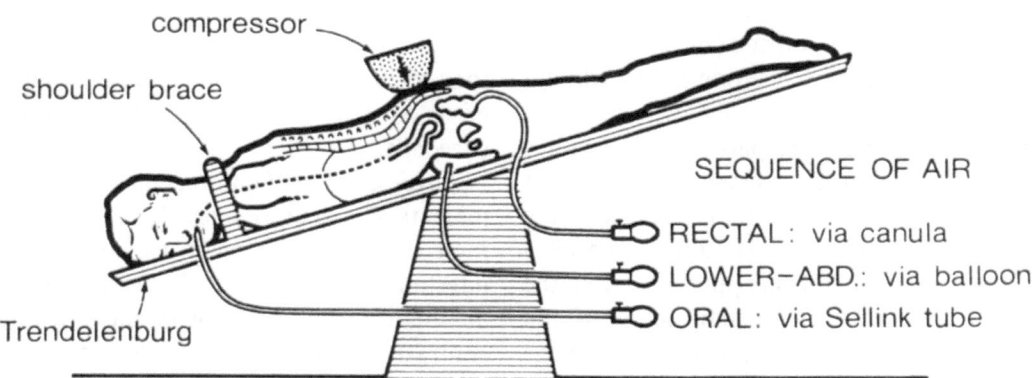

Fig. II.11. Position of the patient during the combined insufflation and special compression technique. The sequence of steps is usually as follows: (1) Place the balloon under the lowen abdomen. (2) Rectal air insufflation. (3) Air insufflation via the duodenal tube. (4) Fill the balloon between the patient and the table with air. (5) Compression on the dorsal side of the patient. (6) If necessary, direct röntgen rays along craniocaudal axis.

der surgeons but also under internists, which have been propagated for nearly 20 years before it could be abandoned, is the use of the contrast medium Gastrografin in ileus examination. Gastrografin is, in fact, here totally unsuitable unless the obstruction is situated in the duodenum or immediate proximal jejunum. Gastrografin is strongly hyperosmotic and dilutes unbelievably rapidly so that the morphological picture obtained is absolutely illusory. Even the presence of stenoses some 1 or 2 mm in diameter are not detected because the Gastrografin passes through them so easily and quickly that it has already reached the colon 15 min after administration. Moreover the strong hyperosmotic properties of Gastrografin cause abdominal cramp, vomiting and diarrhea and can lead to complete disturbance of an already unstable electrolyte balance. Once in the colon the Gastrografin is again concentrated by water absorption so that it is in some measure suitable for visualising the proximal side of a colonic stenosis, which could not be passed by way of the rectum.

There is yet another factor apart from that already described, which has long prevented an efficient

diagnostic technique in case of ileus. The majority of almost all referring colleagues, especially from other disciplines still believe that, when an ileus is suspected, the most adequate approach is an abdominal survey film with horizontal beam. Although there is no danger in this method and even the inexperienced clinician can easily see the fluid levels on such films so that his clinical suspicion is confirmed, their value can be con- can be considered dubious. It is apparently not or insufficiently realized that:

1.1. An ileus can exist without visible fluid levels. As described above this is certainly true in the initial stages when there may as yet be insufficient gas. In other cases the intra-abdominal pressure may be so high that the accumulation of gas is greatly retarded or even prevented.

1.2. Fluid levels form as a result of the presence of gas and thin fluids in the digestive tract. This combination is not at all rare! It is pronounced in patients with diarrhea or retarded resorption. Erect abdominal survey films of patients who for some reason have been allowed to eat before the examination are not often encountered. Therefore it is understandable that experience in recognizing this particular phenomenon is extremely limited.

1.3. Even the presence of fluid levels together with dilated intestinal loops need not necessarily indicate an ileus. This combination can also be seen in a number of diseases such as drug-induced atony, scleroderma, amyloidosis or certain forms of celiac disease.

1.4. An X-ray of an erect patient taken with a horizontal beam may demonstrate the presence of free intra-abdominal air below the diaphragm. Such films should not be considered adequate for this purpose. Often the film is assumed to be satisfactory if the diaphragm is just visible along the upper edge of the röntgenogram. It should be remembered, however, that only large quantities of gas will be seen on such films. Small and therefore narrow sickle-shaped pockets of air between the liver and the diaphragm are not visualized by an oblique beam. It is always necessary to demonstrate the presence of smaller gas accumulations below the diaphragm! The diaphragm should lie at the level of the central beam, thus in the middle of the röntgenogram.

1.5. Dilatation of intestinal loops filled with gas can be established much more easily on an exposure taken with a vertical beam. The gas in the lumen spreads out over a much larger area when the patient is lying down and gives much more information. Experienced radiologists certainly do not need fluid levels to establish a diagnosis of ileus.

A second X-ray taken several minutes later may show that the gas pattern in the intestine has barely changed. This local 'stillness' due to a total absence of peristalsis can occur in a single intestinal loop. This can be considered strongly indicative of a local obstruction or paralysis. At this stage, only a subileus is present which is often clinically unrecognized. However, further investigation of the underlying condition is exceedingly worthwhile. The establishment of a correct or probable diagnosis is almost always possible.

Barium suspension can be regarded as contrast medium sine qua non for the diagnosis of ileus and this is true for all other enteroclysis examinations. The total amount of contrast medium required for the examination is variable. It is highly dependent upon whether the obstruction is in the jejunum or distal ileum, the stage of the ileus and the degree of motility still present. In general much more than an initial dose of 800 ml must be administered; a total dose of 2400 ml is, however, never exceeded.

As the amount of contrast fluid administered to patients with ileus increases, peristalsis decreases in a fairly long segment as stretching of the intestinal wall continues. To retard this so-called 'inhibitory' reflex mechanism, the flow rate of the contrast medium should be decreased gradually during the examination. Here, as in all other cases where large quantities of contrast fluid have to be administered, the specific gravity of each subsequent dose of 800 ml barium suspension is reduced. In practice this gives the following dose schedule:

1) dose of 800 ml
   s.g. = 1.30 or density 40% wt/vol, rate of flow 75 ml/min
2) dose of 800 ml
   s.g. = 1.15 or density 20% wt/vol, rate of flow 40 ml/min
3) 30 ml metoclopramide through tube to enhance peristalsis
4) dose of 800 ml water at body temperature rate of flow 25 ml/min

Obviously it is essential to estimate beforehand the height of the infusion bag required to obtain the correct rate of flow for each phase of the examination. When in doubt, it is preferable to choose for safety a rate that is too low.

In most cases the obstruction site is reached within about an hour, even if it is fairly pronounced and rather distal in the small intestine. It is certainly possible to make compression spot films after administration of this maximum dosage of 2400 ml – but a careful and precise technique is required. If the obstruction has not yet been reached, follow the conservative approach – and wait.

This large quantity of contrast medium usually is in the colon within 6-8 h, even in the presence of pronounced stenoses located in the distal part of the small intestine. In a few patients with an almost total obstruction the colon was not reached until the following morning (24 h later). It can in such cases take one to three weeks before all the contrast medium has disappeared from the large bowel.

Occasionally it is possible to locate the site of the obstruction by means of the gas contours on one or more of the abdominal survey films. In other cases, signs of a space-occupying infiltrate are clearly visible in the lower right quadrant. Partly on the basis of other factors such as age and clinical course, the diagnosis of an 'appendicular infiltrate' can easily be made without using a contrast medium.

It must be stressed that extensive pre-operative diagnostic techniques serve little purpose when the chest and abdominal films have already revealed the diagnosis. The abdominal films may show the presence of extensive bands, an ileus from gall stones, perforation of the digestive tract and indicate urgent surgical intervention.

It should be mentioned that an enteroclysis examination may be carried out only after the obstruction has been determined as not located in the colon. Usually this is easy from the survey films. The abdominal survey films taken before the barium examination should be carefully evaluated, bearing in mind that the site of the obstruction usually lies more distally than is presumed from the gas configurations on these films!

In the case of a stenosis in the colon, dehydration of the contrast fluid proximal to the site of the obstruction where by the barium suspension becomes so thick that barium stones develop may cause a subileus to become a manifest ileus. Where there is doubt about the location of the stenosis, a retrograde enteroclysis examination may also be considered.

When a patient with ileus is examined by enteroclysis, it is important during the first minute of the examination to note whether active peristalsis exists in the proximal jejunum. Important conclusions can be based on this finding! If peristalsis is initially active then a drug-induced non-obstructing ileus can be eliminated.

In the event of a mechanical ileus, peristalsis may be active at first and then gradually decrease during the course of the examination. If there is no peristalsis in the proximal jejunum immediately at the commencement of the examination, then either a paralytic ileus, or a long-term severe mechanical obstruction is possible.

2. In case of babies and small infants

2.1. General

A careful study of the gas shadows on one or more abdominal survey films can sometimes lead to useful conclusions. This certainly does not apply only to children. Air is not a useful contrast medium for visualization of the intenstinal lumen. This is true for both children and adults. Air, however, is no worse than a barium suspension when a conventional follow-through examination is carried out.

Gastrografin also is definitely not a suitable contrast medium for children. In fact, because of its marked hyperosmotic properties, it may even be dangerous. As a result of the rapidly increasing dilution, the mucosal relief in the duodenum and most proximal part of the jejunum may be visualized, but more distally this is impossible.

As in many areas and certainly in radiology, the procedures developed for examination of adults cannot be applied directly to small children. This holds true for enteroclysis. In particular enteroclysis examination of babies and infants between 0 and 3-4 years of age is without doubt much more difficult than examination of adults. Therefore the alternative prerequisites and procedures that have been determined experimentally will be described here.

2.2. Preparation

The younger the child the greater is the tendency towards rapid flocculation of the contrast fluid. The precise reason for this is still unknown, but is possibly related to the larger quantities of mucus and, more especially, lactic acid present in the small bowel. This is particularly true during the period of milk diet, human or bovine in origin. It should be obvious that flocculation can be prevented only by very rapid administration of a large dose of contrast fluid i.e. relative to the rate and quantity required for an adult. The degree of small intestinal filling will thus be relatively greater than in an adult. In addition, there is much less opportunity for obtaining spot films by using compression because of the fragility and minute size of the intestine. The problems arising from excessive filling of the ileal loops in the lower abdomen can be limited by thorough cleansing of the colon, thus ensuring that the contrast medium flows smoothly to the cecum. Here too, as in adults, a rectal cleansing enema is not recommended. A satisfactory oral laxation procedure for children between 1 and 15 years of age is as follows:

7.00 a.m.	– 1 gr magnesium sulfate powder per kg body weight, dissolved in 200 ml water; 1 Dulcolax tablet.
9.00 a.m.	– 300 ml (2 large cups) of tea with sugar; 30 gr (one slice) of white bread with 30 gr (one slice) of cheese; 1 boiled egg.
11.00 a.m.	– 300 ml lemonade.
1.00 p.m.	– 200 ml beef tea; cooked fish or chicken without skin; no potatoes, fruit or vegetables; 200 ml soda water.
3.00 p.m.	– 300 ml lemonade or tea with sugar.
5.00 p.m.	– 200 ml beef tea; 30 gr white bread with one slice of cheese.
7.00 p.m.	– 1 gr magnesium sulfate powder per kg body weight, dissolved in 200 ml water; 1 Dulcolax tablet.
9.00 p.m.	– 300 ml lemonade or tea with sugar.

For the preparation of babies under 12 months of age, the radiologist should contact the pediatrician or the dietician of the childrens's department. The day before the examination the milk diet should contain less fat than usual and the overnight fasting period must be somewhat extended.

There is another aspect in the preparation of the baby and small child that is quite different from that of adults. A child younger than four to five years should be sedated just before the examination. In spite of the unfavorable effect of sedation on intestinal motility, this procedure is essential for succesful intubation and for efficient performance of the examination itself.

If the decrease in intestinal motility is marked, some compensation can be obtained by disconnecting the bag of contrast fluid and administering a few ml. Primperan (metoclopramide) via the tube. This step must be carried out as soon as hypomotility is demonstrated, since reflux into the stomach has by then probably not yet occurred. Most of the Primperan will then enter the duodenum where it achieves its most rapid effect.

2.3. Duodenal intubation

For adults, duodenal intubation is carried out by the staff of the radiology department but for babies and small children the tube should be inserted as far as the stomach by a member of the pediatric staff familiar with the child. The easiest route is via one of the nostrils which gives rise to less resistance than when the oral route is chosen. Furthermore, fixation of the tube with adhesive tape is advisable. For children over two years the Bilbao of Sellink tube can be used. For younger children these tubes are much too rigid. It is better to take a thinner, more flexible, leadrubber tube or a plastic tube with a marker line. In all cases the end of the tube should be closed and rounded. The openings should be situated only in the length of the tube. Manoeuvering the tip of the tube, merely by turning the child, can be facilitated considerably by inserting $\pm$ 1 cm of tin solder wire into the tip of the tube. In this way the tip will sink as a result of its own weight to the lowest part of the stomach.

The lead-rubber tubes with metal olive available today are too thick and unsuitable for babies. The olive does not pass easily through the pyloric canal and certainly not through the child's nostril. When the tip of the tube is somewhere in the stomach, the child is brought to the radiology department. There, under fluoroscopic control and using a thick Seldinger angiographic guide wire, the tube is pushed through the pyloric canal into the duodenum. Only when a child is two to three years old may the much stiffer Bilbao guide wire be used for this purpose. Obviously this second phase of the duodenal intubation of babies may not be carried out a distance (telecommand). The physician should perform this personally

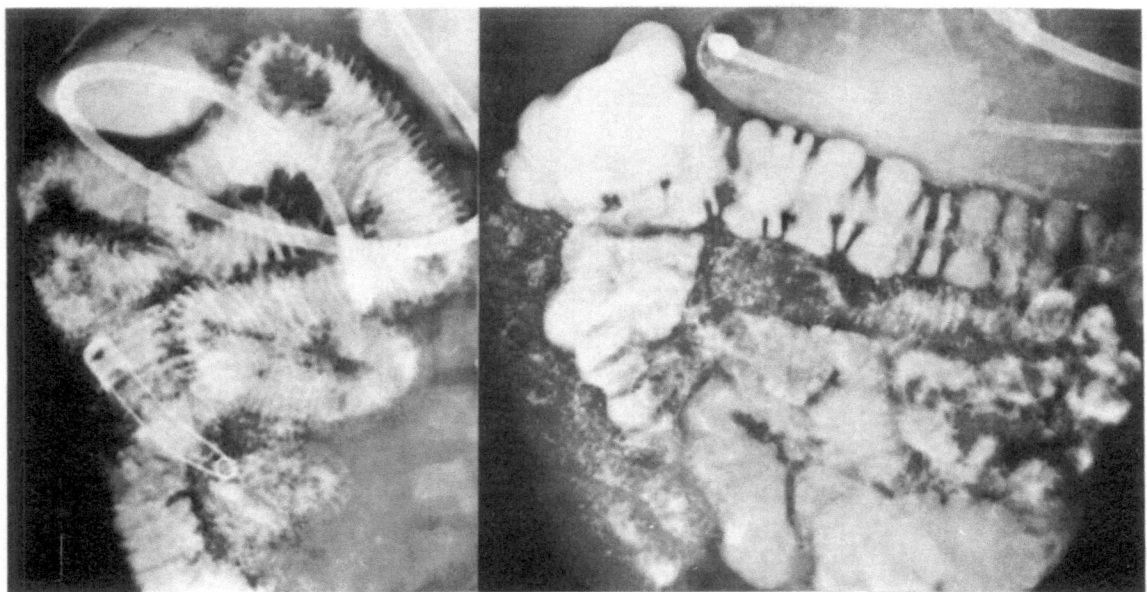

Fig. II.12. Four-year-old child with celiac disease and an unusually marked tendency to flocculation of the contrast fluid. The mucosal folds that are somewhat coarse and bulbous in the jejunum were visible only *during* the infusion.

from the head of the table while fluoroscopy is regulated by a colleague or technician. For fluoroscopy during this procedure, only an exceedingly low radiation dose is required.

2.4. The contrast fluid
It may sound unreasonable but there are radiologists who employ the same contrast fluid for every examination! This produces hopeless results, certainly in babies. We have found that the densities for the contrast fluid listed below are the most suitable.

0-12 months	s.g. = 1.15 = 19% wt/vol (i.e. 1 part 85% barium suspension diluted with 3½ parts water)
1-3 years	s.g. = 1.17 = 21% wt/vol (i.e. 1 part 85% barium suspension diluted with 3 parts water)
3-12 years	s.g. = 1.2 = 24% wt/vol (i.e. 1 part 85% barium suspension diluted with 2½ parts water).

Although doses of 200, 300 and 400 ml, respectively, are sufficient for these age groups, more contrast medium must be prepared. Some usually ends up in the stomach and may or may not be vomited. For all three age groups listed above, the rate of flow is ± 40 ml/min. This may seem fast for a baby but is necessary because of the strong tendency to flocculate. In fact flocculation of the contrast medium begins as soon as the flow decreases or stops. Even more convincing proof of the necessity of a rapid flow is seen in celiac disease. An unusually strong tendency to flocculation of the contrast medium renders reproduction of the mucosal relief virtually impossible (fig. II.12).

2.5. The examination
The flow of the contrast medium is relatively faster in children and in addition there is a greater tendency towards retroperistaltic movements than in adults. Because of this, there will practically always be a more or less pronounced reflux of the contrast medium into the stomach. Frequently the child will vomit the contrast medium that has entered the stomach before the end of the examination and that lasts only 5-10 min! It is therefore wise to turn the child's head to the left or right as soon as the stomach starts to fill. This is best left to a nurse from the pediatric department who, wearing lead apron and lead gloves, should stand at the head of the table. A good

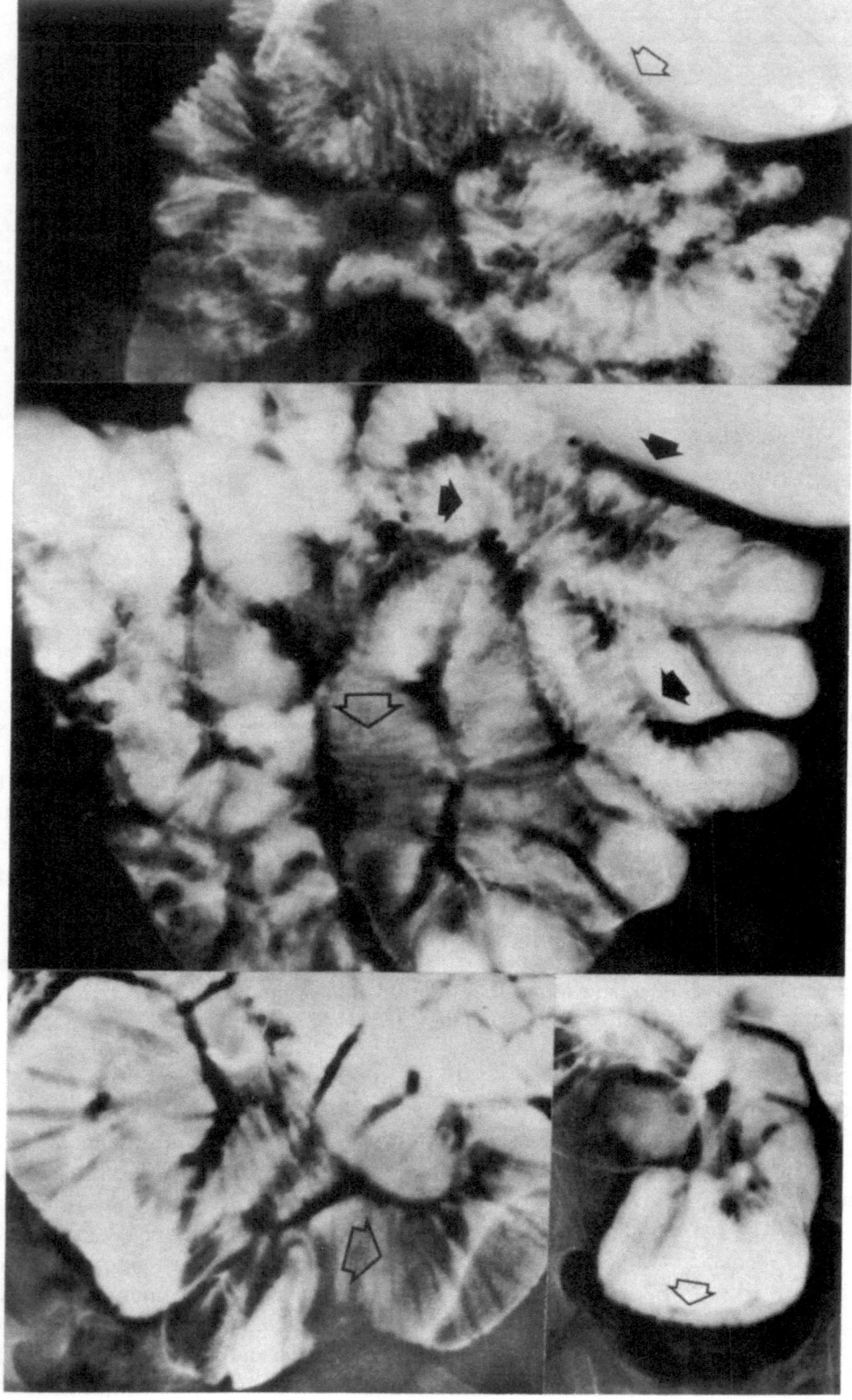

Fig. II.13. Shallow but easily recognized mucosal folds in an eight-week-old baby. In the ileum in particular the folds are only visible as minute ridges. For some unknown reason the ileum shows adhesions and is therefore dilated.

alternative is to insert a second tube via the other nostril into the stomach, which can be kept empty with a hypodermic or a suction pump. This prevents vomiting and the danger of aspirating the barium suspension. During adminstration of the contrast fluid, children must always lie on their backs. This is because it is absolutely necessary to make spot films as quickly as possible, whether compression is used or not.

Disintegration of the contrast fluid begins as soon as the flow of fluid decreases due to reflux or vomiting, or is terminated for any reason. Further exposures are then no longer possible!

It should be emphasized that compression must be carried out with the greatest possible care. Adequate compression in the minor pelvis can be considered an illusion in babies of less than one year. A röntgen examination for the purpose of demonstrating a Meckel's diverticulum, in particular in babies of this age, is absurd. Since compression of the lower abdomen is impossible, it is equally ridiculous to attempt double-contrast exposures with air, as this results only in a large number of extremely confusing curved lines yielding absolutely no diagnostic information. As soon as enough contrast fluid has reached the cecum for the desired degree of filling and several survey as well as spot films have been taken, the examination can be terminated. In children less than one year old there is, because of rapid distintegration, no further opportunity for supplementary exposures after the first have been evaluated. The tube is retracted until the tip lies in the cardia of the stomach. After the contrast fluid in the stomach has been suctioned off, the tube is removed entirely.

2.6. Results

All claims that the small intestine does not show mucosal relief in the first months of life, or that the mucosal relief cannot be visualized, can now truly be regarded as mythical. The enteroclysis examination has demonstrated that, although thin, these folds can certainly be visualized (fig. II.13).

Autopsy studies have shown that the mucosa slides easily over the underlying layers. The folds disappear quickly when the intestinal lumen is slightly stretched.

3. Retrograde administration of the contrast fluid

Miller found that the appearance of the ileum in particular is determined by tone and peristalsis to such an extent that constricting lesions in an early stage and smaller mucosal lesions are definitely missed during a transit examination. The functioning of the pylorus causes intermittent, irregular and incomplete filling so that the elasticity of the intestine cannot be determined. Furthermore, flocculation and segmentation often completely distort the evaluation. Miller was then of the opinion that enteroclysis was a good method of examination, but duodenal intubation beforehand too troublesome. He therefore proposed retrograde filling of the entire small intestine. Although it was possible to reach the stomach in nine out of ten patients, he advised terminating the filling of the small intestine as the duodenum was approached. It is obvious that this filling must occur under fluoroscopic control and that care must be taken that the contrast fluid does not enter the lungs by way of the stomach and esophagus.

In many patients it is possible to pass Bauhin's valve easily but sometimes this is difficult or impossible. This difficulty can be overcome in most cases by oral administration of 1 mgr atropine or 0.5-1.0 mgr glucagon i.v. prior to the examination; this may also cause a decrease in the secretion of intestinal juices and in forward peristalsis, thus greatly facilitating retrograde filling.

The amount of contrast medium required to fill the colon and small intestine is normally less than 3 litres but sometimes considerably more. More than 4.5 litres are never given, even if the duodenum has not yet been reached.

Miller later changed his method slightly by replacing the barium suspension with a physiological salt solution as soon as the ileum began to fill. The striking advantage of this latter method is that the recto-sigmoid, descending and transverse colon are rendered transparent and cause no hindrance to small bowel exposure by superimposition.

When the infusion of the contrast medium has been terminated, the colon is emptied by first

24

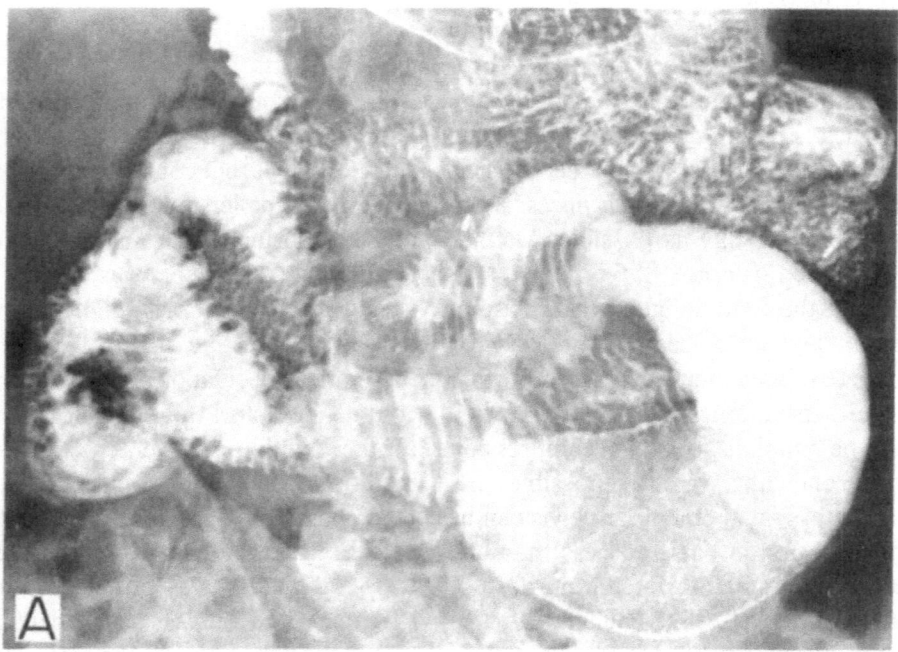

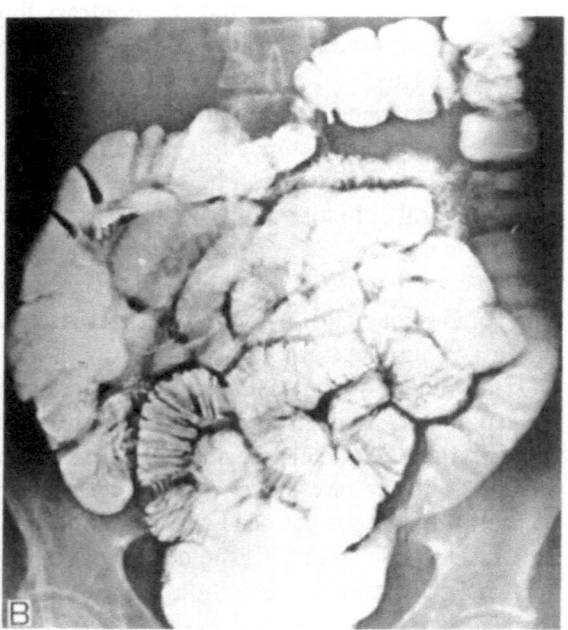
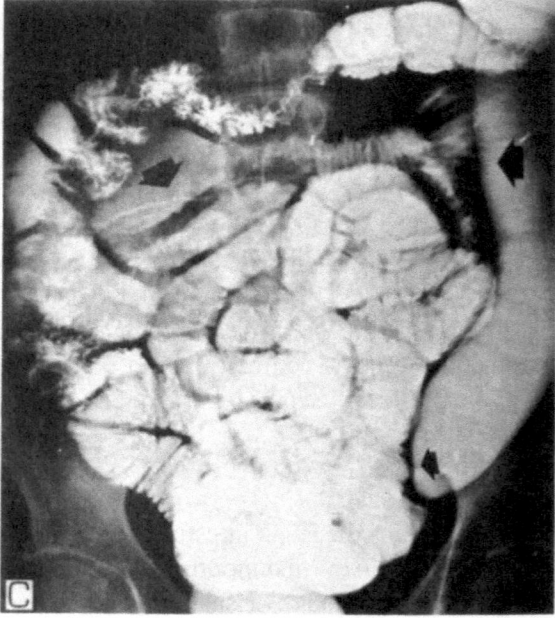

Fig. II.14A-E. (A) As a result of a stenosis in the jejunum due to radiation enteritis, it was not possible to obtain adequate filling of the ileum. (B) Filling of the ileum via the colon appeared possible without administration of a hypotonic agent. (C) The exposure after defecation showed edematous mucosal folds in the left upper quadrant, extensive fusion and obliteration of the mucosa in the right upper quadrant, and a stenosis in the sigmoid. (D) The mass of ileal loops in the minor pelvis became accessible for compression after filling the recto-sigmoid with air. (E) Spot films using compression reveal a skip lesion in the right lower quadrant.

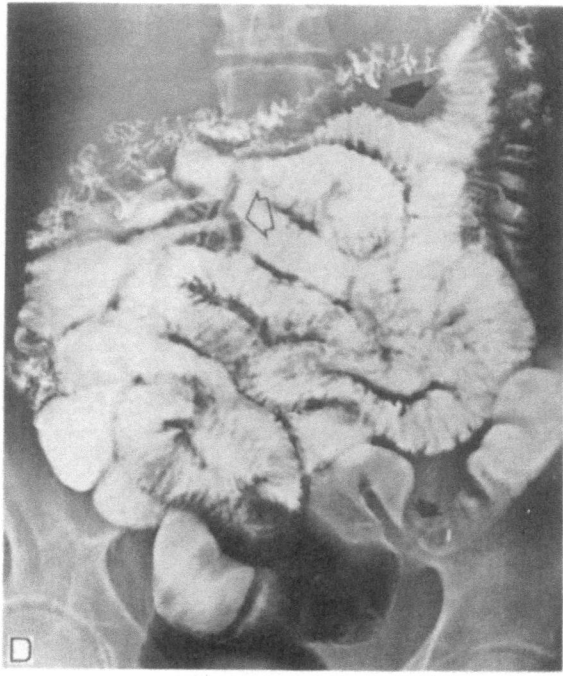 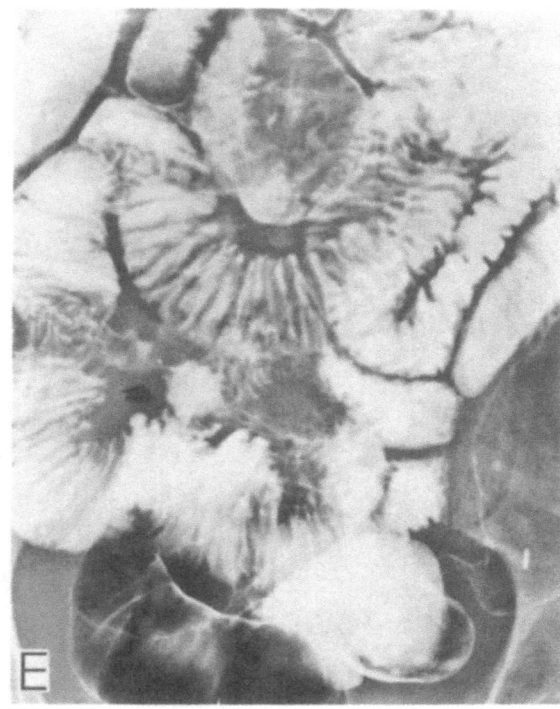

Fig. II.14D-E.

lowering the plastic infusion bag below the level of the table and then sending the patient to the toilet. Frequent but short periods for evacuation can also easily be accomplished by lowering the bag under the level of the table regularly. If retrograde filling of the small intestine is not possible without atropine or Buscopan, then the patient must be allowed much longer periods for evacuation. Films of the small intestine are subsequently made; films of the colon, if desired, can be made at the beginning of the infusion period.

The contrast fluid is naturally not that for a colon enema but is the barium suspension normally used for oral enteroclysis. If it is possible to pass Bauhin's valve and fill the small intestine without medication to induce hypotonicity, the time available for making röntgen films is quite short since the small intestine will empty quickly. Small intestine films are best made as soon as peristalsis resumes.

An enormous advantage of Miller's method is that stenotic processes in the small intestine can be approached very quickly from their distal side (fig. II.14A-E). Proximal approach in these cases costs more time, and moreover, a troublesome dilution of the contrast medium can occur in the dilated loops.

4. *Visualization of fistulous tracts*

Fistulous canals are usually of small calibre, have an irregular track and occasionally form a complicated network that is neither easy to fill adequately, nor to visualize. It is selfevident that while a thin fluid contrast medium is better for filling such fistulas, a more viscous fluid on the other hand, is better retained. Gastrografin is well known for its ability to penetrate a fistulous tract from which it just as readily disappears. The best contrast medium for abdominal fistulas suspected of opening into the bowel lumen is a slightly viscous barium suspension as used in enteroclysis. Filling of the fistulous canal should be enhanced, where possible, by increase of intraluminal pressure in the bowel. The administration rate of the contrast medium and peristalsis should therefore preferably be above normal limits, stimulated if need be by metoclopramide. In addition emptying of the small intestine should be inhibited by pressure

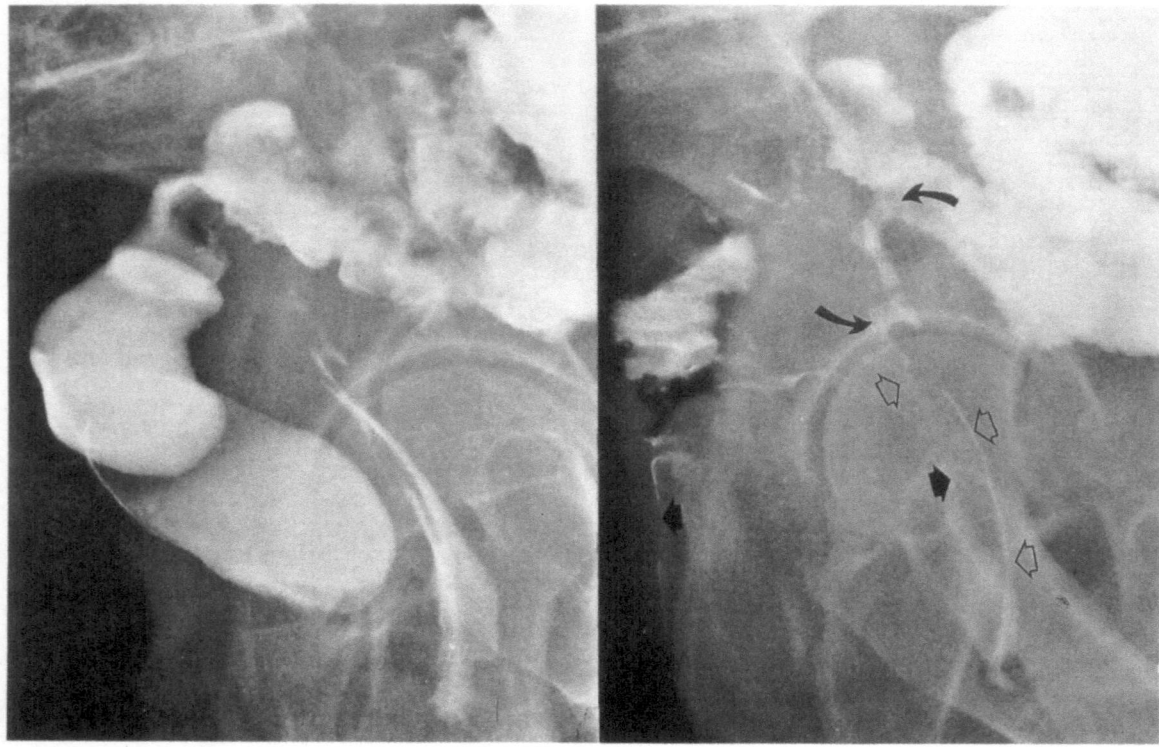

Fig. II.15. Case of Crohn's disease. A fistulous canal (curved arrows) between ileum and vagina (open arrows) could only be visualized by hindering evacuation of the contrast fluid via the rectum. This was achieved by introducing an inflatable cannula into the rectum (short closed arrows) whereby closure could be accomplished by means of water instead of air.

over the ileocecal region or by introduction of a water filled balloon into the rectum (fig. II.15). Improvisation is frequently necessary, depending on the type and site of the fistula.

Even when fistula canals have been adequately filled, visualization can still produce problems. Fixation of the fistula in an inflamed or infiltrated area makes adequate compression often impossible. Filling of troublesome superimposed bowel loops with air or water can here offer a solution (fig. II.16).

Stomata of the fistulous process opening onto the external abdominal wall should be occluded with inflated Foley catheters. In this latter case it is preferable to fill the fistula complex through one or other of the abdominal openings, the other canals being occluded. Thereby sufficient contrast medium must be introduced to ensure that an adequate number of bowel loops are filled to provide orientation. Barium suspension is the contrast medium of choice here but Dionosil aquosum is possible.

5. Marshak's technique

In very exceptional cases administration of contrast medium by drinking is unavoidable. The patient is here given 1 litre barium suspension to which 30 ml metoclopramide has been added. The first exposures are made immediately after drinking is completed and further as required. Between exposures the patient is allowed to lie on his right side. The results are unpredictable, usually the degree of filling of the bowel is insufficient (fig. II.17).

H. Common errors and failures

There are numerous ways to ruin an enteroclysis examination completely and the results are then such that it would have been better if a conventional follow-through examination had been carried out.

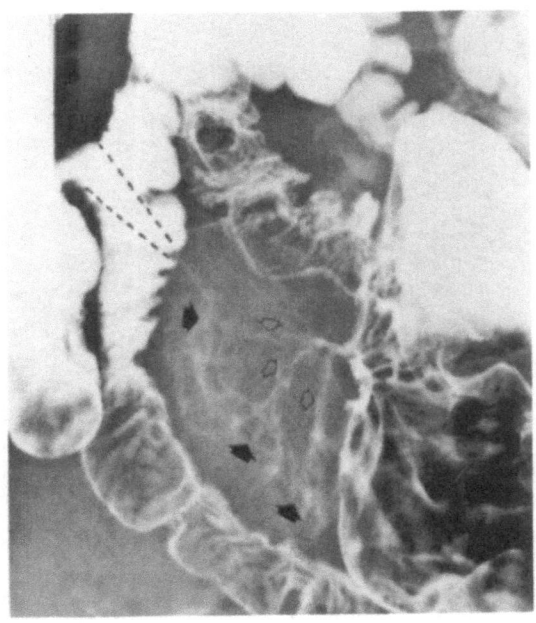

Fig. II.16. Three fistulous tracts between the ileum (barely visible) and the recto-sigmoid, visibility improved after rectal air insufflation. Crohn's disease.

Frequently these poor results originate in a marked lack of interest and an unwillingness to change routine procedures that have been in use for years.

Clumsy attempts at duodenal intubation, a result of not carefully studying the available literature, is likewise a fairly common reason for condemning the infusion technique.

The most common errors and their causes will be discussed systematically.

1. Preparation

1.1. Colon not thoroughly cleansed

In numerous cases it has been found that the colon was not cleansed before the examination (see fig. II.23). The extreme importance of this step has been explained. It is striking that in these patients passage proceeds quickly through the jejunum but becomes greatly retarded more distally as the contaminated cecum is approached. The examination then takes long and the contrast fluid thickens in the ileum so that exposures of this region are poor in quality. A water infusion after administration of the contrast medium can force filling of the distal ileum, but the calibre of the loops then increases so much that good compression spot films are no longer possible.

1.2. Colon cleansed by means of a rectal enema

This method is definitely not to be preferred as there is frequently reflux of clyster fluid into the ileum and therefore considerable mixing occurs with the contrast fluid entering proximally. The troublesome disadvantage of clyster fluid in the small intestine can be avoided by postponing the enteroclysis examination until 1 or 2 h after the clysma. A 'quick' examination is then out of the question.

1.3. Drugs not discontinued

Another frequent error is that treatment with tranquillizers, sedatives and antispasmodic drugs has not been discontinued before the examination. The resulting reduction in motility leads to a marked increase in the amount of contrast medium required and therefore prolongs the examination. Furthermore there is less chance of obtaining good spot films by using compression.

1.4. Temperature of the contrast fluid

The technician should be fully conversant with the requirements. Cold suspensions reduce the chance of reflux into the stomach but icy fluids cause nausea and vomiting with reflux into the stomach. As pointed out in chapter II.D1 the contrast medium should be administered at room temperature.

1.5. Specific gravity of the barium suspension

All too often the technician asks the radiologist what the dilution of the contrast fluid should be before he has even seen the patient, believing apparently that this factor is dependant upon the physicians personal whims. The radiologist should more or less comply with the specific values listed in chapter II.D.1. If the contrast fluid is either too dense or too radiolucent, the results will be unacceptable. If the specific gravity is too high, much more radiation will be required to obtain exposures that are only just acceptable. In fact this compensation is more usually an illusion

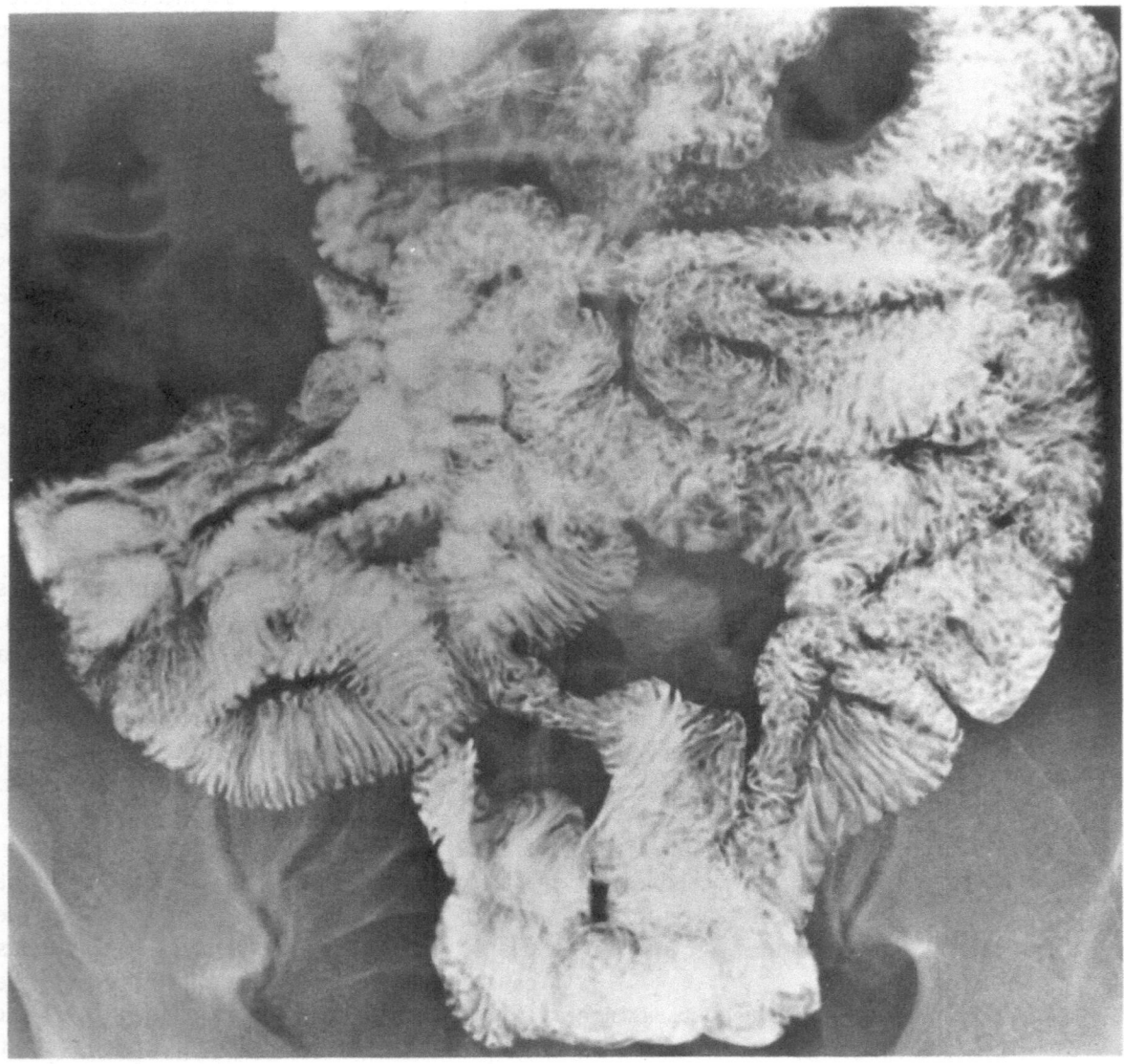

Fig. II.17. Although satisfactory result of a conventional transit examination, the amount of contrast fluid in the bowel is not sufficient and the mucosal folds are disorderly arranged.

illusion rather than reality (fig. II.18). If the specific gravity is too low, the contrast medium will generally be fairly thin and fluid. It will run in too fast and there will be excessive filling of the intestinal loops. The contrast will not be sufficient to visualize details such as aphthoid ulcers. In particular if the specific gravity is too low and the voltage too high, the films are easily overexposed (fig. II.19).

2. Performance of the examination

2.1. Tube not far enough into the duodenum

This fault can often be attributed to nonchalant technical handling or supply of Bilbao tubes that are too short for some patients. It has been pointed out that longer (125-135 cm) Bilbao tubes have been produced for enteroclysis. Furthermore, these new tubes are safer because the guide

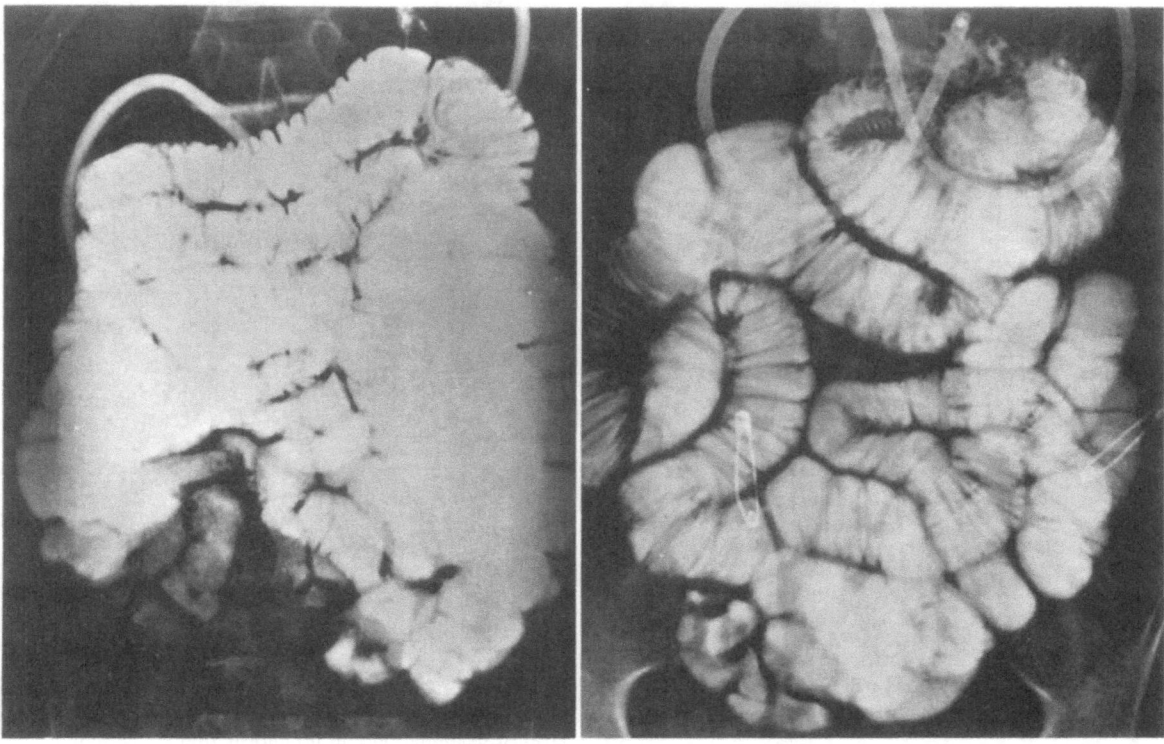

Fig. II.18. Inadequate survey film of an enteroclysis examination, submitted for comment (left). Despite rather high background density, the information attainable is only marginal; no evidence of low kilovoltage; presumably contrast medium of too high specific gravity employed. Repetition (right) gave better results from use of a barium suspension with lower specific gravity requiring less background density and thus lower dosage of X-rays.

wire cannot pass through the side openings. Once the tube is in the duodenum, it is usually easy to push the tip further towards the ligament of Treitz. If problems should arise, for instance in extra thin patients, no attempt should be made to push the tube further. The tube will then most probably curl up in the duodenum. Should the tip end up in the duodenal bulb, the inevitable result will be reflux of the contrast medium into the stomach.

2.2. Too slow administration of contrast medium

If the flowrate of the barium suspension is less than 75 ml/min, there will be insufficient stretching of the duodenum, peristalsis will not be strong and the examination thus prolonged. In addition, the degree of small intestine filling will be similar to that of a conventional transit examination and the advantage of forced flow will be lost (fig. II.20 and II.17). Mild cases of celiac disease will certainly not be recognized. Prestenotic dilata-

tions will not develop as easily and the differences between hypermotility and hypomotility will nearly disappear. A sluggish flow can produce an almost identical pattern in the small bowel as hypermotility when the flow is too fast. The importance of a correct flow rate is pointed out in chapter II.D2.

2.3. Too rapid administration of contrast medium

In practice the flow is commonly too fast rather than too slow. The rate of flow is determined not only by the height of the contrast medium bag above the table but by several other factors such as the length and minimum bore of the infusion system and composition, dilution and temperature of the barium suspension. Therefore, the flow rates of the different densities of barium suspension at various levels above the examination table should be determined within every radiology department.

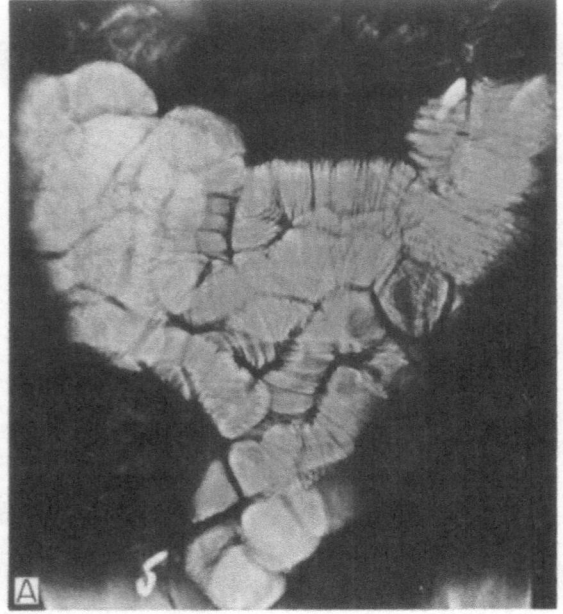

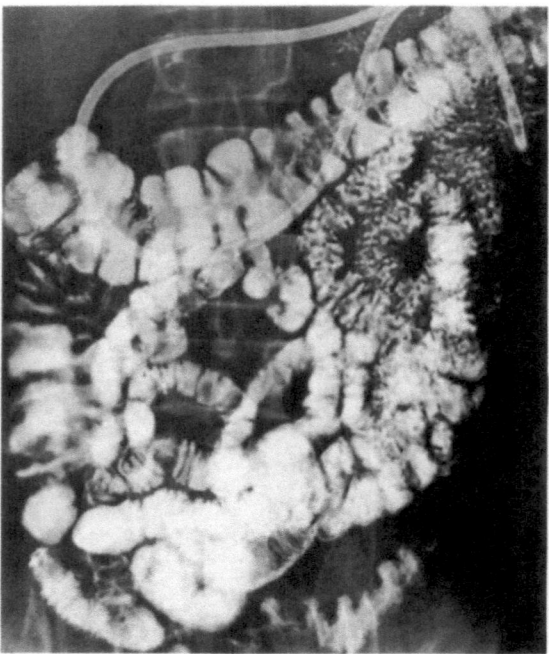

Fig. II.20. If the speed of administration of the contrast fluid is too low, then the result resembles that of a regular transit examination and no information concerning motility will be obtained.

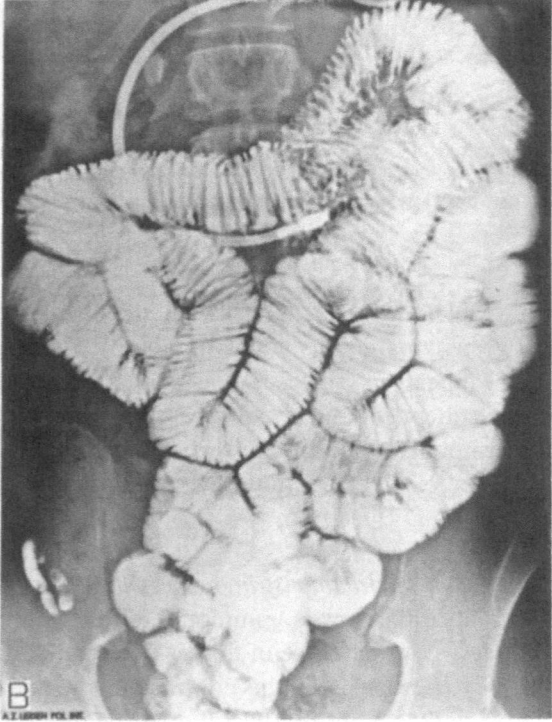

Fig. II.19. Overexposured film and density of the contrast medium too low (above). Moreover. 150 kV was employed! In an attempt to compensate the low specific gravity of the contrast medium, a better result would have been obtained in this case with 90 kV. The degree of filling of the bowel is excessive and must have been the result of too rapid administration of the contrast fluid, probably from use of too dilute barium suspension. A completely different result was obtained with a repeat examination a few days later (lower).

Only standard equipment and contrast media should be used. If the flow rate of the barium suspension is too high, reflux into the stomach is promoted.

In addition, a long segment of the jejunum will be stretched too fast and paralyse the entero-enteral reflex mechanism, resulting in a temporary disappearance of motility. Therefore, evaluation of motility, which is based on conditions in the jejunum, becomes impossible. Disturbed motility is a direct cause of about 10% of small intestinal complaints and is also an important indicator of many diseases. The consequencies of this lack of diagnostic information should not be underestimated.

Reflex hypomotility, together with frequent reflux into the stomach resulting from too rapid flow of contrast medium, cause prolongation of the examination. Moreover as a result of the much larger dose of contrast medium required and the high degree of filling of the intestine, it is much more difficult to make good compression spot films.

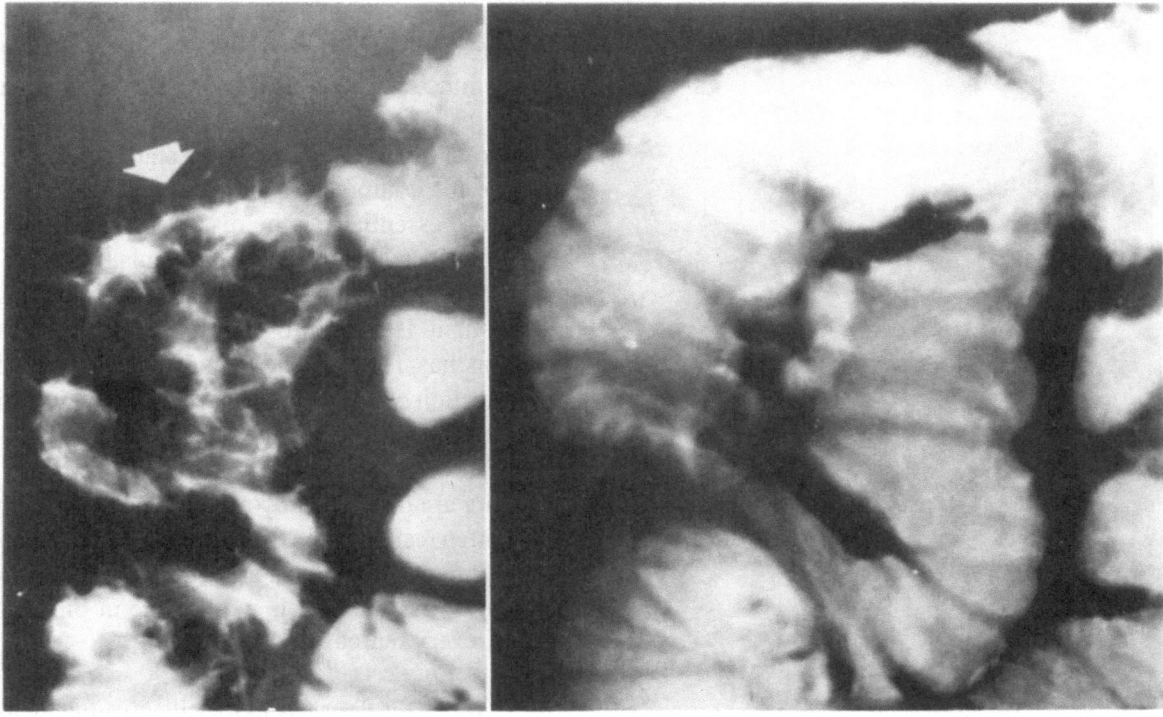

Fig. II.21. Recurrence of Crohn's disease after an ileocecal resection. The swollen mucosal folds are clearly visible when the intestinal loops are only moderately filled, but are difficult to see when the loops are well filled.

2.4. Contrast fluid dose too low

On occasion a dose of 600-800 ml is administered and the tube removed whether the cecum has been reached or not. Further developments are then awaited as in a conventional examination. If the flow rate is correct and all the prescribed preparatory measures have been performed, in most cases the cecum will indeed have been reached. However, this is not so if preparation has been inadequate or in the presence of a stenosis or hypomotility. With inadequate preparation the examination, like a conventional one, produces absolutely no result.

In the event of stenosis or hypomotility, the examination is greatly prolonged and the contrast fluid shows troublesome thickening in the ileum. The best course in this situation is to try to complete the examination as soon as possible by means of an i.v. injection of 1-2 ml metoclopramide (see fig. II.22).

2.5. The routine use of aircontrast technique only

If aircontrast films are wanted then, even in case of hypomotility, not more than about 600 ml contrast fluid must be administered. The cecum must also be reached with only this amount before air insufflation can begin. This is often time consuming, so that the examination can no longer be considered as short. Because the amount of contrast fluid is limited, prestenotic dilatations, especially in the distal intestine, will seldom or never develop. Ulcers, adhesions and tumors can thus easily be overlooked. This disadvantage might be minimized or even eliminated if the double-contrast films provided sufficent compensation; unfortunately this is not the case. A prestenotic dilatation is much less likely to develop when air is used instead of barium. It is also easily missed in the complex of lines. This confusing pattern will also hinder identification of polyps and Meckel's

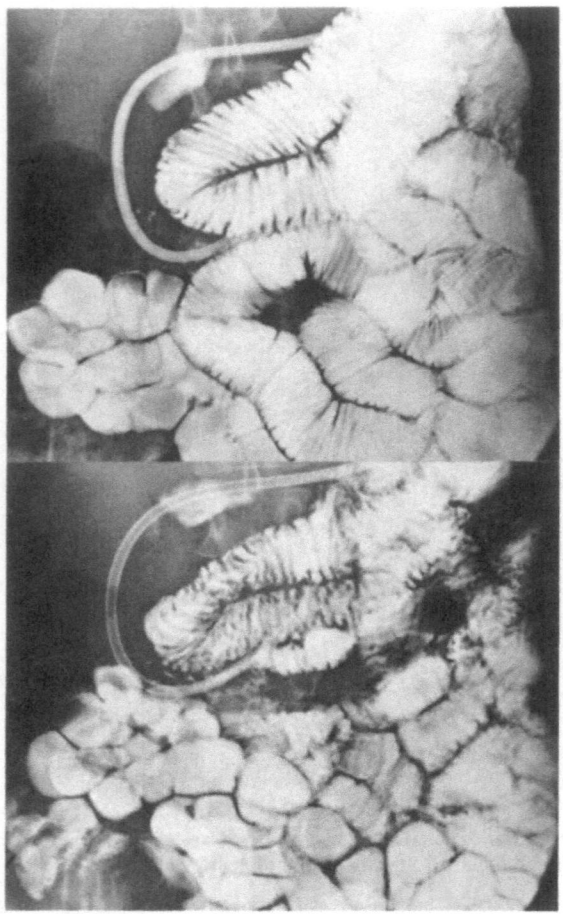

Fig. II.22. Hypomotility and dilatation due to long-term use of antispasmodics. Cecum not yet reached after 1200 ml contrast fluid (above). Within 2 min after the i.v. injection of Primperan (metoclopramide) there is an increase of muscular tone and peristalsis and the cecum is reached (lower). It will be clear that it is much easier to make compression details under these latter circumstances because it is less full in the abdomen.

diverticula unless the loops can be projected free from mutual interference. Constrictions caused by bands are visualized much more clearly when the intestinal loops are filled with barium suspension only (figs. III.17B and IV.63). Reproduction of subtle abnormalities of the mucosa is better in aircontrast, especially if a dense contrast fluid is used (figs. II.8 and IV.161). However, a double-contrast examination means a reduction in total diagnostic information. The only exception is when air is used to facilitate visualization of the mass of ileal loops deep in the minor pelvis.

2.6. Routine use of the water-push technique only

Stenosis of the intestine as well as constrictions and impressions are most easily discovered when the intestine is well filled. An edematous swelling of the mucous membrane is, on the other hand, much better seen when the degree of filling is moderate (fig. II.21). This latter state is also preferable for compression of individual loops and therefore essential for the discovery of aphthoid ulcers and small Meckel's diverticula.

If a water infusion is to follow the barium suspension, it is better to wait until the contrast column has reached the cecum. Too early administration of water renders evaluation of intestinal motility impossible, the intestine may even be more or less paralysed. Furthermore, many patients are distressed by a rapid water infusion. This often results in the development of reflux into the stomach with nausea and vomiting. Administration of air or water is worthwhile in only one out of every ten cases.

2.7. Incorrect decisions during the examination

Frequently the reasons leading to a decision to use air insufflation or a water infusion are completely wrong. Often the contrast medium infusion is terminated too soon. In case of hypomotility or obstruction, the radiologist frequently does not dare administer more contrast fluid. He believes erroneously (usually from incorrect information in the literature) that the total dose would be too high.

Occasionally the contrast medium infusion has been allowed to run too long. If the colon is well cleansed, excessive filling of the recto-sigmoid can occur quickly. Adequate compression of the ileum is then out of the question. The only alternative in such cases to try to save the situation is by emptying the recto-sigmoid using a cannula or by allowing a quick, short defecation! Air then is insufflated with the patient in the prone position.

Finally, a much too common error is omitting to give Primperan (metoclopramide), once hypomotility has been established. This is especially true after a large quantity of contrast fluid has already been administered. When Primperan is given as an injection or via the tube, it is essential to wait 5-10 min before proceeding further. The useful effect of metoclopramide (Primperan) injection is illustrated in fig. II.22.

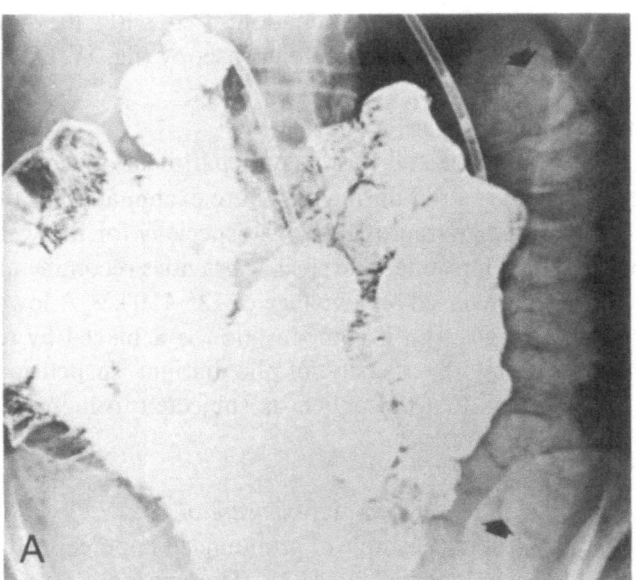

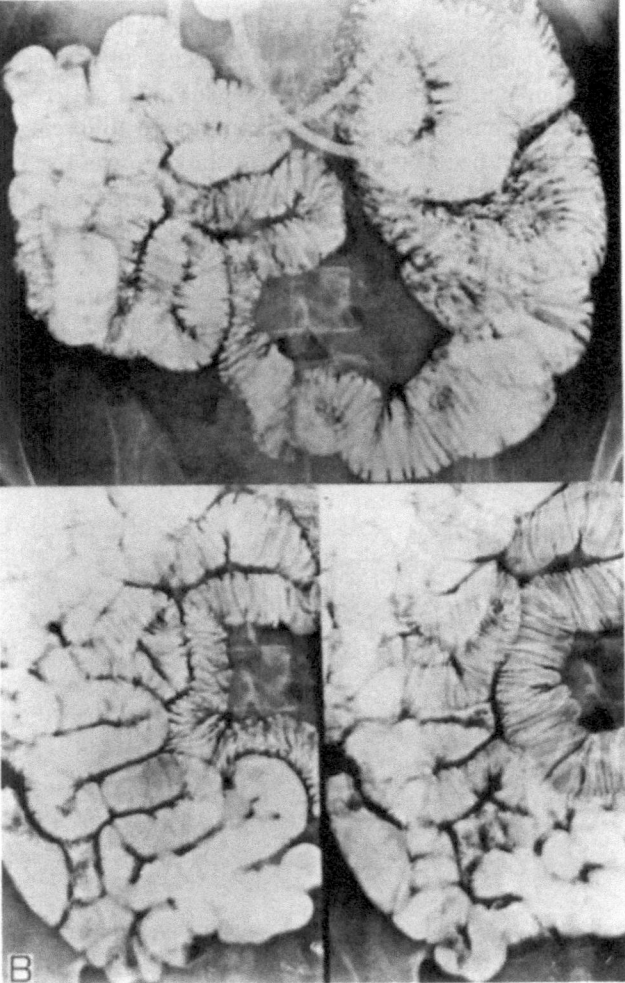

Fig. II.23. (A) Useless and misleading enteroclysis examination, showing an obvious underexposure. The colon was in no way cleansed and therefore a considerable amount of contrast fluid was needed to reach the cecum. Finally air was insufflated through the tube without any chance of success. (B) The result of the repeat examination, performed one week later. There were indeed no abnormalities.

34

3. General faults and failures

3.1. Not enough exposures
Unusual or suspect configurations of the mucosal relief or the contrast column should be recorded at least twice or more if possible. This should be done especially in cases of doubt. It is therefore useful to take two exposures of the same region with a short interval routinely, as the position of the intestinal loops has then not yet changed and comparison is facilitated. It is astonishing to see cases in which the entire small bowel was covered by only two survey films!

3.2. Omission of or too few spot films with compression
The most common of all faults is the assumption that compression is of value only in the distal ileum. It is incorrectly believed that abnormalities will seldom be found elsewhere. Experience with thousands of patients has shown that many more abnormalities are found in the much longer segment proximal to the 20 cm-long distal ileum. Eight compression spot films, spread out over the entire small intestine may be considered as the absolute minimum. Spot films of a mass of ileal loops in the minor pelvis do not necessarily form a satisfactory examination; frequently they are made without careful fluoroscopy (fig. IV.125).

3.3. Voltage too low
There are still radiology departments where the voltage used during the entire examination of the digestive tract is too low, especially for the well-filled intestine. The specific gravities recommended are based on a voltage of 125-150 kV. A lower voltage, even if compensation is achieved by reducing the density of the barium suspension, means that the patient is subjected to increased exposure.

3.4. Under and overexposure of films
A striking example of pronounced underexposure can be seen in fig. II.23. The examination was evaluated as normal. These films show that no attempt had been made to cleanse the colon before examination. Furthermore, without reason or any chance of obtaining good results, possibly in desperation, air was insufflated. A repeat examination produced completely different results because the correct technique was used. Overexposure is less serious than underexposure

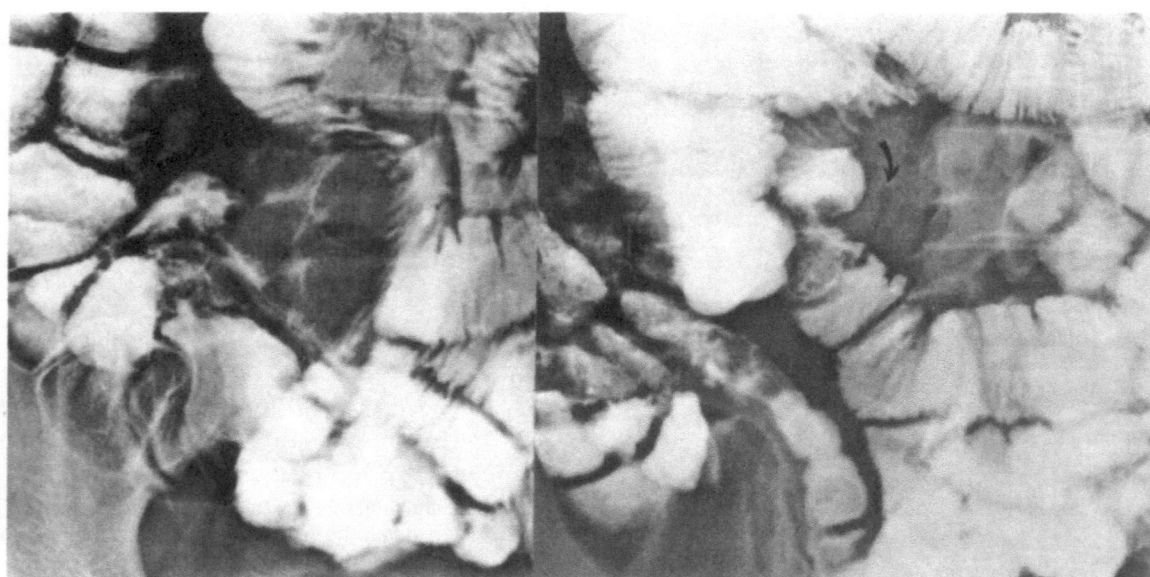

Fig. II.24. Space-occupying defect in the ileocecal region attributed to an infiltrate or mesenteric tumor (left). A repeat examination was necessary to convince the radiologist conducting the examination that the colon was causing an impression on the intestinal loops (see the haustra pattern on the right film).

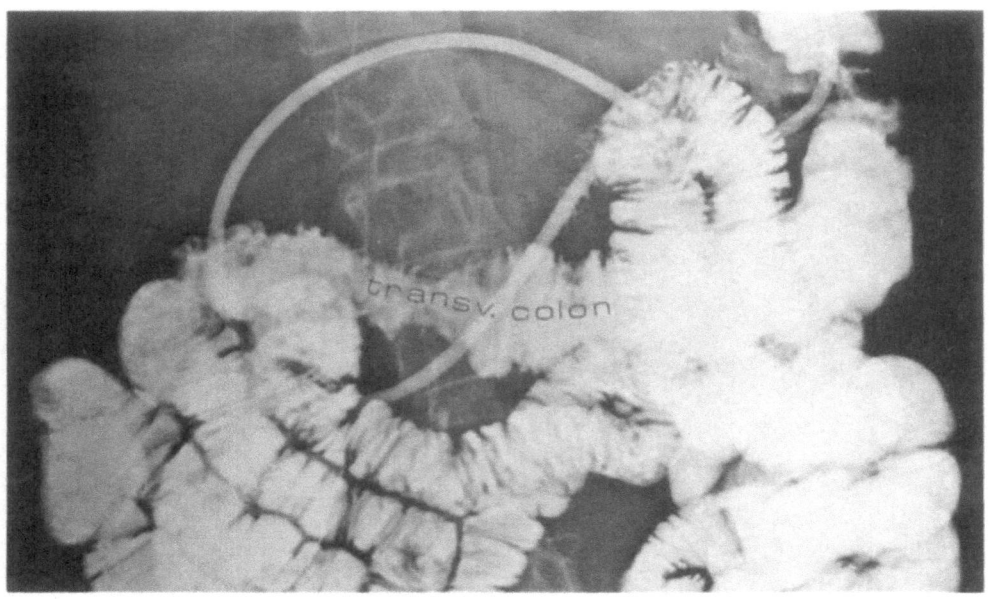

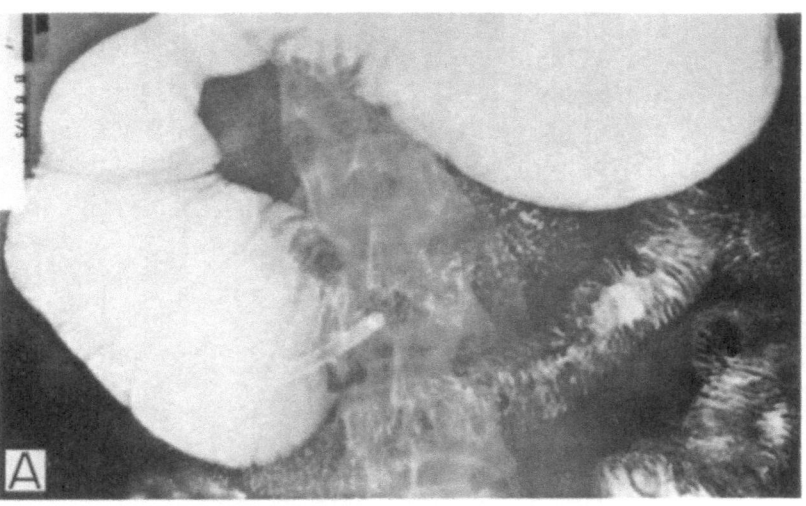

Fig. II.25A. Completely normal small bowel examination of a patient with loss of blood from the digestive tract. The gastric examination, however, clearly showed tumor growth in the duodenum. Apparently it was possible to pass the stenosis with the infusion tube.

since a bright viewing box can compensate for this to some extent. If, however, in addition to overexposure, the specific gravity of the contrast fluid is too low and the voltage is 150 kV, then the problems of evaluation will indeed be enormous (fig. II.19).

3.5. *Errors in evaluation*

All too often, abnormalities present but unkwown remain unobserved on the röntgenograms. Common examples are edematous swollen folds, mucosal atrophy and disturbed motility. The tendency is to keep to traditionally correct interpretations of patterns hallowed by years of use and still persistent in the literature. Unfortunately these incorrect evalutations are not based on reality but on misleading patterns. A good example of this are those conventional examinations that, according to many radiologists, show coarse and 'certainly pathological' mucosal folds. A subsequent enteroclysis examination not showing these coarse folds may be regarded as

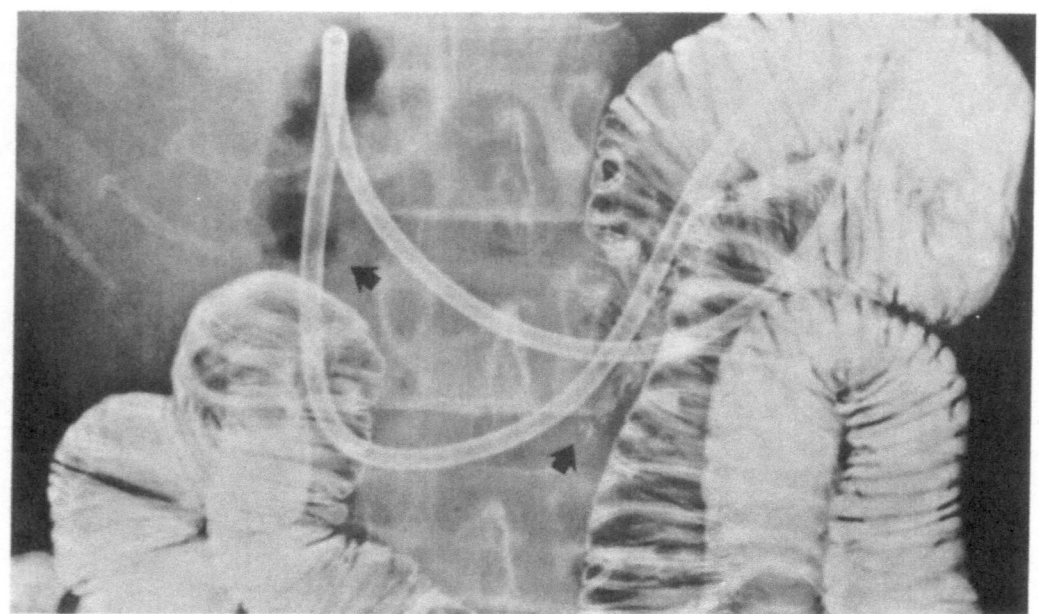

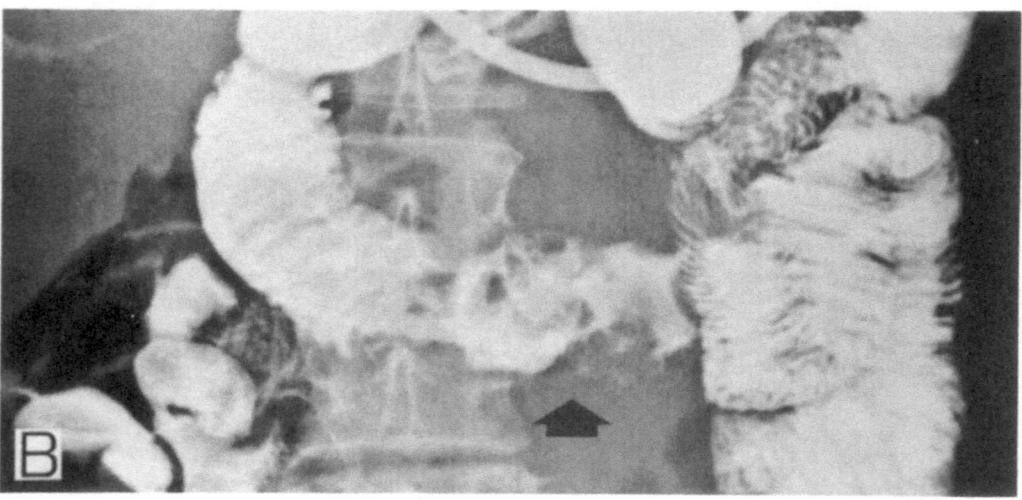

Fig. II.25B. Duodenal tumor that was not visualized because the tube extendend beyond the tumor (above). In this case, the examiner should have noted that, in spite of marked filling of the jejunum and total absence of motility, reflux into the duodenum did *not* occur. Moreover the air configuration ends abruptly in the proximal duodenum. During a second examination carried out shortly after, the tumor was demonstrated because the tube could no longer be pushed past it (below).

inadequate because it does not reproduce this 'pathology'. The cause of this so-called fold coarsening (see figs. IV.145AB and IV.146) is described in chapter IV.E1.

Frequently the radiologist does not even know the most basic and characteristic signs of pathology. Moreover he is liable to report abnormalities in the presence of purely normal patterns (fig. II.24).

It is none the less most important to be aware of the limits of an enteroclysis examination. The duodenum is certainly not always visualized. In such cases the report should contain the explicit statement that only the jejunum and the ileum were evaluated, good examples of this are seen in fig. II.25AB, where the infusion tube passed a duodenal tumor that consequently was not visualized on the films.

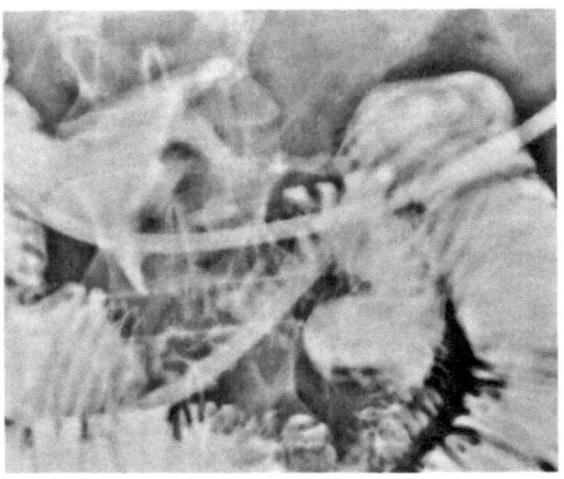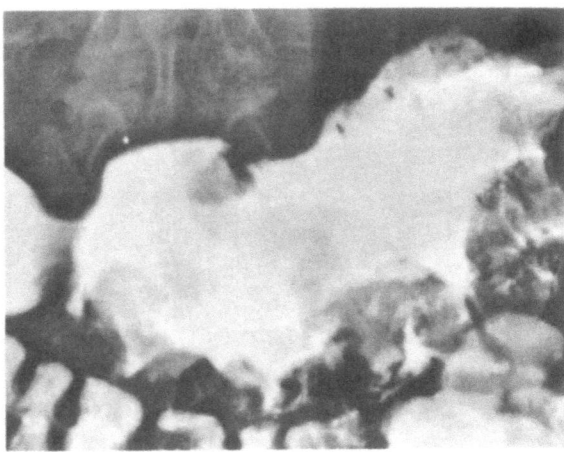

Fig. II.26. One of the films of an otherwise normal enteroclysis examination showed that reflux of the contrast fluid into the stomach caused a configuration indicative of a tumor; this was almost overlooked. A gastric examination carried out several days later confirmed the findings of the enteroclysis examination. The tumor was a lymphoreticular malignancy.

When evaluating a series of X-rays, every radiologist has the tendency to think only in terms of the patient's complaints. Regularly therefore, abnormalities located elsewhere or of an entirely different nature are completely overlooked, even when clearly visualized on the films. A striking example of this is the enteroclysis examination shown in fig. II.26, which was evaluated by several radiologists as being normal. None of them noted that reflux of the contrast fluid into the stomach caused a configuration in that organ that was highly suggestive of tumor growth, a diagnosis confirmed a few days later during gastric examination.

Finally, deficiency in the radiologists knowledge of small intestine pathology is sometimes manifest.

III. The normal small intestine

A. Length and position of the small bowel

The length of the small intestine varies between 5 and 7 m and this is assumed to be 3/5 of the total length of the digestive tract. The distance from nose or mounth to the duodeno-jejunal flexure varies only slightly around an assumed 90 cm. It is known that both length and diameter of the small intestine are very largely dependent on its tone, so that results of measurements postmortem or under anesthesia give too high a figure. The intestine shortens around an ingested tube, the so-called 'telescope effect'.

In 90% of adults, the jejunum is located in the left upper quadrant and the ileum in the right lower quadrant (fig. III.1). According to Zimmer, a small convolution usually lies in the middle, forming the transition between these two segments of the intestine. Lack of this 'intermediate convolution' may be the most common anomaly. The small intestine usually leaves the retroperitoneal space and enters the abdominal cavity to the left of the spinal column, this site is called 'Treitz ligament'.

B. Calibre of lumen

For the jejunum, the diameter is normally assumed to be 2.5-3.0 cm and for the ileum 2.0-2.5 cm. Values have also been reported of 1.0 and 0.5 inch respectively, which probably represent a closer approximation to the diameter in vivo or during a conventional transit examination. During an enteroclysis examination, as a result of the more active peristalsis, the diameter of the loops of the small intestine is generally greater and more variable than during a conventional examination. With infusion of 600-900 ml and a flow rate of 75 ml per minute, the maximum diameter of the

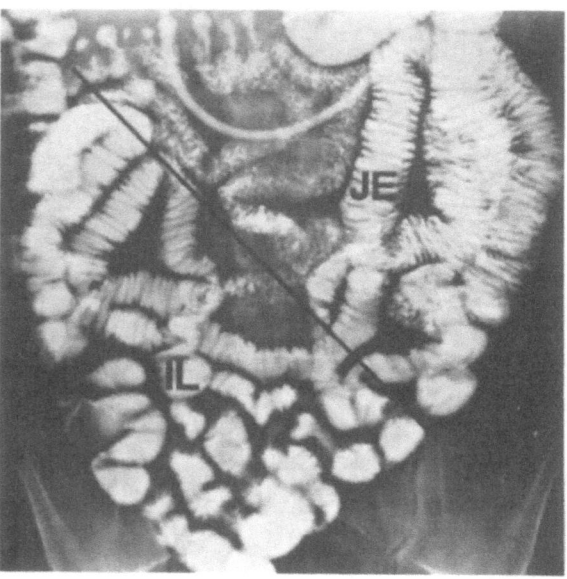

Fig. III.1. Most common position of the small bowel. Jejenum in left upper quadrant; ileum in right lower quadrant. The line separating these two convolutions is diagonal, running more or less perpendicular to the root of the mesentery which extends from the upper left to the lower right.

proximal jejunal loops is 4 cm in normal cases. Generally the diameter of the distal ileal loops depends to a large extent on the counterpressure caused by a fecal-filled cecum.

A diameter of 3 cm for segments in resting phase is normal in this region. During a conventional transit examination, the diameter of the contrast column in the distal ileum depends partly on the degree of increased viscosity of the contrast fluid, which in turn is determined by the duration of the examination. At the transition between jejunum and ileum, the diameter of the intestinal lumen differs only slightly from the standard values for a conventional transit examination. Of course with a greater flow rate, an increased amount of contrast medium or transit retarding

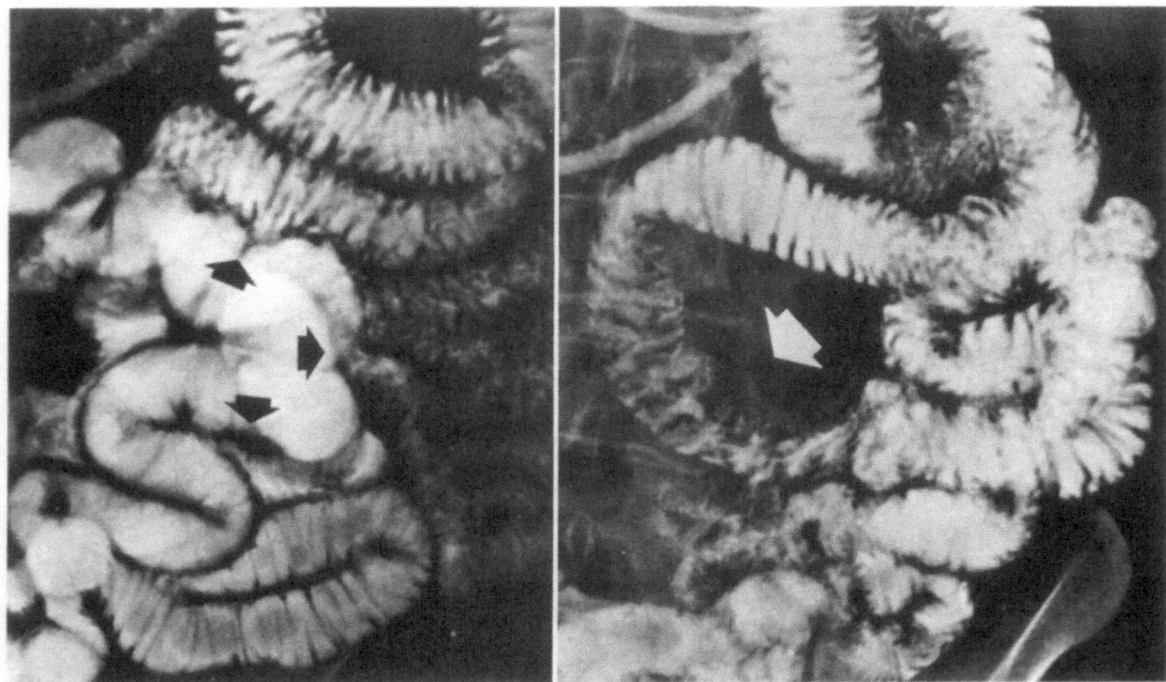

Fig. III.2A. Impression on the jejunum from other intestinal loops not yet filled with contrast fluid.

factors, the diameter of the intestinal lumen will increase.

C. Intestinal interspaces

1. Impressions on the intestine

Impressions can be caused by other intestinal loops, adjacent organs, vessels, inflammatory infiltrates, tumor tissue and fat. In enteroclysis, the degree of filling of the intestinal loops is greater than in a conventional follow-through examination so that mutual compression of these loops occurs much more frequently.

1.1. By other intestinal loops
In the jejunum, indentations in the contrast column may be seen, which on later films are shown to be caused by other small intestinal loops (fig. III.2A). In general, these impressions are most clearly visible on the largest loops, which usually have the lowest tone or are at that moment in a resting phase. Fewer impressions are seen on an intestine with active peristalsis, thus with good

tone, than on an atonic intestine. Since atony usually affects the proximal sooner than the distal intestinal loops, the most distal are more likely to indent the most proximal. An impression produced by ileal loops on the jejunal is therefore likely and the contrary is probably never seen (fig. III.2B).

It is not always possible to explain an impression even though later films prove without a doubt that it is temporary (fig. III.3).

The most frequently encountered impression of one intestinal loop on another is that of the colon on the small intestine (fig. III.5). The most likely explanation for this is the considerable difference in the viscosity of their contents. The most common impressions are of the cecum or sigmoid on the ileum (fig. III.4ab). Occasionally an impression of the descending colon on the jejunum is noted (fig. III.6).

1.2. By vessels
The pressure in the veins is so low that indentation by a vein on an intestinal loop is not conceivable. On the other hand, the large arteries frequently cause an impression on the small

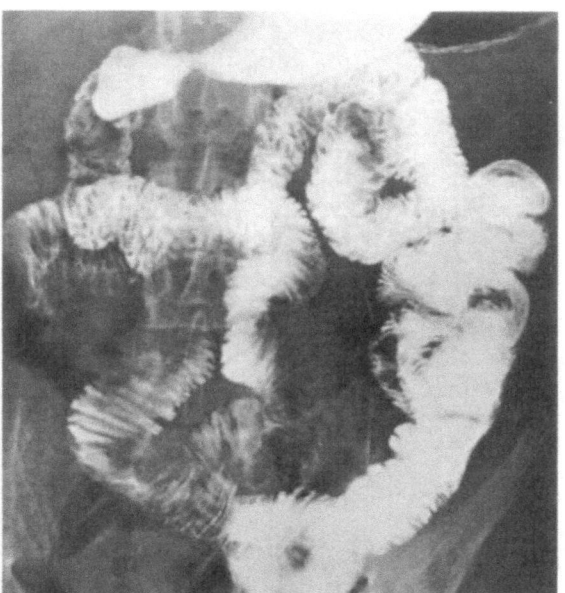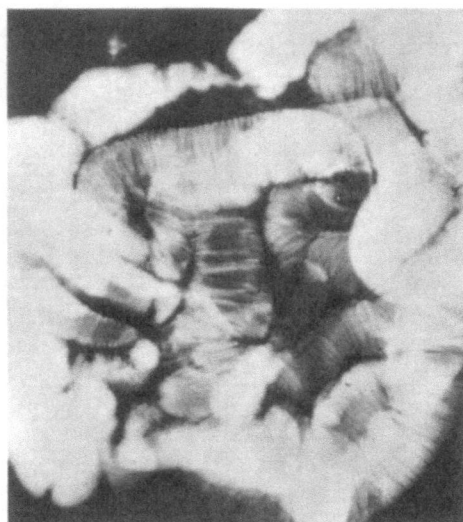

Fig. III.2B.   Regular follow-through examination first revealed a large defect between the intestinal loops which was assumed to be a tumor or cyst in the mesentery. A second examination, using enteroclysis, showed no abnormalities. Impression caused by dilated ileal loops in a female patient suffering from atony, a result of longstanding sedative therapy.

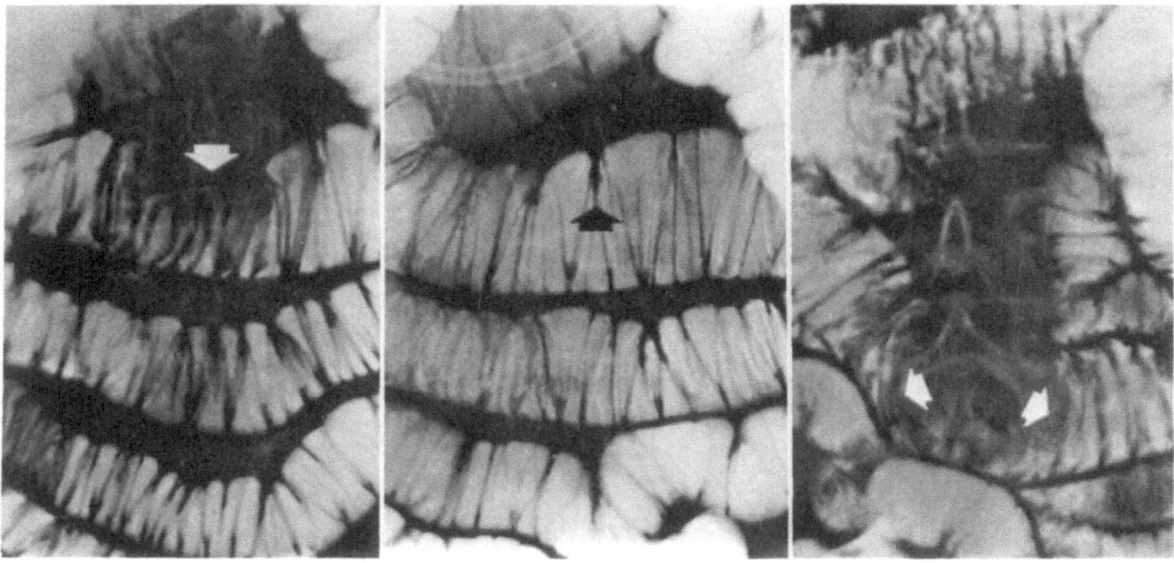

Fig. III.3.   Temporary impression of unknown origin (abdominal aorta?) on the jejunum.

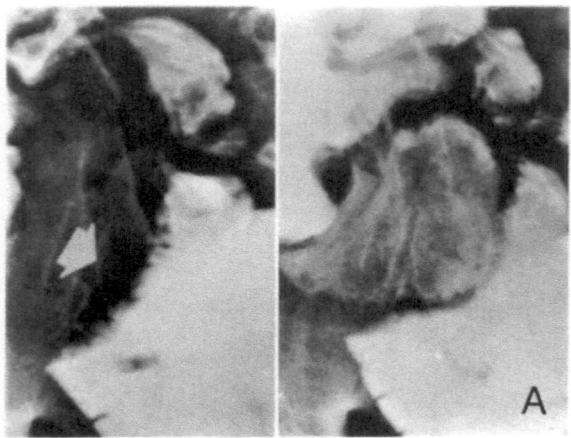

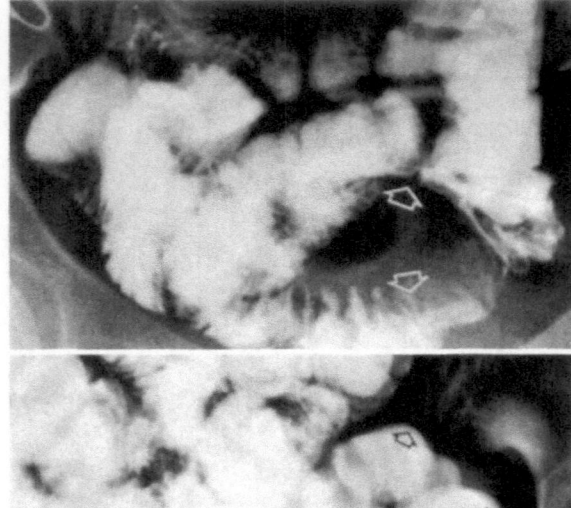

Fig. III.4AB. Impressions of the colon on the small intestine: (A) the cecum on the ileum; (B) the sigmoid on the ileum.

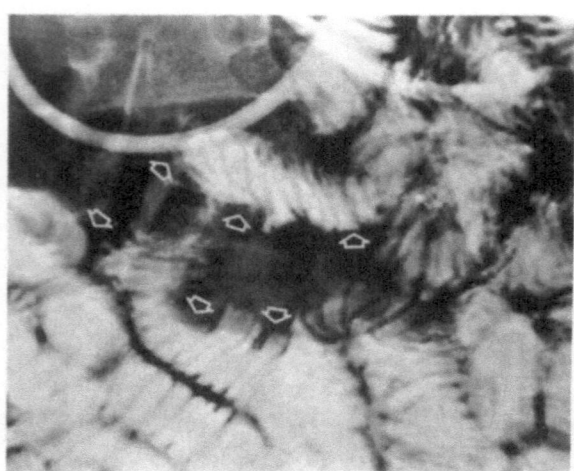

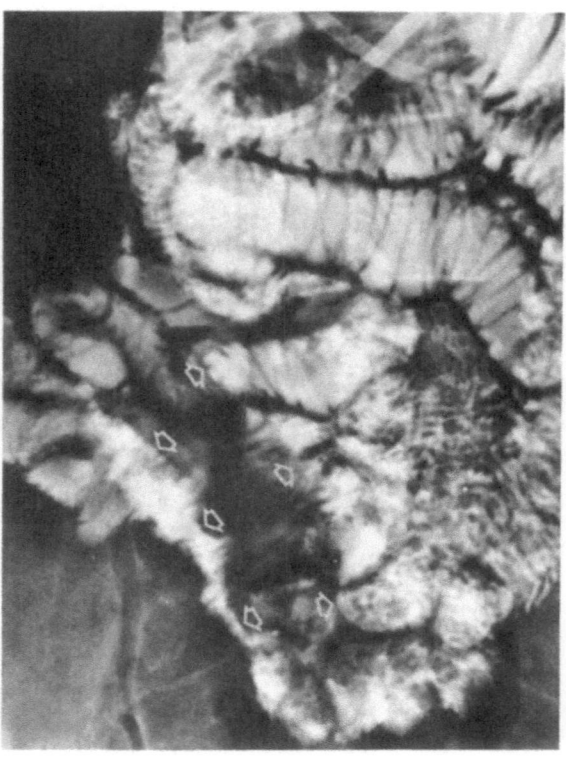

Fig. III.5. Translucency between the intestinal loops in the mid and right lower abdomen, caused by the transverse colon.

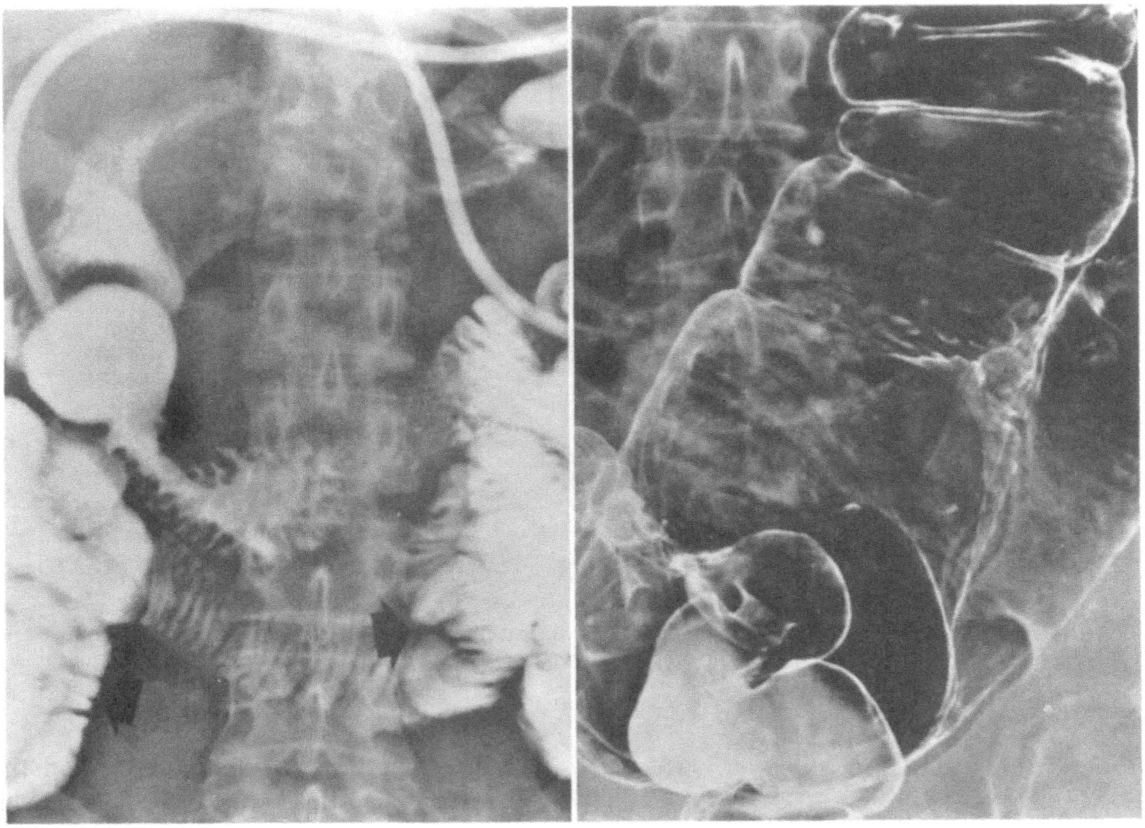

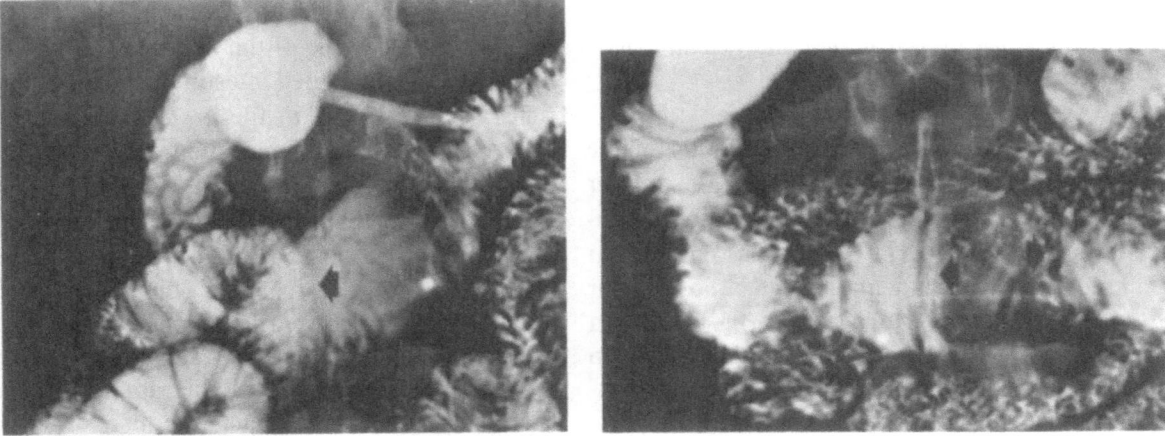

Fig. III.6. Impression from megasigmoid on the jejunum.

Fig. III.7. Impression of the abdominal aorta on the duodenum.

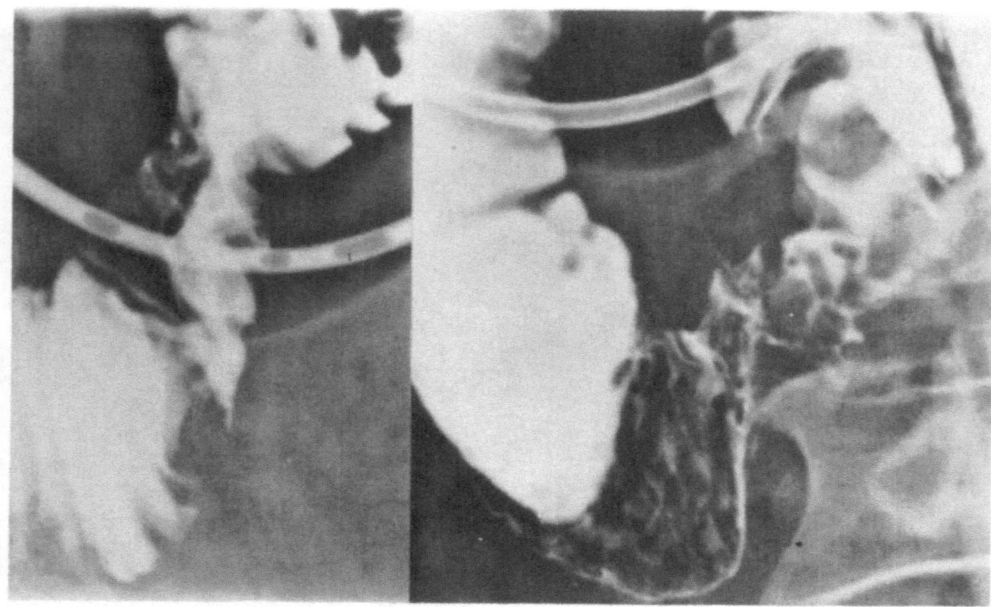

Fig. III.8. Highly irregular mucosal relief in the duodenum where it crosses the aorta in a patient with complaints of frequent vomiting and a history of atony inducing drugs. Endoscopic examination revealed a completely normal mucosa.

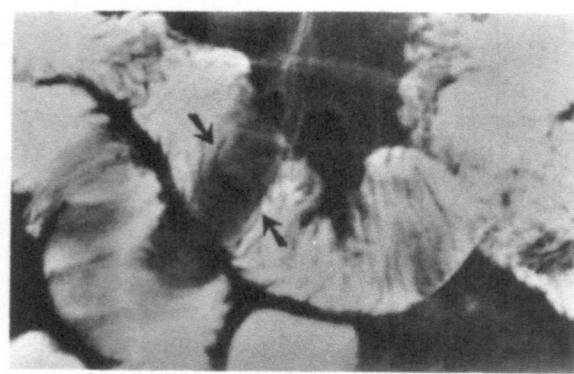

Fig. III.9. Impression of the iliac artery on the ileum.

intestine. Usually we see an indentation in the duodenum due to the aorta where the former passes between the aorta and the superior mesenteric artery (fig. III.7). The mucosal pattern caused by an aortic indentation can be so irregular that it even mimics tumor growth (fig. III.8). An impression of the superior mesenteric artery on the duodenum is rarely visible; it is probable completely 'overshadowed' by the much larger impression of the aorta. Another common indentation on an intestinal loop by a large vessel is that of the iliac artery on the ileum at the somewhat narrow pelvic outlet (fig. III.9). Here too, as in the duodenum and the jejunum, it is striking that such cases involve a fairly wide and abundantly filled intestinal loop, usually as a result of an iatrogenic atony.

2. Filling defects between the intestinal loops

2.1. Caused by other organs

Exactly in the middle of the abdomen an abnormality in the convoluted intestinal loops is sometimes seen, but only in the prone position and caused by a sagging loop of the transverse colon filled with feces (figs. III.5 and II.24).
A phenomenon that is hardly to be considered as abnormal or 'pathological' is the appearance of an abnormality in the convolution of intestinal loops in the lower left or lower right abdomen due to the pressure of a heterotopically transplanted kidney (fig. III.10). Recognition of this abnormality is exceedingly important since the use of compression in this region could cause severe damage to the transplanted kidney.

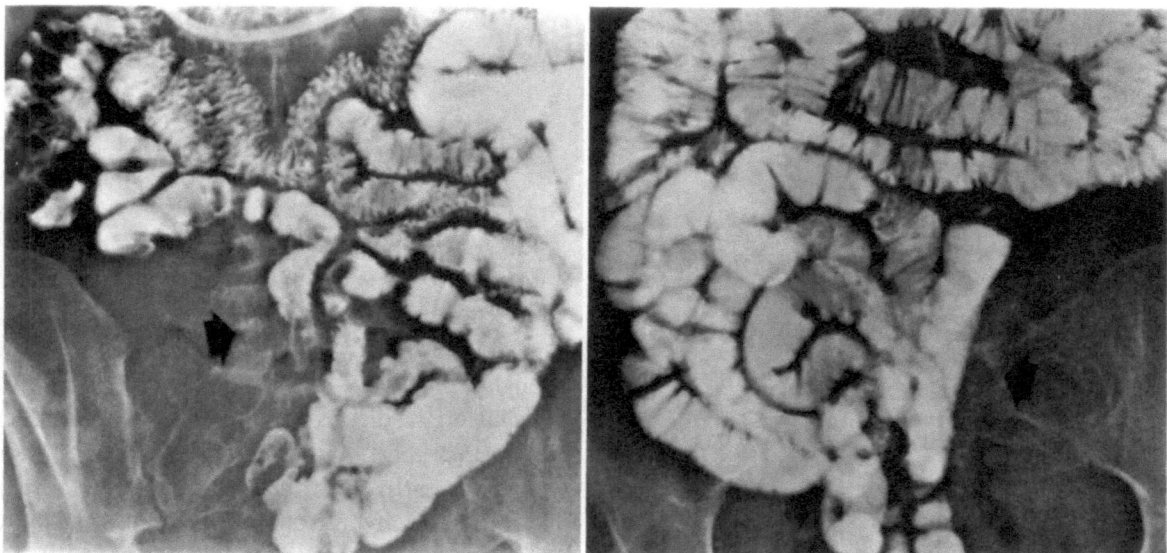

Fig. III.10. Translucency in the right or left lower abdomen, caused by a heterotopically transplanted kidney.

2.2. *Caused by other tissue structures*

This is not considered a normally occurring phenomenon. For instance, although impressions on the intestinal loops caused by the psoas muscles could be expected fairly frequently, they are – for some unknown reason – rarely observed (fig. III.11). In so far as it can be determined, marked lordosis of the lumbar spine, hypertrophy of the psoas musculature, pronounced ptosis of the kidneys or a clear-cut atony of the intestine do not significantly enhance the development of this phenomenon.

A voluminous omentum and degeneration or

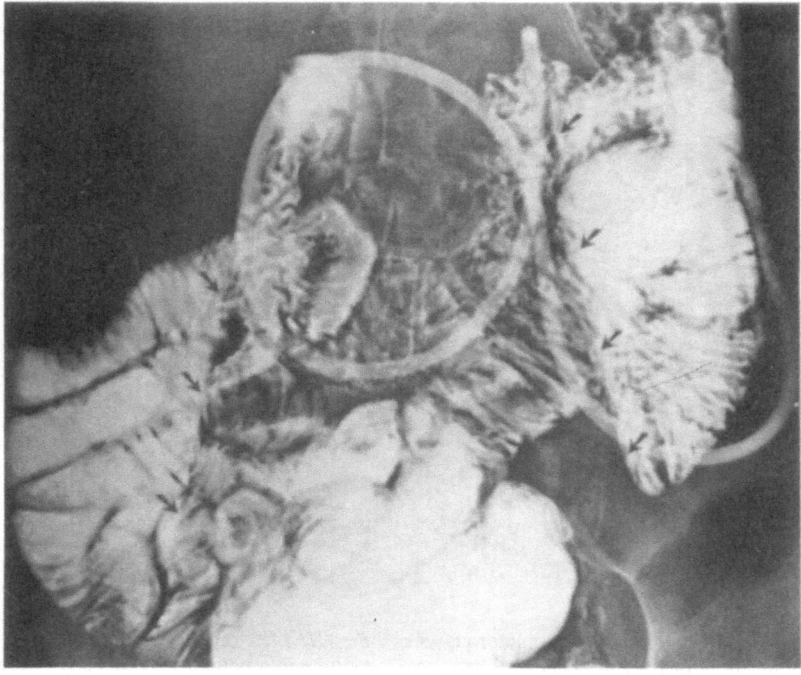

Fig. III.11. Bilateral sharp lines (arrows) caused by impression of the psoas muscles on the small intestine.

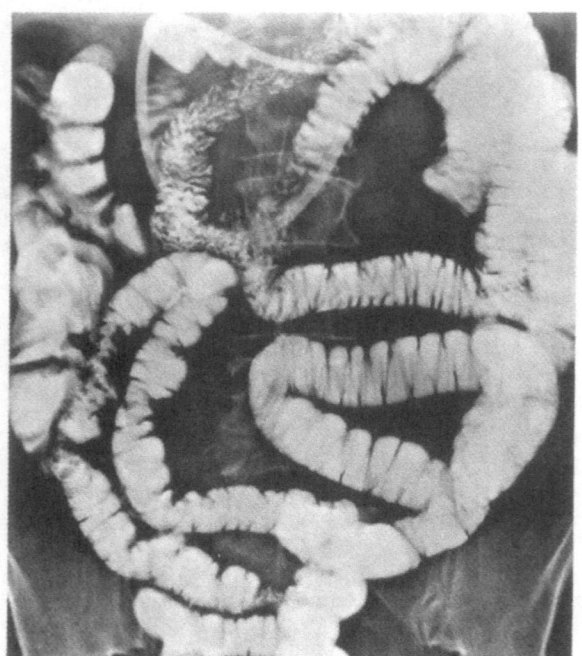

Fig. III.12. Unusually large translucent spaces between the intestinal loops in the centre of the abdomen, possible from a voluminous greater omentum.

contracture of the mesentery can result in empty spaces in the mid-abdomen or scattered among the intestinal loops (see figs. IV.5 and IV.8B); these defects are even more striking than those in pyknics (fig. III.12). In pyknics, there is hardly ever a convolution of intestinal loops in the minor pelvis.

D. Mucosal relief

1. Height, separation and thickness of folds

The folds of Kerkring begin 3-5 cm beyond the pylorus in the proximal part of the jejunum, they are 3-6 mm high and 1-6 mm apart. Occassionally folds 7-10 mm high and local separations of 7-12 mm have been seen in an enteroclysis examination under normal conditions. A separation of 1 mm is encountered only when the tone of the intestine is high or in children, where active motility is also present. In the distal jejunum the folds are smaller and farther apart. In the ileum the number of folds can vary greatly. With hypermotility (fig. III.13) or compensatory hypertrophy as a result of atrophy of the jejunal mucosa (fig. III.14), they can be as numerous as in the jejunum. On the other hand, in patients with atony of the bowel, fold relief may be barely visible in the ileum (fig. III.15A).

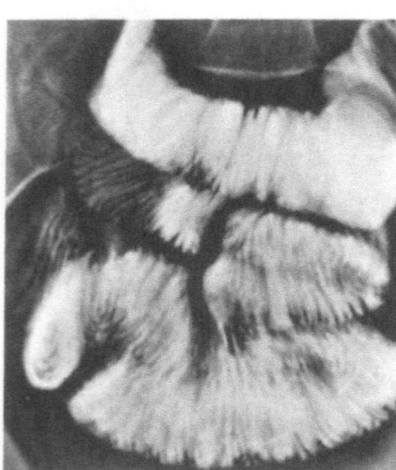

Fig. III.13. The folds in the ileum are more numerous as a result of high muscular tone of the intestinal wall from too rapid infusion.

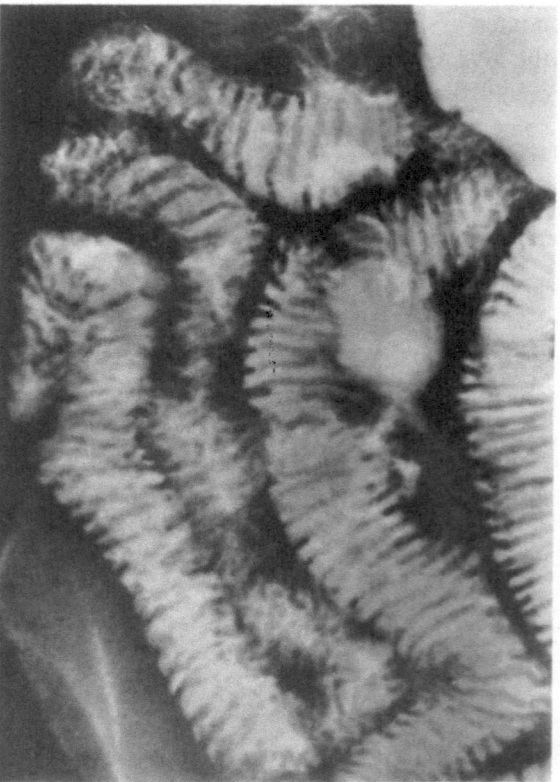

Fig. III.14. Increased number of folds in the ileum ('jejunization') in a patient with atrophy of the jejunal mucosa as a result of celiac disease.

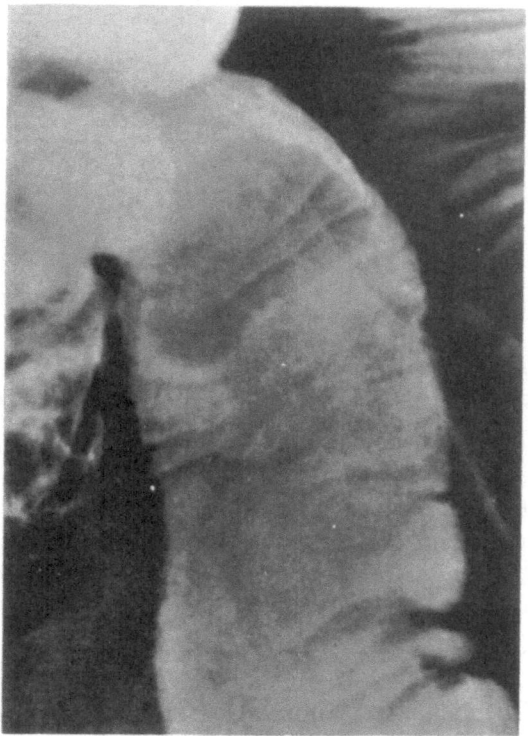

Fig. III.15A.   When the ileum is stretched, the fold relief is barely visible.

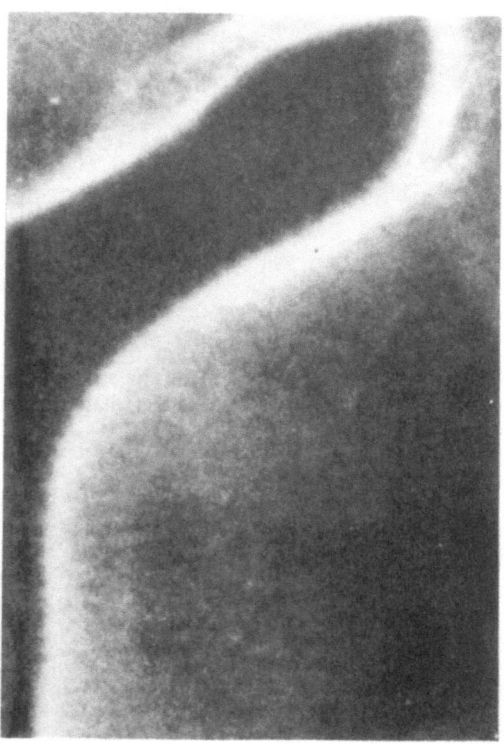

Fig. III.15B.   Sawtoothed margins of the wall of the distal ileum due to contractions of the muscularis mucosae. Similar configurations can also occur in the colon, especially if a laxative is added to the contrast fluid, and in the esophagus and stomach.

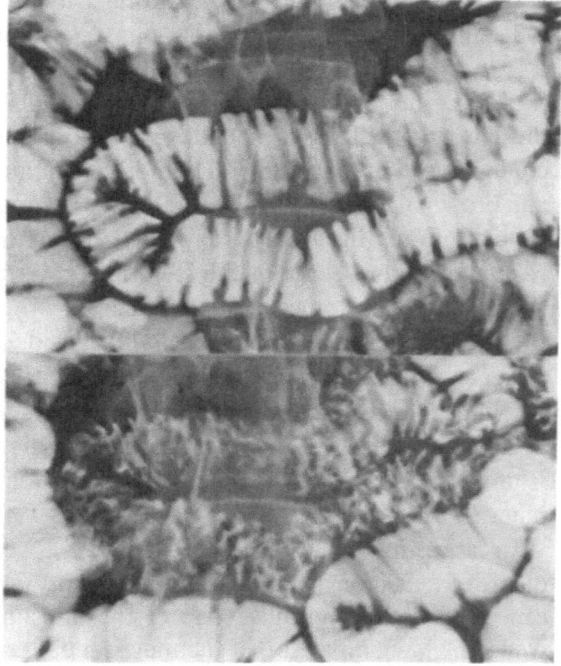

Fig. III.16.   Circular course of the mucosal folds in the proximal part of the jejunum. Evaluation is much easier when the intestine is stretched (upper) than during the resting phase (lower).

In comparison with a conventional examination of the small intestine, the height of a fold may therefore be somewhat less on an enteroclysis film, but the thickness will barely change. Evaluation of the height of a fold is much easier with enteroclysis because the more active peristalsis induces stronger contractions in conjunction with more pronounced dilatations during the rest phases (fig. III.16). When the intestine is in a state of dilatation, the folds are stretched and of quite orderly arrangement so that they are easy to measure. In addition, minor anatomical abnormalities are less likely to be overlooked (fig. III.17).

Thickness of the folds is fairly constant and is therefore not influenced by the different phases of contraction. Whatever the degree of stretching of the intestine, the folds are about 2 mm thick in the jejunum and about 1 mm in the ileum. In the first

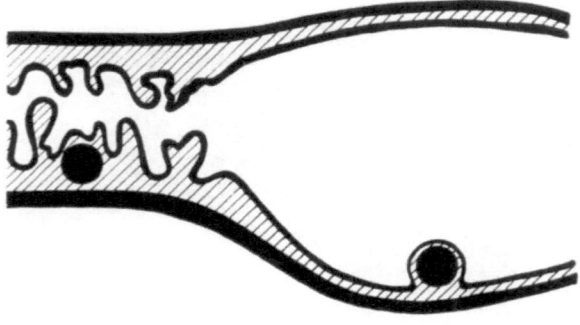

Fig. III.17A. An abnormality of the mucosa is more clearly visible when the intestine is in a state of dilatation than in a state of contraction.

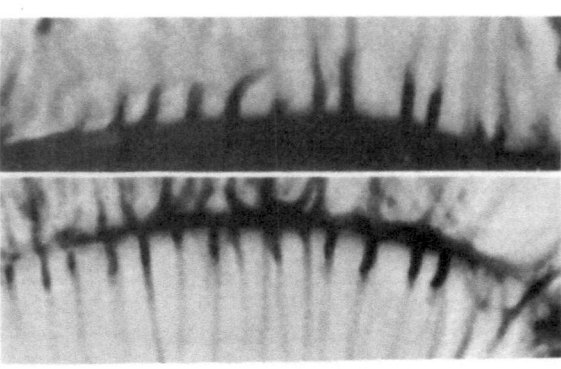

Fig. III.18. The margins of a fold of Kerkring extend approximately in parallel; the transition from fold to intestinal wall has the shape of a rounded corner.

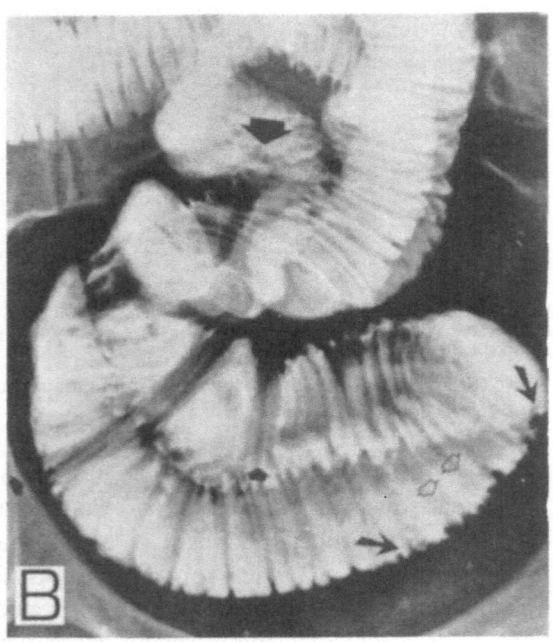

Fig. III.17B. Mild inflammatory-like changes in the wall (between the long arrows) and impressions in the intestinal lumen due to bands (short solid arrows) are only visible because the course of the folds is orderly and the intestine is well filled. The short open arrows show how far these abnormalities extend along the length of the folds.

part of the jejunum, however, the folds can sometimes be 2¹/₂-3 mm thick – although no visible cause can be found. If these folds are normal in shape, they problably have no pathological significance. Even if there is marked stretching of the intestinal wall, the folds of Kerkring retain their thickness fairly well. The folds do become somewhat shorter and smoothed out, which implies

that the shorter and thinner ileal folds may be visible only as minute ridges (fig. III.15A).

2. *Appearance of fold pattern*

The margins of a normal fold of Kerkring extend in parallel into the intestinal lumen; the transition from fold to intestinal wall can best be described as a rounded corner (fig. III.18). On the röntgenogram, the space between two intestinal loops is 2-3 mm, depending upon the phase of contraction; the thickness of the intestinal wall is therefore only 1-1¹/₄ mm. In the proximal half of the jejunum, the folds lie in a more or less circular configuration but in the distal half of the jejunum and proximal half of the ileum, the course assumes a spiral form (figs. III.16 and III.19). In this region it can be seen that the folds follow a true spiral course in some segments while in others they resemble more or less a chain of tridents along each wall meshing together in the centre of the lumen (arrow) (fig. III.19). The latter configuration seems to be more common in the distal jejunum while that of the spiral course predominates in the proximal ileum.

In a resting phase, the folds lie in a very disorderly fashion if the intestine is empty and especially if the muscular tone of the intestinal wall is high. Comparison of the mucosal patterns of an intestinal segment in various stages of contraction (figs. III.16 and III.20) illustrates this quite clearly. A fine circular sawtooth pattern, like that often seen in the mucosa of a colon influenced

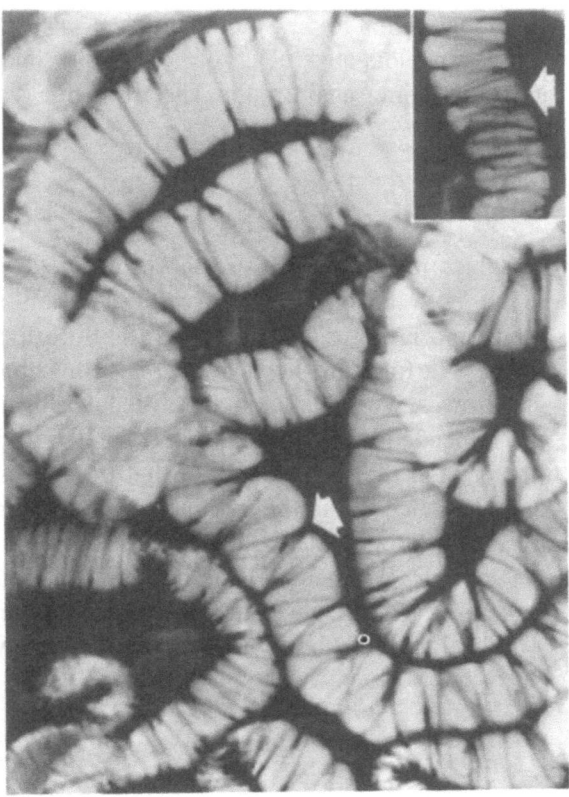

Fig. III.19. Trident-shaped mucosal folds which mesh together in the region of the jejuno-ileal transition.

by laxatives, may also be found in the distal ileum. This presumably is a result of contractions of the muscularis mucosae (fig. III.15B).

3. Longitudinal folding

It is generally stated that the folds in the distal ileum often follow a longitudinal course. This is, however, not true. The configuration of the folds is just as circular as in all other parts of the small intestine. The ileal folds are in fact smaller, thinner, and farther apart and do not contribute significantly to the fold relief, irrespective of the state of contraction of the intestine.

The longitudinal folds frequently seen on X-rays of the ileum are obviously wider and higher than the circular. Like those on the evacuation films of a colon with few haustra, they must be explained as puckering caused by collapse of the intestinal wall, possibly enhanced by contractions of the circular muscle fibres (fig. III.21AB). During contraction, the folds in the jejunum seem to extend also in a more longitudinal direction, but in fact circular folds of Kerkring which really extend in a longitudinal direction, do not exist! The mucosal pattern can, depending upon the state of

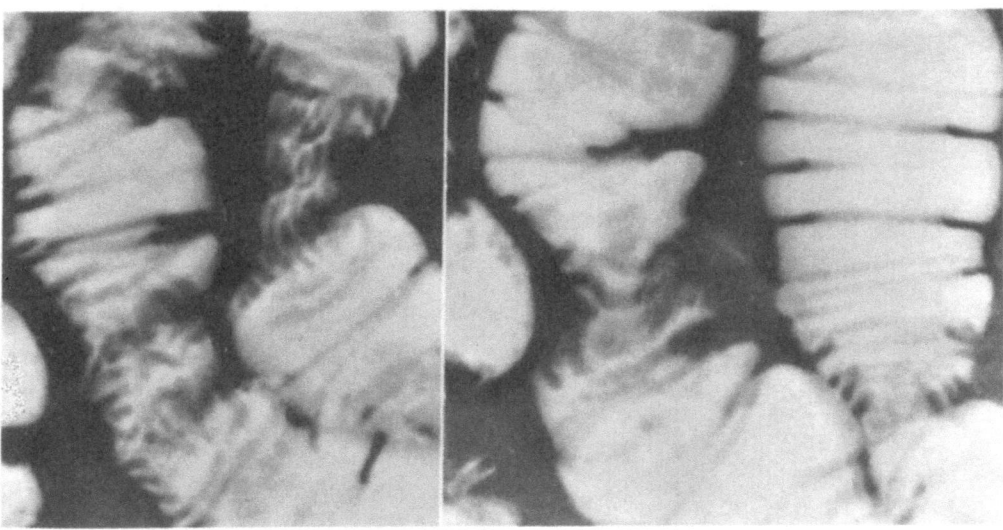

Fig. III.20. Various phases of contraction of the same intestinal loops in the distal part of the jejunum. Disorderly arrangement of the folds in the resting phase, orderly in the dilated phase or when well filled.

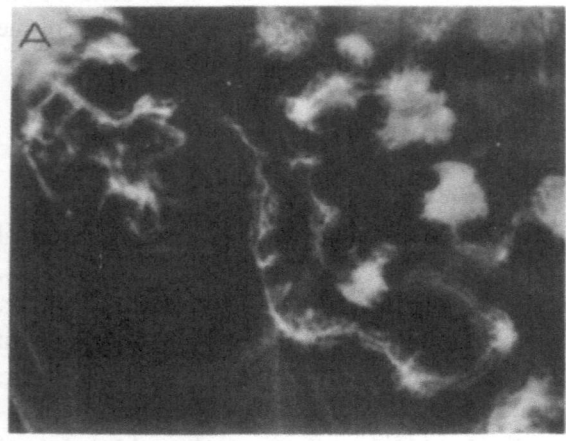

Fig. III.21A. Longitudinal folds in the ileum in a contracted intestinal loop.

upon the state of contraction or dilatation, show very pronounced changes. (see also figs. III.20 and IV.145AB.) Occasionally in the most distal part of the ileum, the folds have a longitudinal

course on the mesenteric side and a circular course on the other side of the loop (fig.III.22A). This longitudinal folding can sometimes even resemble an elongated ulcer or a partially filled appendix lying against the distal ileum (fig. III.22B).

4. Fold pattern in babies

In babies mucosal folds are more highly developed, both absolutely and relatively, than in adults and are present as early as the third fetal month. The folds are, however, thinner and somewhat lower. Vascularization and cellularity are pronounced in the mucosa. The submucosa is thinner than that in an adult so that the muscularis, the mucosa and the submucosa of an infant are all of approximately equal thickness. The relative underdevelopment of the muscularis and mucosa can cause the mucosal folds to be flattened completely by the barium column in a follow-

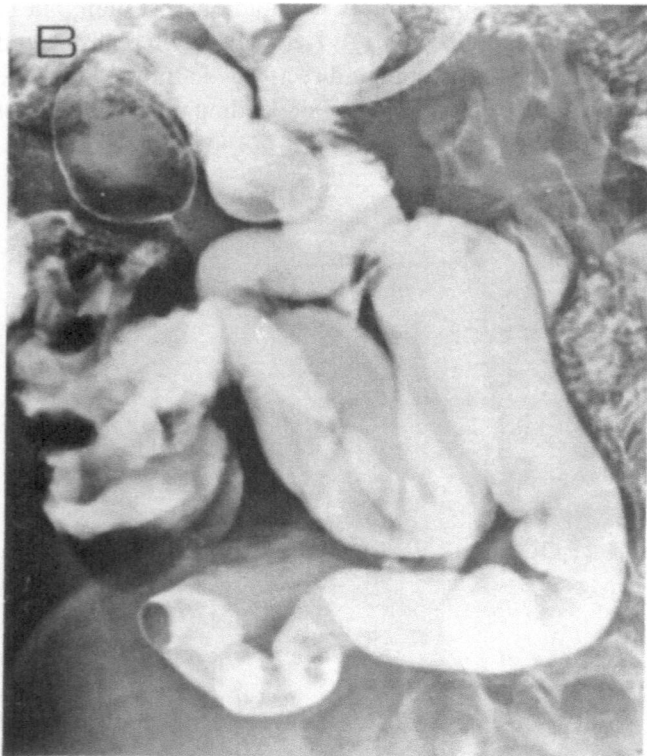
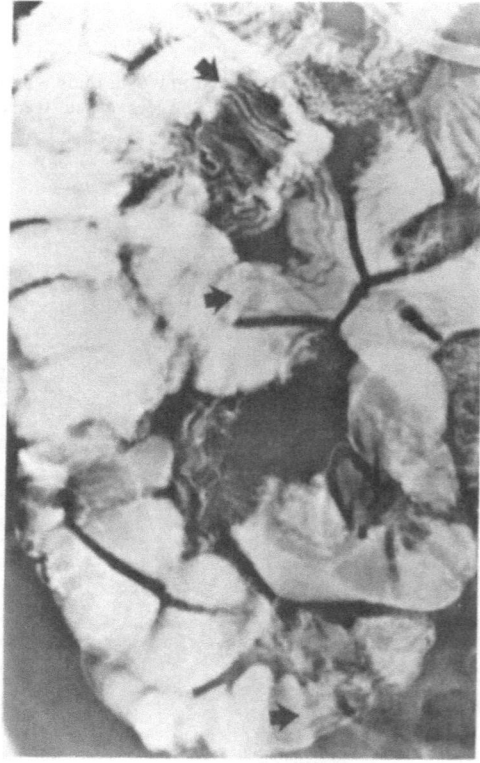

Fig. III.21B. Quiescent Chrohn's disease. When the intestine is well filled, the longitudinal folds disappear entirely (left) leaving a completely smooth intestinal wall devoid of mucosal relief. In case of collapse (right), only longitudinal folding is seen. Circular folds have disappeared.

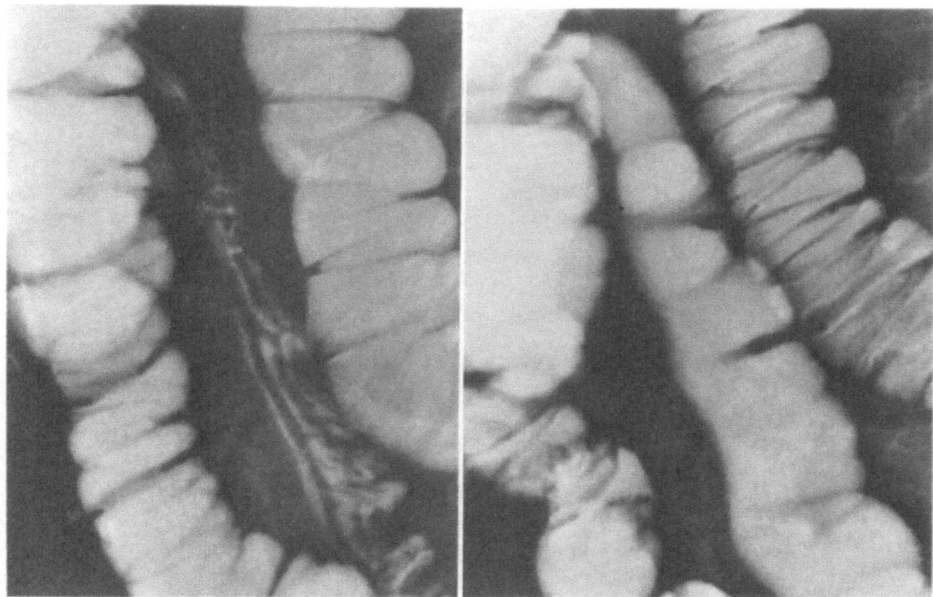

Fig. III.22A.   Fold relief occasionally seen in the distal ileum. Longitudinal folds on the mesenteric side of the intestine.

through examination of a baby, 3-6 months old. The appearance of a baby's small intestine on these X-ray films is strikingly similar to that of an adult with a severe malabsorption or 'deficiency state'. This is due to the contrast medium being less stable whereby flocculation occurs from mucin and lactic acid. Although the stability of modern contrast fluids has been greatly improved, it is still impossible to demonstrate mucosal folds in young babies on follow-through examinations. The enteroclysis technique with its ability to administer a large amount of contrast fluid very rapidly, has completely changed this incompetence.

E.   Intestinal contents

1.   Lymphfollicles and Peyer's patches

If the jejunum is in a resting phase and there is only moderate filling with contrast medium, evaluation is difficult. Because the folds intersect frequently, particularly in a highly contractile intestine, multiple small round bright spots appear in the mucosal patterns which are highly suggestive of lymphfollicles. Since dilatation and a high degree of filling are difficult to achieve in a contractile intestine, it may be necessary to induce hypotonicity to facilitate evaluation (fig. III.23). Because there are fewer folds in the distal ileum, the presence of true lymphfollicles is there easily demonstrated. These follicles are frequently encountered under normal circumstances in small children but disappear when the children are 10-14 years of age. The much larger Peyer's patches can be seen in the distal ileum in older patients. They are recognized by the cushion-like configurations that occur mainly on the mesenteric side of the intestine (fig. III.24).

Fig. III.22B.   Longitudinal ileal fold resembling a fissure-like ulcer or appendix in unusual position.
(Courtesy Prof. Schütte – Rotterdam)

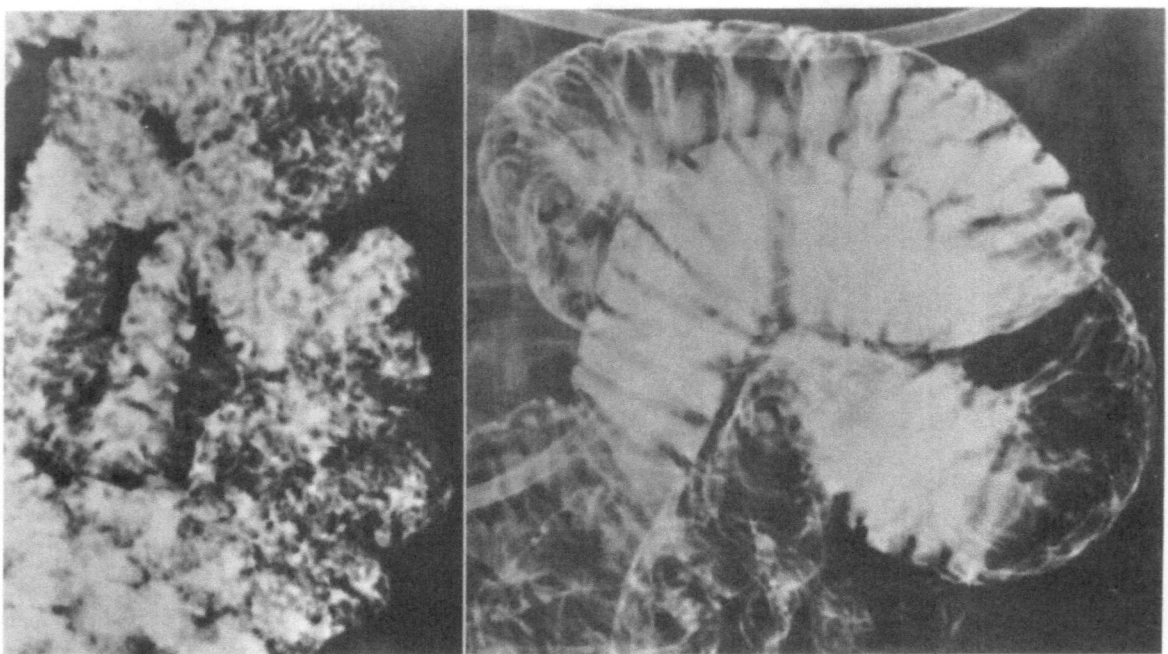

Fig. III.23. Translucent spots in the mucosal pattern, from intersection of multiple loops, that resemble enlarged lymphfollicles. After administration of a hypotonic agent, this illusory pattern disappears completely.

2. Food residues

The specific gravity of food residue is usually lower than that of the barium suspension; it is therefore visible as a filling defect in the contrast fluid. Food residue is seen almost exclusively in the distal half of the ileum since transit is most

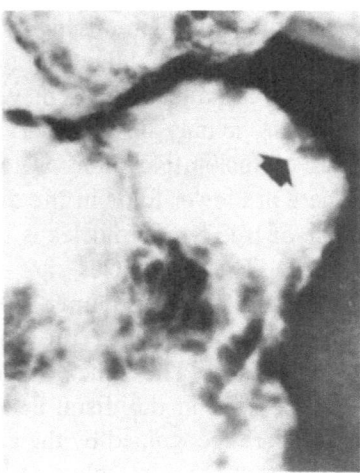

Fig. III.24. Cushion-like configurations in the mucosal pattern, caused by Peyer's patches in the distal ileum.

likely to be disturbed in this section from a full cecum. Food residue can also be found when the patient has eaten shortly before the radiological examination, gastric emptying is mechanically impeded, or where motility is disturbed from chronic use of tranquilizers, sedatives or antispasmodics. Food residue usually causes a conglomeration of relatively small bright spots in the barium suspension (fig. III.25). Sometimes an undigested bean pod for example can produce a sharply defined filling defect and it will then be necessary to examine the feces carefully for several days (fig. III.26). The pattern caused by the food residue after rice has been eaten is particularly misleading (fig. III.27). These filling defects are small and round and have to be differentiated from those caused by lymph follicles or air bubbles (fig. III.28).

3. Foaming of the contrast fluid

Troublesome foaming, especially in the lumen of bowel, constantly in movement, can occur with poor contrast media to which too little anti-

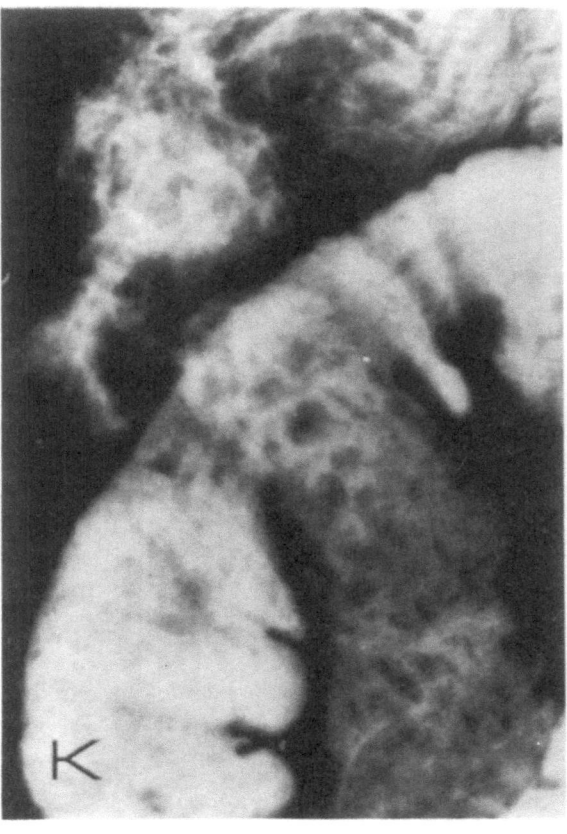
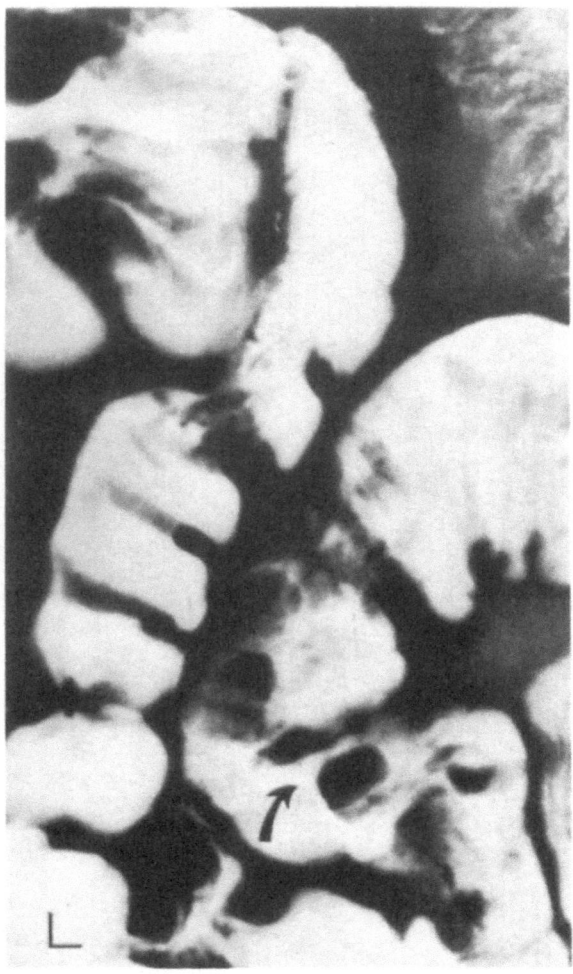

Fig. III.25. Most common appearance of food residue in the distal ileum (K). Filling defects resembling fruit stones (L).

foaming agent has been added (fig. III.29). The constituent gas bubbles can be of varying size and thus sometimes difficult to differentiate from cobblestones (fig. IV.74) or lymphfollicles (figs. IV.165 and IV.171). In other cases they may mimic a candida infection (fig. IV.172) or the swollen villi of Whipple's disease (fig. IV.92). A distinguishing feature of gas shadows is that the contour of the bowel wall is uninterrupted; a feature not seen with villi, lymphfollicles or cobblestones.

F.   Motility of the bowel

The enteroclysis technique, whereby the rate of flow of the contrast fluid is identical for all patients, has permitted comparison of the ability of various patients to propel this fluid stream in a distal direction. It has been found that if peristalsis is normal, the cecum is reached in 7-11 min with some 600-900 ml (average 700 ml) contrast fluid. During fluoroscopy peristalsis appears most active in the jejunum, particularly in the proximal half. Furthermore when these peristaltic movements are abnormal, whether overactive or diminished, this is most easily seen in the jejunum. A change in the motility of the intestine is easily diagnosed, not only under fluoroscopy but also on the röntgenograms. On the survey films taken during the enteroclysis examination, it appears that in normal patients about one-third of the

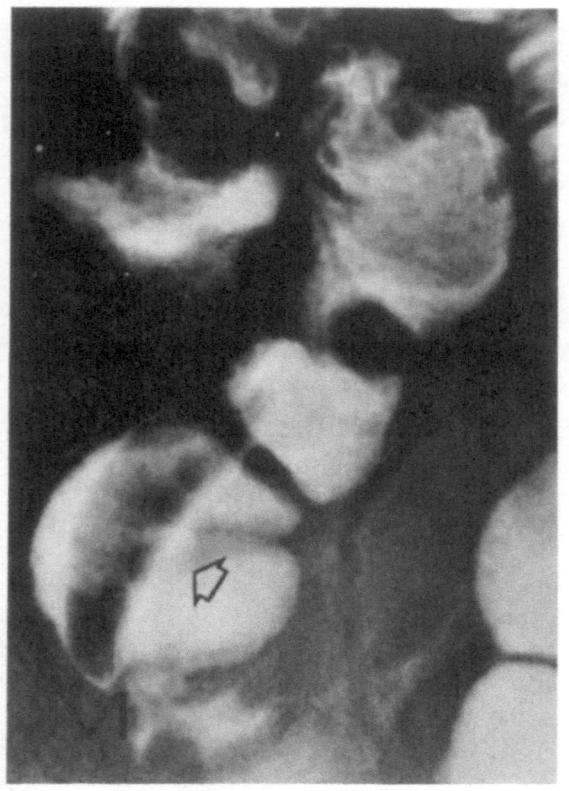

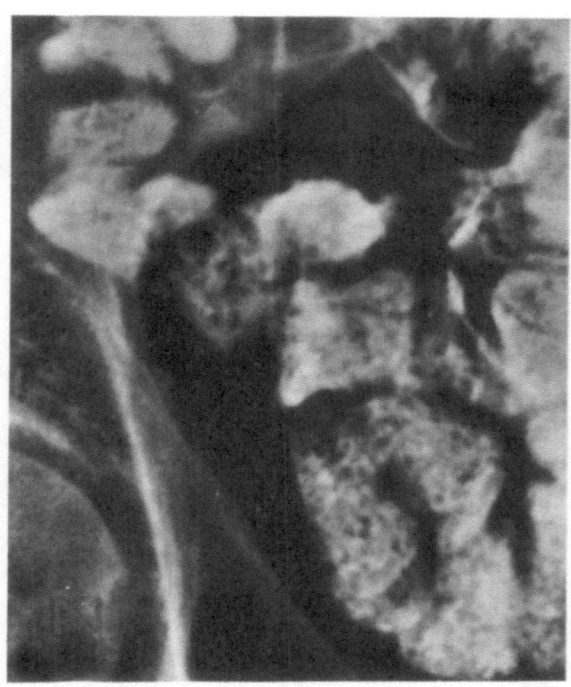

Fig. III.27.   Round filling defects due to undigested rice.

Fig. III.26.   Undigested bean pod.

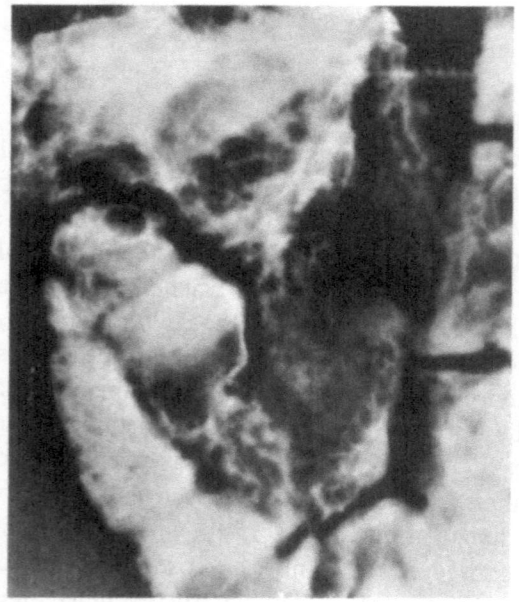

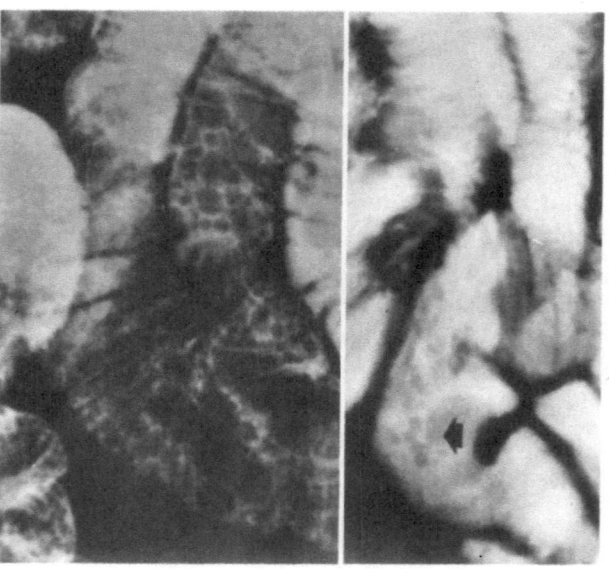

Fig. III.28.   Lymphfollicles (left). Filling defects 2-3 mm across in the contrast fluid due to gas bubbles (right).

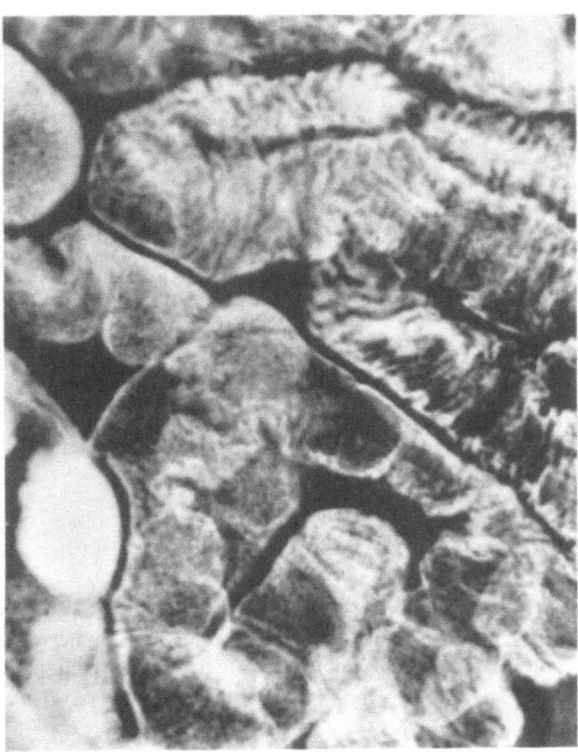

Fig. III.29. Inadequate antifoaming characteristics of the contrast fluid have permitted the formation of tiny gasbubbles.

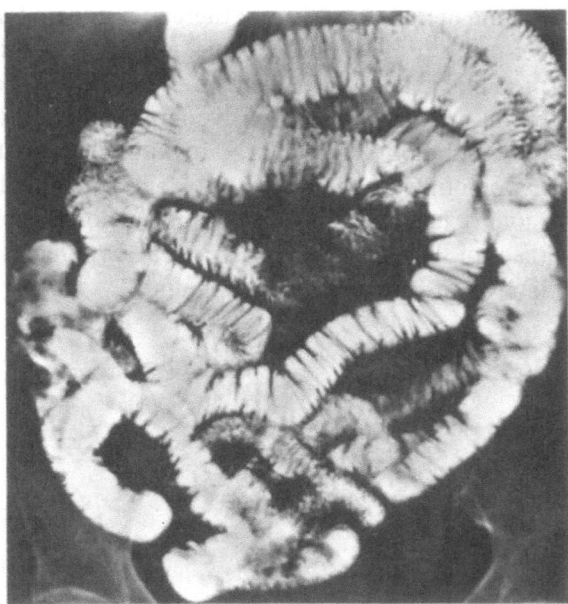

Fig. III.30. In normal patients about one-third of the loops visualized on a survey exposure are in a state of contraction.

jejunal loops are in a state of contraction (fig. III.30).

In cases of so-called 'intestinal hurry' the cecum is reached in much less than 6 min and frequently less than 500 ml of contrast fluid is required. In these cases numerous contractions are seen and the average calibre of the intestinal lumen is 1/2-1 cm less than normal. Because of increased tonus in the muscle wall the intestine is shortened and the circular mucosal folds brought closer together (fig. III.31RS). The reverse, decreased motility and a somewhat larger average diameter of the intestinal lumen, is more often seen than intestinal hurry (see also chapter IV.G3). It then takes much longer for the contrast medium to reach the cecum and the amount required is also considerably larger. On the X-ray it is obvious that only a few loops are in a state of contraction (fig. III.32).

Quite obviously, decreased peristalsis with dilated intestinal loops and highly contractile intestine with narrow calibre, will usually be found concurrently.

It is of the uttermost importance for judgement of intestinal moitility that, as explained in chapter II.D2, the recommended infusion speed of 75-80 ml/min be very strictly maintained during the course of the enteroclysis.

Notwithstanding that with a slower infusion rate of 50ml/min visualisation of disturbances in motility is still quite readily feasible, this lower rate is not so desirable. The filling grade of the intestine approaches that of the conventional transit (c.25ml/min) and the forming of an opinion on the mucosal folds is made sensibly more difficult by a more tortuous and chaotic course (compare figs. II.17 and II.20).

With an infusion rate higher than 75-80 ml/min the bowel motility becomes artificially paralysed and thus certainly no proper impression of motility obtained. The amount of contrast medium employed increases to a litre or much more, examination time is significantly prolonged and producing compression spot films is more difficult. Troublesome reflux into the stomach also often appears.

In case of a too high infusion rate the presence of hypermotility can be observed by the very

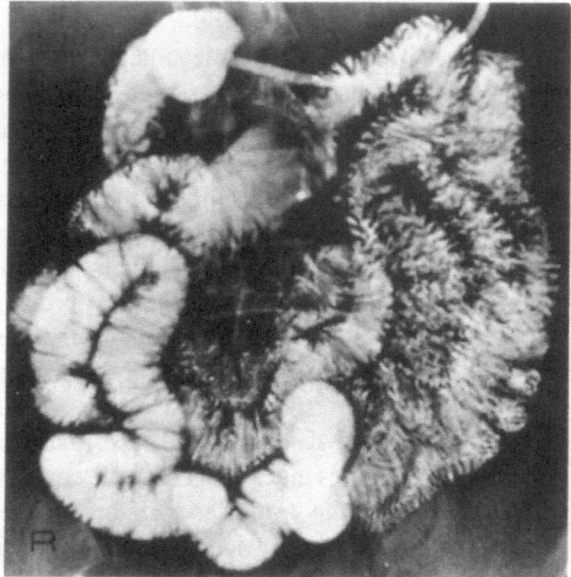

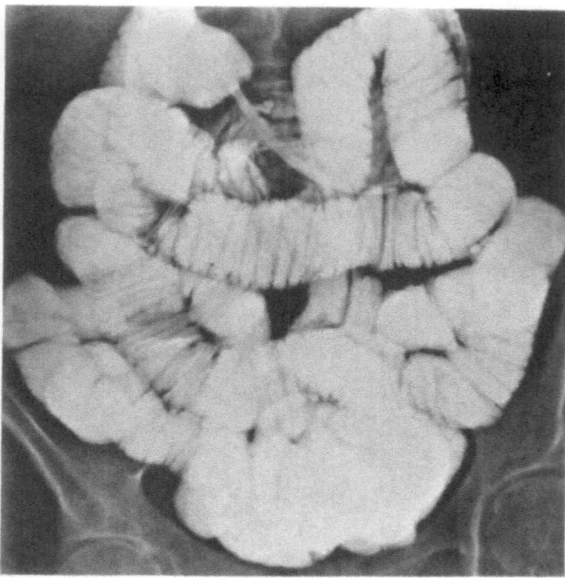

Fig. III.32. In hypomotility of the intestine, very few loops are in a state of contraction and in addition, the lumen of the intestine is obviously dilated. Patient had used vagotonics for years.

Fig. III.31. In the event of hypermotility of the intestine, about two-thirds of the loops (R) and sometimes even more (s) are in a state of contraction and the diameter of the intestine is usually somewhat smaller than normal.

experienced radiologist during only the first half minute of the examination; thereafter it is no longer possible. This fluoroscopic appearence of the proximal jejunum, which can naturally be recorded on an X-ray, is of decisive importance in the differentiation from a real hypomotility. With hypomotility induced by too rapid infusion the motility is very briefly normal at the commencement of the examination but a 'real' hypomotility is present from the very beginning.

IV. Pathological patterns

A. Changes in the length of the intestine

1. Shortening

1.1. Presence of a catheter or tube in the lumen

A very noticeably shortened intestine is presented where the small intestine has formed a 'concertina' over a tube or catheter, inserted for therapeutic or diagnostic ends to a considerable length within the lumen. The circular folds then lie closely approximated while the mucosal pattern appears uniformly intact.

1.2. Entero-enteral fistula

A noticeable but only apparent shortening of the intestine can occur where a considerable segment of the bowel has been short-circuited by a fistula. Visualisation of a fistulous canal, where accompanying adhesions frequently hinder an adequately free projection, can be extremely difficult. It is important here to have exposures made early in the examination, as further filling of the loops renders visualisation and localisation of the fistula increasingly more difficult. Complementary infusion of water offers more chance of clarification than air insufflation. Extensive adhesions are not always present and then the only sign may be the absence of a considerable length of the jejunum or ileum, as recognized by their different mucosal pattern.

1.3. Hypermotility and hypertonicity

Slight shortening of the intestine is evident when these two states are present. The diameter is generally somewhat less than normal while the mucosal pattern is uniformly intact and the circular folds closely approximated. When hypermotility or spasm is greatly exaggerated, circular folds may be absent in short segments of several centimetres. Then only tightly bundled longitudinal folds may be visible (fig. IV.1).

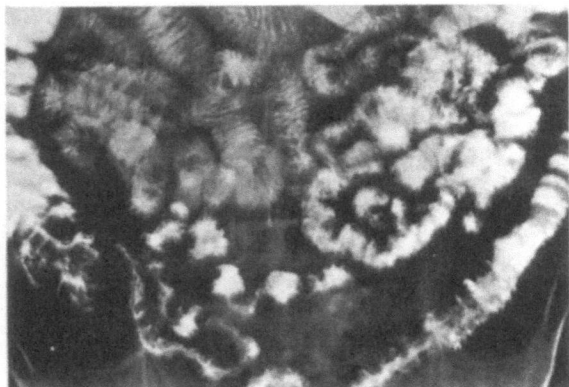

Fig. IV.1. Longitudinal fold relief in the distal ileum in case of severe hypermotility.

1.4. Short-circuit for bypass in treatment of adiposity, or post-resection in case of ischemia, venous thrombosis, tumor or local Crohn's disease

In the case of a bypass operation (fig. IV.2) a large portion, of mainly the jejunum, is short-circuited and thus made non-functional, while in Crohn's disease a part of the ileum is usually removed. Recognition of Crohn's disease gives no difficulty where a recurrence (generally mucosal edema), not necessarily in relation to the anastomosis, is present or skip lesions are seen elsewhere. Frequently, resection has been repeatedly performed and sometimes only a metre of bowel remains, resulting in the so-called 'short bowel' (fig. IV.3). Resection for tumor or vascular accident can occur anywhere, but the resected segment in case of tumor is as a rule much shorter than in vascular lesions where sometimes more than a metre is removed. The remaining bowel generally shows no further abnormalities. The anastomosis (fig. IV.4) is not easy to find and here, a higher flowrate of the contrast fluid or double contrast using methylcellulose, can be very useful. In the case of

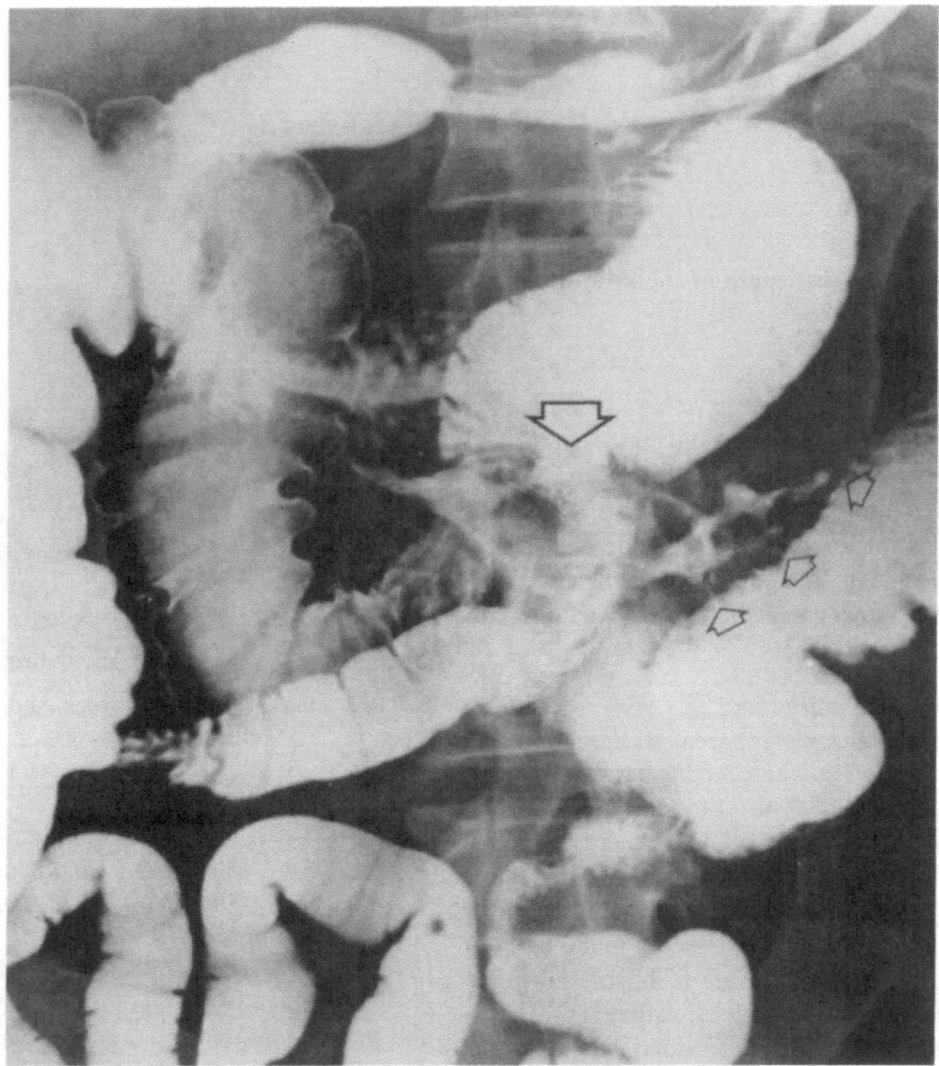

Fig. IV.2. Enteroclysis examination of a patient weighing 450 pounds who underwent bypass surgery, whereby the jejunum and the ileum were anastomosed, to combat obesity. Physical examination was impossible. It appeared that at the site of the anastomosis (arrow), fistulization including three canals to the transverse colon had developed.

a tumor attention should be paid to the possible presence of recurrence or metastases.

1.5. *Extensive adhesions*
These can be found where one or more resections have been performed, resulting in a varying but usually marked shortening of the bowel. Frequently fibrous bands remain or local adhesions that can be recognized by pointed protrusions of the bowel wall (fig. IV.57). The X-ray films may show pre-stenotic dilatations, local bizarre

changes in the course of the bowel (fig. IV.5 and IV.59) and local hypermotility (fig. IV.115).

1.6. *Mesenteric fibrosis*
One or often more bowel resections have occurred in this rare condition in which, as a result of mesenteric contracture, the intestinal loops are located very centrally in the abdomen. The calibre of the bowel is irregularly dilated because of several stenotic areas arising from this condition. The position of the loops of the bowel has an

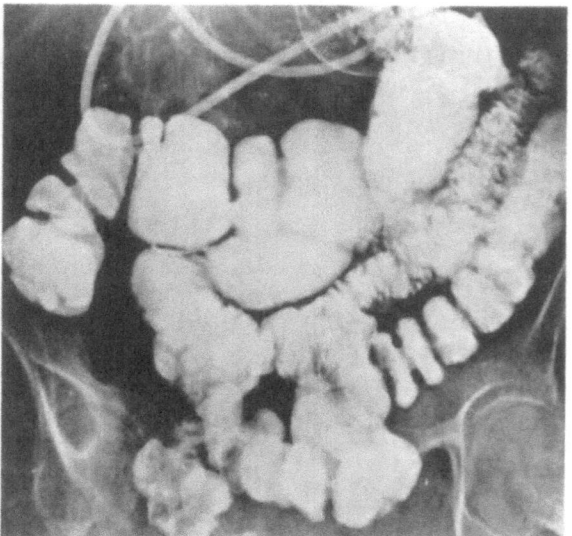

Fig. IV.3. So-called 'short-bowel': after multiple resections the small intestine is at the most 1 m long.

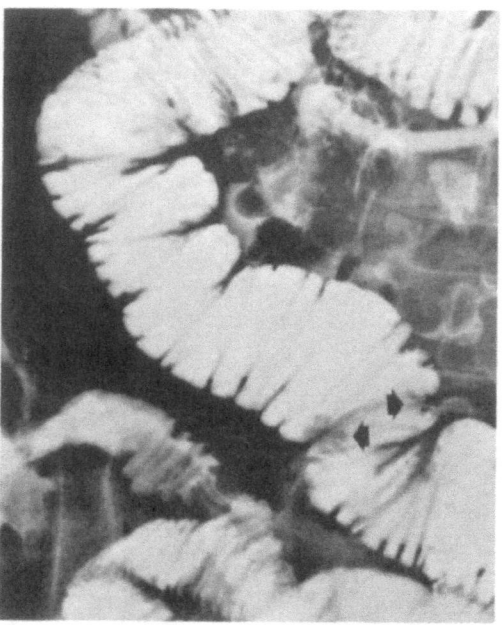

Fig. IV.4. Locally very irregular but intact mucosal relief causing moderate stenosis at an intestinal suture line after tumor resection.

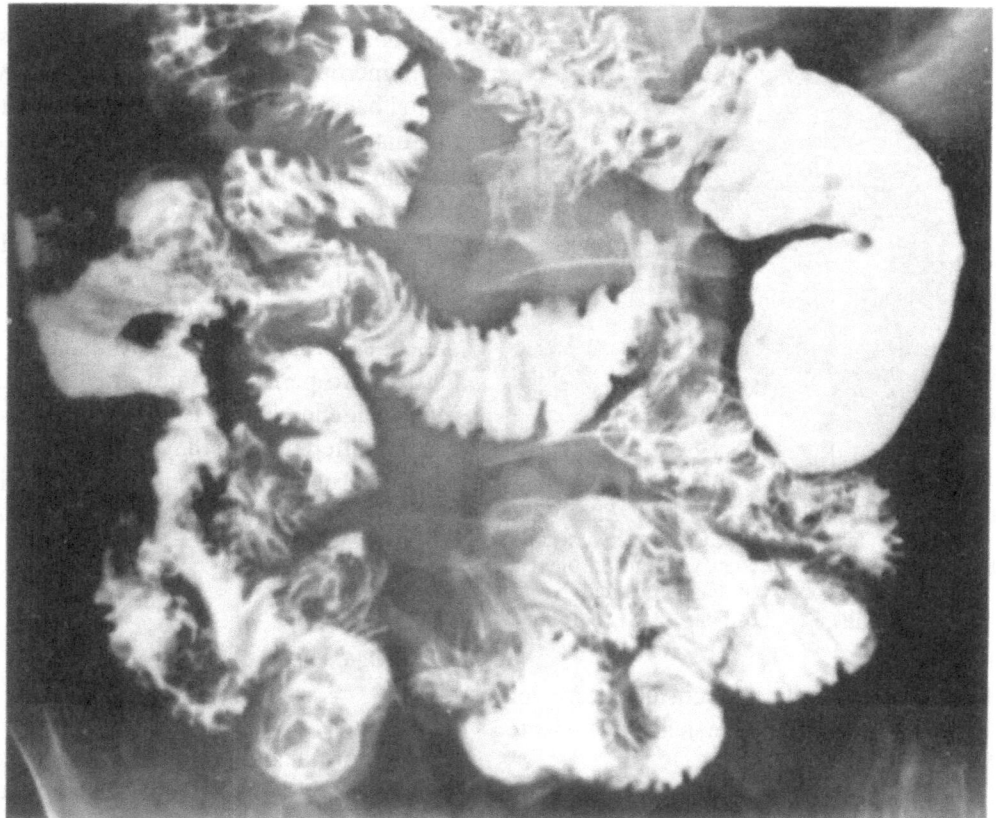

Fig. IV.5. Proven case of mesentric fibrosis. There are stenotic areas and kink-like configurations with an empty space in the middle of the abdomen. Bowel shortened by resection a few years previously.

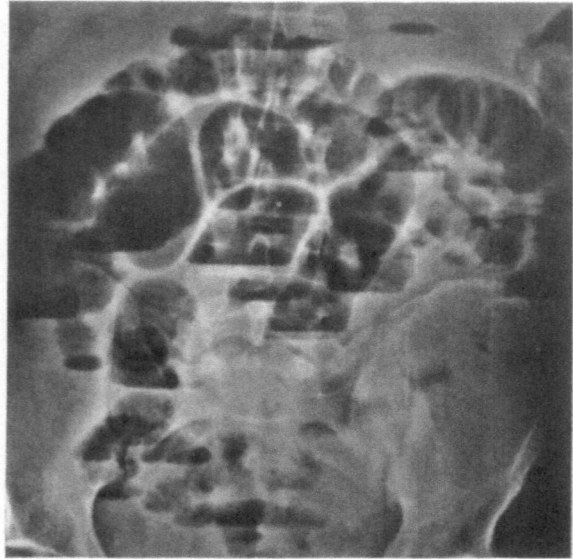

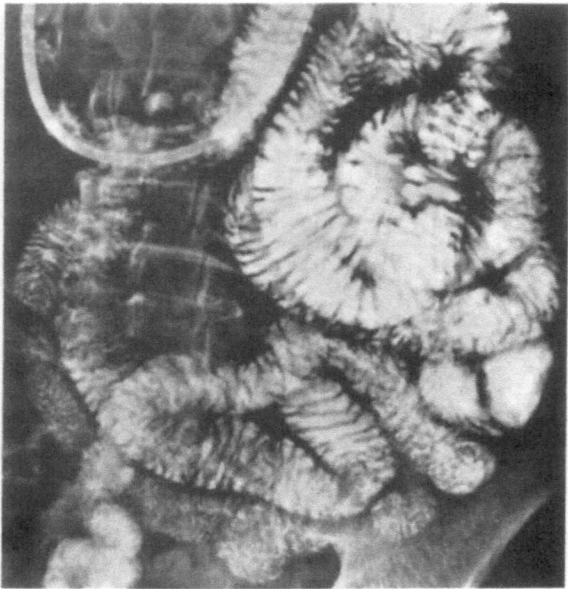

Fig. IV.7. 10 year old child with celiac disease. Markedly dilated loops, rapid transit and tendency to flocculate.

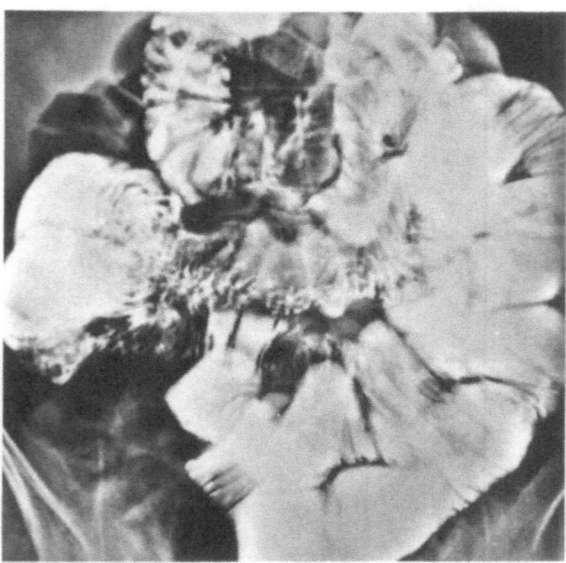

Fig. IV.6. Patient with degeneration of the nerve cells in the wall of the bowel (Naish's syndrome). Although the intestinal loops are markedly dilated, contracted segments can still be seen. During fluoroscopy, vigorous retroperistaltic movements could be observed. Numerous fluid levels in the erect position.

irregular appearance. The mucosal pattern may show bizarre changes but is basically not affected (fig. IV.5).

1.7. Naish's syndrome

In this equally rare disease multiple resections are unjustly performed, based on the presumtive and erroneous diagnosis of ileus. Wide loops containing numerous fluid levels, as visualised with horizontal beam (fig. IV.6), were the fundamentals for this diagnosis. Peristalsis is in fact good but uncoordinated with much retro-peristaltic movements and signs of pseudo-obstruction.

Recognition of this condition demands nothing less than the most careful fluoroscopy. A useless operation, as a rule leading to deterioration in the patient's condition, can be avoided. The vigorous, partly retro-peristaltic movements with a generously widened lumen is such an impressive view and so diffferent from that of paralytic or mechnanical obstruction that recognition of this disease during fluoroscopy is utterly simple (see chapter IV.A1.7, fig. IV.98).

2. Lengthening

Lengthening of the bowel is confined to about 30% of normal and is a more or less physiological variation as in Negros, vegetarians or subjects of leptosome habitus and also accompanies several conditions associated with a more voluminous and wider bowel.

For example:

2.1. Intestinal hypomotility

This is almost always the consequence of chronic use of antispasmodics, soporifics or sedatives and is thus frequently encountered under psychiatric patients and epileptics. Characteristic are dilatation and loss of motility, present most markedly in the proximal jejunum and becoming less pronounced more distally (fig. IV.182).

2.2. Celiac syndrome

Lengthening of the intestine is encountered in the form of this condition that is associated with hypermotility, wide loops and tendency to flocculation of the barium suspension. These patients have many complaints and respond poorly to treatment (fig. IV.7).

2.3. Zollinger-Ellison disease

The tendency to flocculation of the contrast fluid under influence of the high gastric acidity level as well as the dilatation is here strongest in the proximal jejunum. Hypermotility may be present but is no essential part of the picture (fig. IV.100).

2.4. Tropical sprue

This condition is distinguished by dilatation predominantly in the ileum and increasing distally. Ileal mucosal pattern is well-nigh or completely absent and the motility normal (fig. IV.104).

3. Alterations in length summarised

Shortening
    non-functioning as result of:
        fistula
        bypass operation for adiposity
    resection for:
        adhesions and bands
        tumor
        Crohn's disease
        ischemia or thrombosis
        mesenteric fibrosis
        pseudo-obstruction
    hypermotility and increased tonicity:
        collagen disease
        carcinoid lesions
    'concertina' effect around a catheter or tube

Lengthening
    physiological variations
        Negros
        vegetarians
        leptosomal habitus
    coupled with widening
        with decreased motility (dilatation mainly proximal)
            soporifics, sedatives and anti-spasmodics
        with increased motility
            1/3 of celiac patients
            Zollinger-Ellison disease
        with normal motility
            tropical sprue (dilatation mainly distal).

B. Deviation in course or position of part or whole of the bowel

1. Positional abnormalities of the entire small intestine

An iatrogenic cause is the condition resulting from use of the beta-adrenergic blocker Practolol and associated with skin conditions suggestive of psoriasis or lupus erythematosis. The pathogenesis of this disease, which is called 'sclerosing peritonitis', is probably based on the occlusion of small vessels. As a result of this progressive occlusive process, both parietal and visceral peritoneum show a gradually increasing degree of fibrous contracture. The entire mass of intestinal loops is, as it were, caught in the meshes of a strong net which slowly contracts towards the base of the mesentery, thus forcing the intestinal loops into a position central in the abdominal cavity. Although transit can be seriously impeded, the loops are not able to dilate and the radiological diagnosis of 'ileus' is thus masked.

It has been noted, however, that the affected loops show numerous widely scattered indentations suggesting bands or abrupt kinking from which the diagnosis, if considered, can be deduced (fig. IV.8AB).

Occasionally is a considerable part of the small intestine encountered in the sac of an *abdominal wall hernia*, or *post-traumatic in the thoracic cavity*. Positional abnormalities of the bowel are further

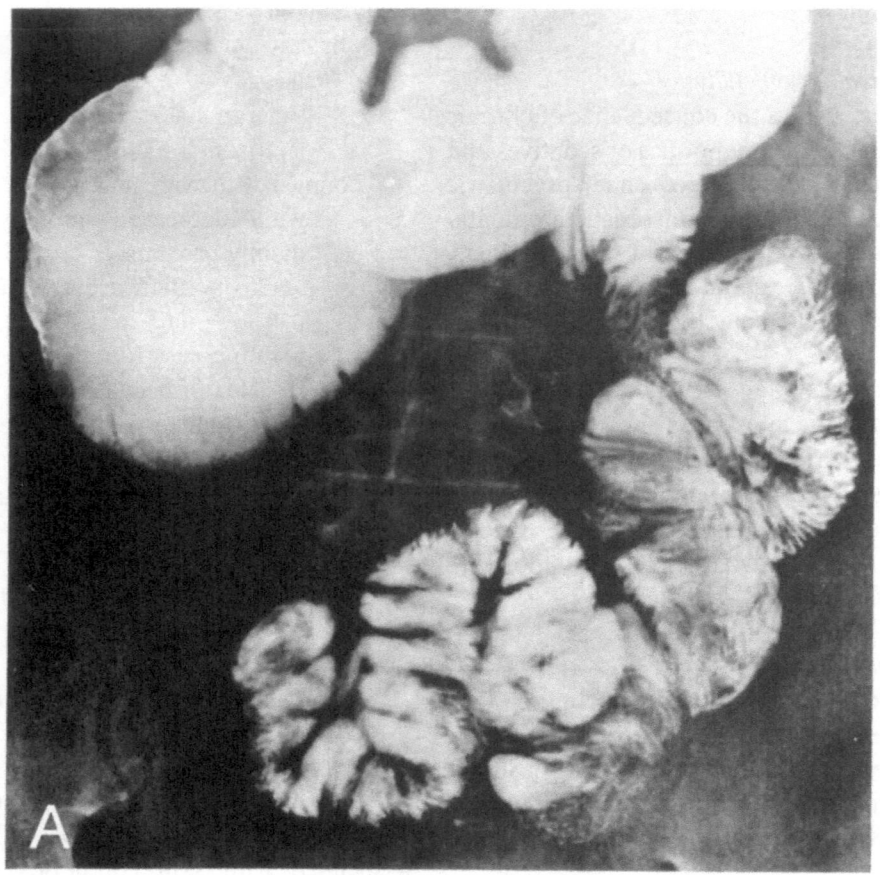

Fig. IV.8A. Two examples of so-called 'sclerosing peritonitis' whereby the mass of intestinal loops becomes more or less wedged in a continuously shrinking peritoneal sac. The intestinal loops show multiple indentations. Markedly dilated duodenum in patient A, only slight dilatation in patient B (see page 63). The normal ileus pattern is masked because the intestinal loops are not able to dilate.

almost exclusively congenital. These *congenital malpositions* are of importance only if they are combined with disturbance of fixation or abnormal mobility and can thus give rise to a, mostly intermittent, volvulus. It can also be advantageous if a patient is aware of an abnormal position of his appendix in situs inversus or other transpositions.

A fairly frequently encountered variation in the position of the mass of small intestinal loops is when the jejunum lies more of less centrally in the upper abdomen with the ileum almost directly below (fig. IV.9).

If during embryonal development the jejunum

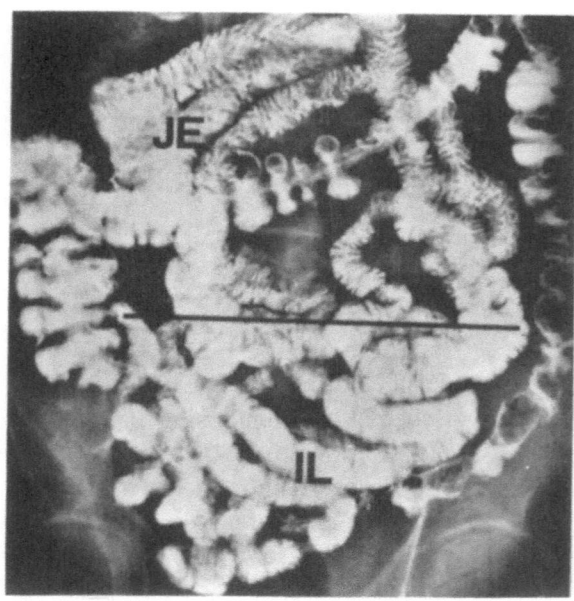

Fig. IV.9. A fairly frequently encountered variation in the position of the mass of loops of the smal intestine is when the jejunum lies more or less in the middle of the upper abdomen with the ileum directly underneath.

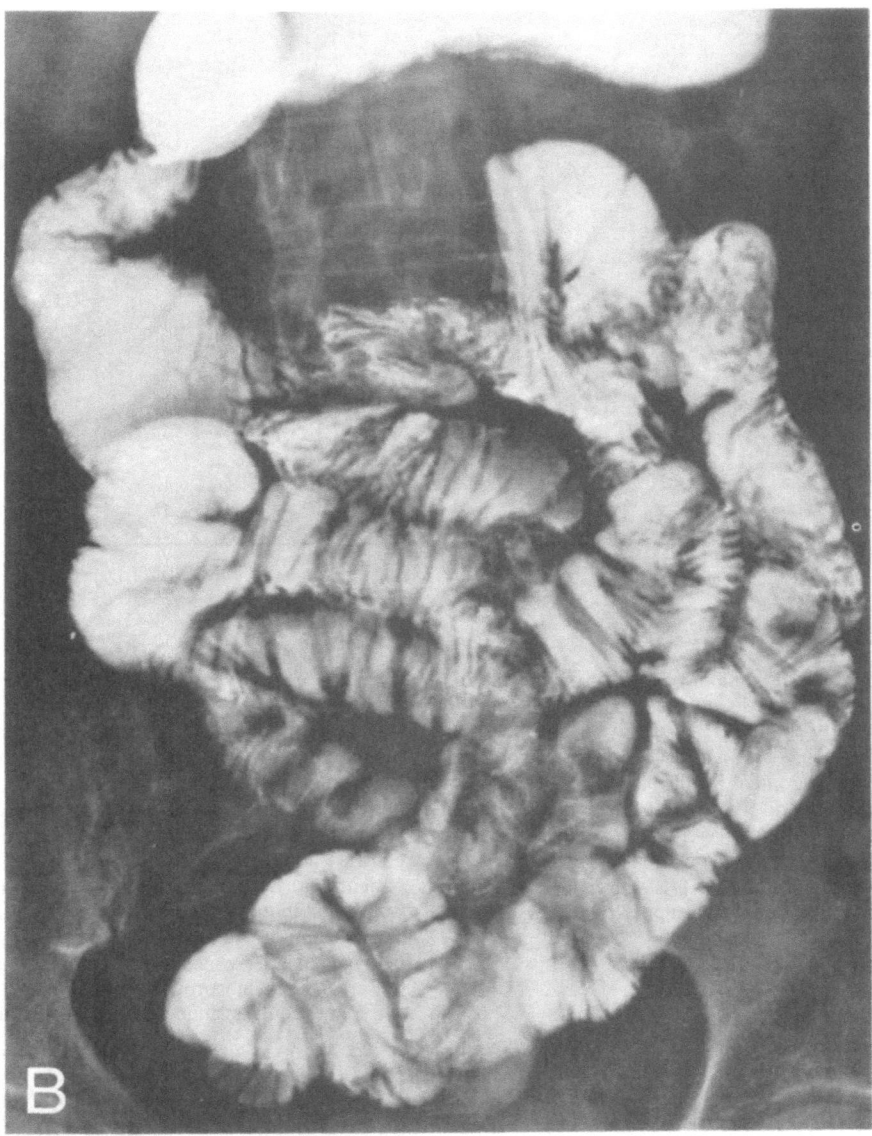

Fig. IV.8.

remains on the right side, we are then confronted with an inversion of the small intestine. In these cases the ileum lies in the middle or to the left in the abdominal cavity (fig. IV.10). If the ileum is found on the left side, the distal segment can lie in the lower, middle or upper abdomen. It is therefore possible that the last ileal loop coming from the left will cross the abdomen diagonally to terminate in the cecum in the lower right quadrant (fig. IV.11). If the entire colon is found in the left half of the abdomen, then the second stage of the rotation phase has not occurred and the base of the mesentery will lie more or less vertically. Usually the entire mass of jejunal loops is then located in the right half of the abdomen and the duodeno-jejunal junction is approximately in the centre (fig. IV.12).

If the omphalo-enteric duct is far removed from Bauhin's valve, most of the ileal loops may come to lie in the right half of the abdomen during the second stage of rotation and if the ascending colon fails to descend, the cecum may also be found in the upper right quadrant. The relationship between the failure of the ascending colon to descend and a distal ileum high in the right upper quadrant is not clear. It is in any case striking that this combination is regularly encountered (fig. IV.13).

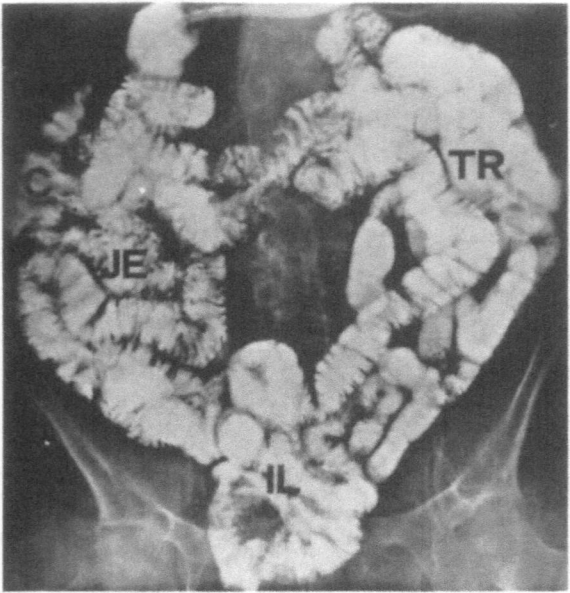

Fig. IV.10. If after reduction of the physiological herniation the jejunal loops do not pass behind the superior mesenteric artery to the upper left quadrant but remain on the right, then the ileal loops are forced to lie more or less in the left half of the abdomen. In this case the transition (TR) between the jejunum and the ileum is in the upper left quadrant. In contrast to a total inversion, the duodenum and the cecum are here in their normal position. Furthermore in this patient, the ascending colon has barely descended so that the cecum (C) is in the right upper quadrant.

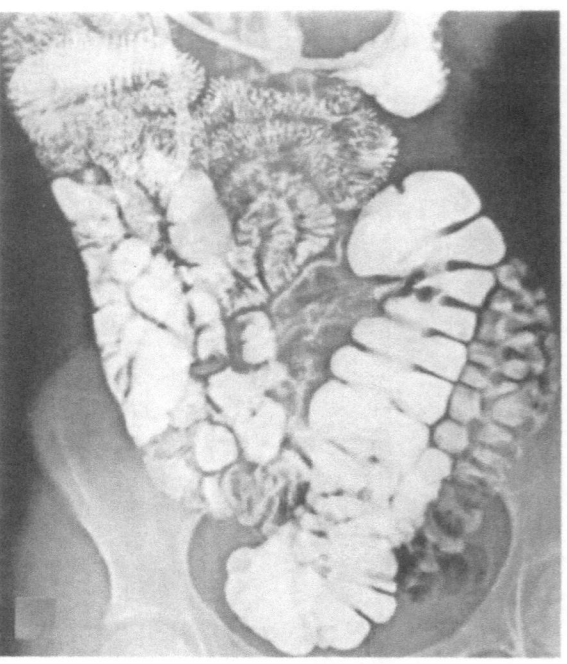

Fig. IV.12. Patient with vague abdominal complaints and periodic cramps. There is a rotational anomaly of the large and the small intestine. The appendix is located near the navel. There was pronounced hypermotility so that the small intestine and the entire colon could be filled with 600 ml contrast fluid within 6 min. Hypermotility is not unusual in patients with a rotational anomaly. Presumably hypermotility can be attributed to anoxia of the small intestine resulting from a (temporary) disturbance of the blood flow. The rapid passage and decreased oxygenation of the intestinal wall often cause malabsorption with quick flocculation of the contrast fluid, as seen in this patient.

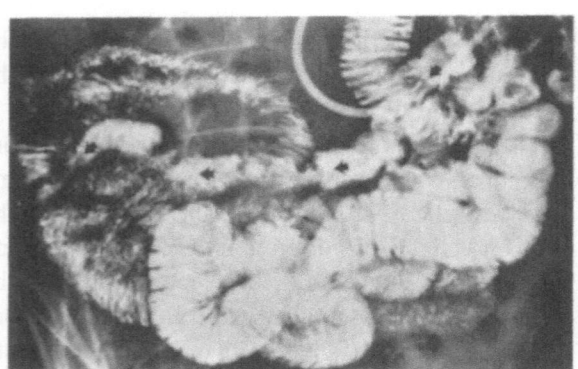

Fig. IV.11. The jejunum is in the right half of the abdomen and the ileum in the left. The distal ileum crosses the abdomen diagonally from left to right (arrows).

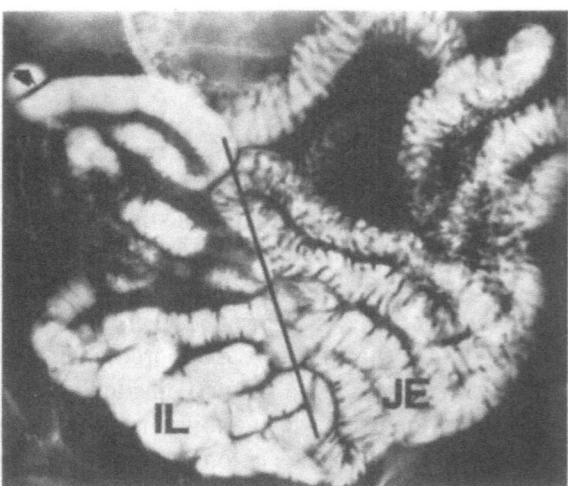

Fig. IV.13. The jejunum is to the left in the abdomen, the ileum to the right. Since the ascending colon has failed to descend, the cecum (here not yet filled) and Bauhin's valve are situated under the liver in the upper abdomen.

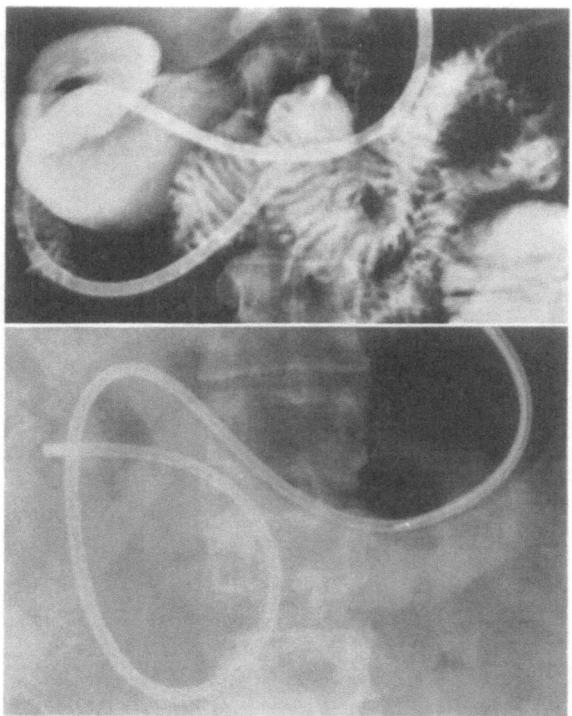

Fig. IV.14. Treitz's ligament may also be found centrally in front of the spinal column (upper) or next to it on the right (lower).

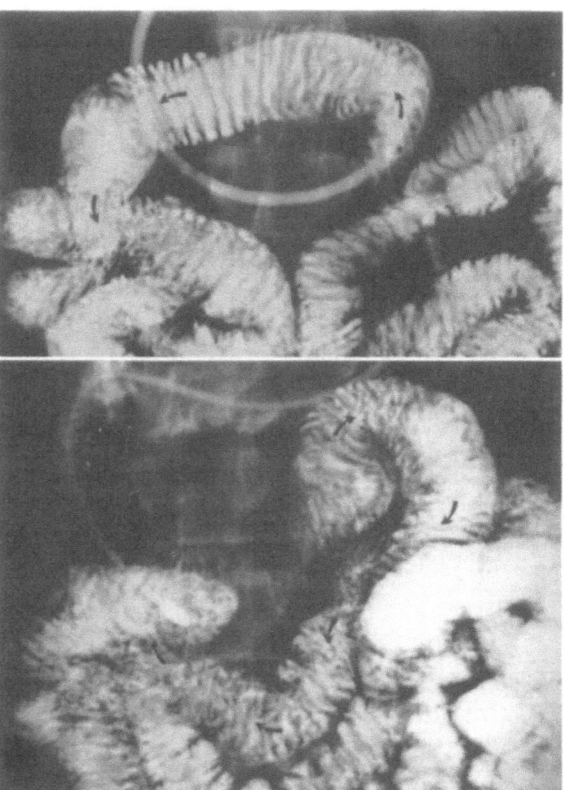

Fig. IV.15. Temporary inversion of the most proximal part of the jejunum. During the first examination this loop was located in the right upper quadrant (above); in a subsequent examination it was approximately in the middle (below).

Quite rare are cases of total stomach-intestine inversion or the anomaly whereby the jejunum lies in the middle of the upper abdomen, the ileum in the middle of the lower abdomen and stomach and cecum to the left.

Although it is a very striking abnormality, malrotation during embryonal development is often overlooked, or is at least not included in the reports. Fortunately this negligence seldom has consequences since most developmental anomalies do not give rise to complaints. This is, however, not always true since some inversions can be reduced quite easily and can cause intermittent complaints.

2. Partial transpositions and herniation

2.1. Congenital

In rare cases the ligament of Treitz can lie centrally, in front or even to the right of the spinal column (fig. IV.14). This may cause problems during intu-

bation if this possibility is not kept in mind. Further distally a temporary inversion of the most proximal jejunal loops sometimes occurs (fig. IV.15). Here, slight vascular disorders may develop, probably as a result of some torsion of the involved intestinal segment. The ease with which temporary inversions can occur is aggravated by increasing length of the intestinal mesentery and concomitant decrease in that of the mesenteric base.

A very common feature is a lack of fixation of the cecum after descent, which can lead to excessive mobility of this organ and eventually to a lateral Bauhin's valve (fig. IV.16). When fixation of the cecum is retarded, it may show pronounced growth in length. A very low cecum may develop if in the final stage descent of the ascending colon is excessively prolonged. In all of these cases the cecum can come to lie deep in the pelvis minor

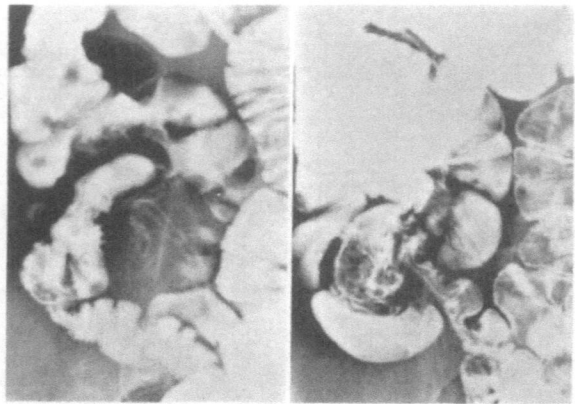

Fig. IV.16. Excessive mobility of the cecum; Bauhin's valve then sometimes assumes a lateral position.

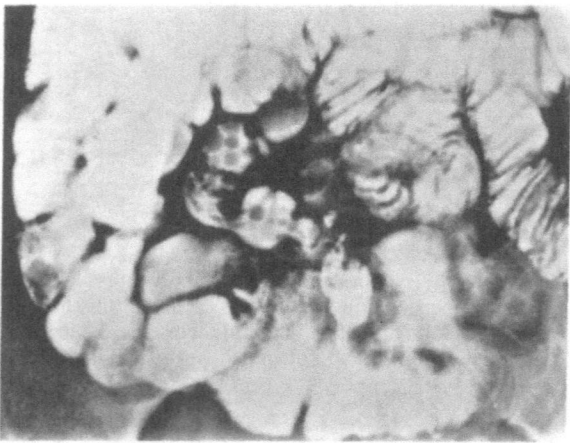

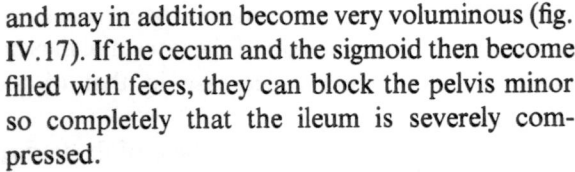

Fig. IV.17. Excessive lengthwise growth of the cecum from tardy descent of the ascending colon, this may sometimes be accompanied by abnormal fixation.

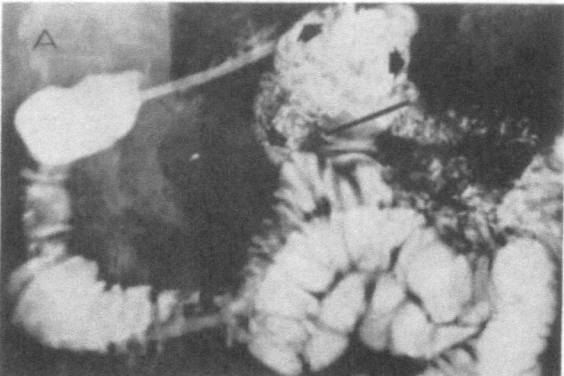

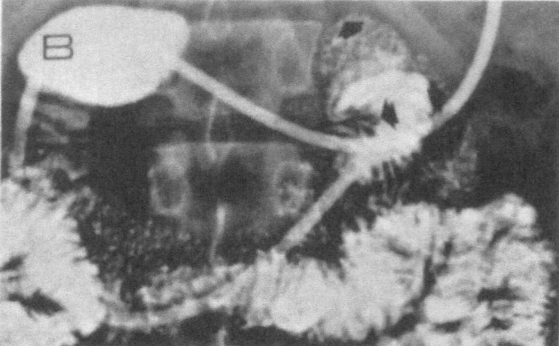

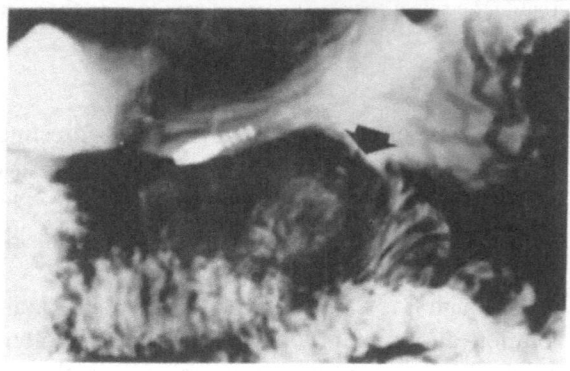

Fig. IV.18. Two cases of paraduodenal herniation. (A) There were only slight intermittent complaints so that surgery was not necessary. (B) The hernia is small but the complaints were quite severe (above). During complaint-free periods, the herniation was not visible (below).

and may in addition become very voluminous (fig. IV.17). If the cecum and the sigmoid then become filled with feces, they can block the pelvis minor so completely that the ileum is severely compressed.

An incomplete or partial fixation can be such that intestinal loops may herniate. Such hernias are found in the region of the ileocecal valve, the so-called retrocecal hernia and in the duodeno-jejunal flexure, where left and right paraduodenal hernias develop (fig. IV.18AB). The latter type in particular accounts for half of all internal hernias; it can become quite large and cause alarming clini-

cal symptoms which resemble those of obstruction in the proximal intestine.

In the region of the ileocecal valve, a fairly deep sac behind and underneath the cecum can develop. Especially if the mesentery of the distal ileum is long, a mass of ileal loops can easily become fixed within such a sac (fig. IV.19). Differentiation between a hernia, a fake pattern (fig.

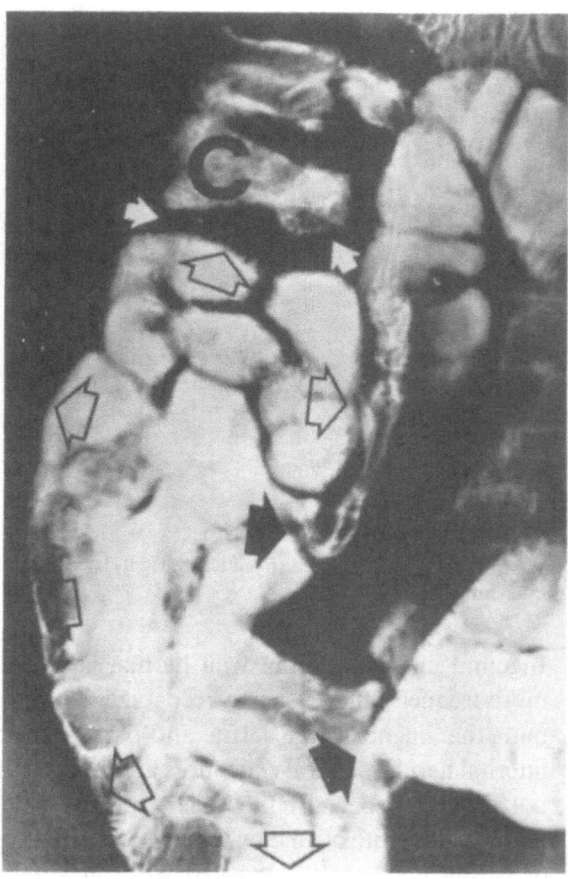

Fig. IV.19. Large sac (open black arrow) containing fixed ileal loops filled with air on a preceding plain X-ray. The afferent and efferent ileal loop indicated by black arrows. C = cecum.

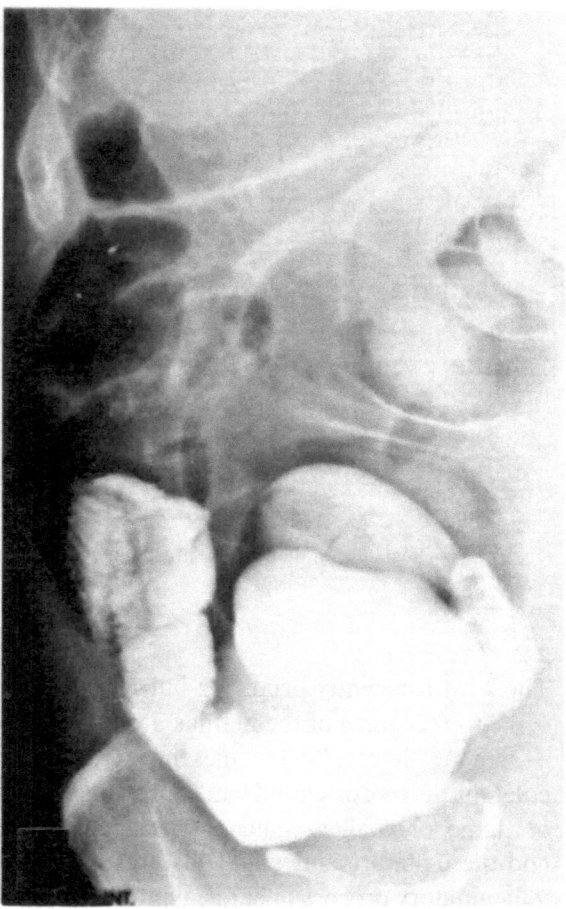

Fig. IV.20. The last meter of the ileum is located on the lateral side of the ascending colon under the liver in the right upper quadrant. Usually, as here, this is not the result of herniation whereby the ileum passes behind the colon. It is the result of a long mesentery that passes *in front* of the colon. This condition is quite different from that shown in fig. IV.19.

IV.20) or a deep retrocecal fossa is radiologically not always possible. Sometimes the fossa is so small that the intestinal loop trapped within it can be forced free by increasing the degree of filling (fig. IV.21). In general it is not possible to use compression or palpation to force loops out of a hernia or deep fossa. Herniation of the small intestine through defects in the mesentery can be left- or right-handed and may become so large that practically all the loops of the small intestine are included.

Another common type of herniation is that through the transverse mesocolon whereby the intestinal loops, part of the omentum or both, come to lie behind the stomach and cause an obvious impression on the antral region (fig.

IV.22). In addition the foramen of Winslow may be so large that the intestinal loops pass easily into the lesser sac of the peritoneum.

Some patients may have colic-like attacks of abdominal pain whenever they assume an abnormal position, such as bending over, climbing (or descending) the stairs quickly, etc. In these patients their pain can be elicited by sharp thrusting movements during the X-ray examination. In such cases fluoroscopy of the patient by the radiologist is essential and the diagnosis may well be missed if reliance is placed solely on films taken by a technician.

68

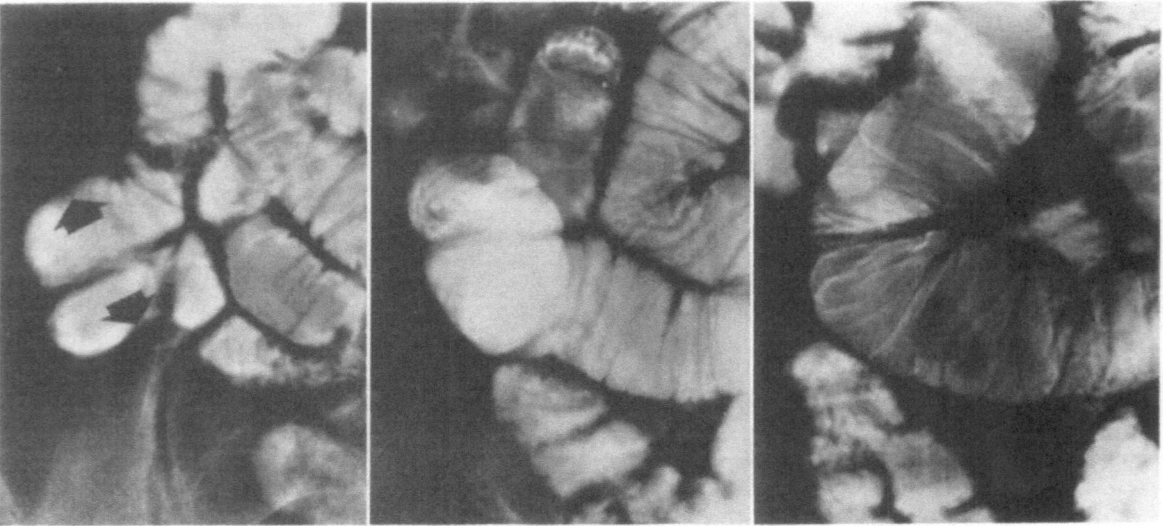

Fig. IV.21. Segment of ileal loop in shallow retrocecal fossa (arrows) that was freed (from left to right) by means of maximum filling (water infusion).

2.2. Acquired

The least frequently occurring but most trouble-some to recognize of the hernias are the internal. Traumatic defects in the mesentery, the meso-colon or the mesosigmoid can cause compression of a larger or smaller segment of the small intestine and these abnormalities may also result from an inflammatory process or surgical interference (fig. IV.23).

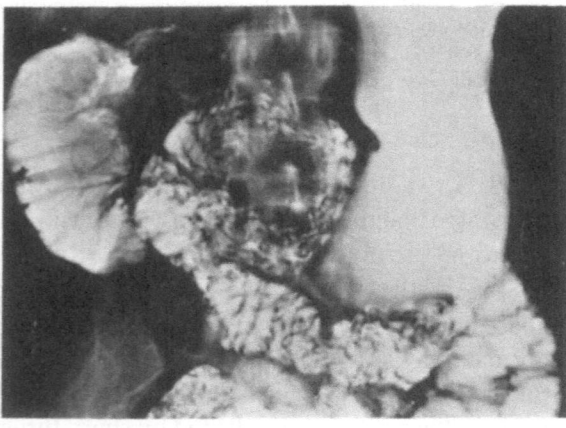

Fig. IV.22. Compression effect of proximal jejunal loop on the posterior pars antralis of the stomach. This is encountered in cases of herniation through the transverse mesocolon (or through a dilated foramen of Winslow into the lesser sac). In this case there were no complaints and therefore surgical confirmation was not available.

Inguinal and abdominal wall hernias are much more frequent and easier to recognize. To determine the diagnosis in external and particularly in internal hernias, lateral exposures are often essential. This is especially the case with abdominal hernias at the site of an old surgical scar. This type of hernia may not be revealed with an anterio-posterior exposure since in this view the orifice can be rather easily overlooked. It is important to follow the contrast column under fluoroscopy since intestinal motility in and in front of the hernia is often very locally but quite definitely disturbed. Obstruction or locally reduced motility may exist but usually there is pronounced hyper-motility and the patients complain of attacks of coliky abdominal pain precisely localised to the site of the hernia.

Another characteristic is that the afferent and efferent loops of the compressed intestine taper slightly at the hernial orifice which is in itself invisible. They also lie closely approximated and so absolutely fixed that they cannot be moved by palpation. If survey photographs of the abdomen are made before the contrast medium examination, it will be noted that several intestinal loops consistently lie close together and are filled with air. Moreover, when the patient stands upright, these loops show fluid levels.

According to the numerous reports in the literature, a pre-operative radiological examination hardly ever yields a diagnosis of 'internal hernia'. We have found, however, that this disorder with its fairly classical history is easily recognized if this diagnostic possibility is at least considered and if the röntgen examination is carried out using the enteroclysis technique and intermittent fluoroscopy.

If the hernial opening is small, an incarcerated hernia can develop which requires immediate surgery (fig. IV.24A). It will be clear that when constriction occurs, the venous circulation will be the first and most severely disturbed. If the obstruction of the venous flow is incomplete or intermittent, it is possible that the hematomata in the mucosa will not so enlarge that they cause acute obstruction. Moreover a transient and increasingly pronounced fibrosis during the recovery phase can apparently prevent the development of necrosis. After some time the results of a disturbance of the venous circulation can no longer be differentiated radiologically from those of a disturbed arterial flow, from Crohn's disease, or conditions resulting from radiotherapy.

A good example of an obstruction of the venous flow (in the rest phase) which proceeded so gradually that the history was in fact 'clean' is seen in fig. IV.24B. There is a large hernial sac which developed in the abdominal scar of a previous

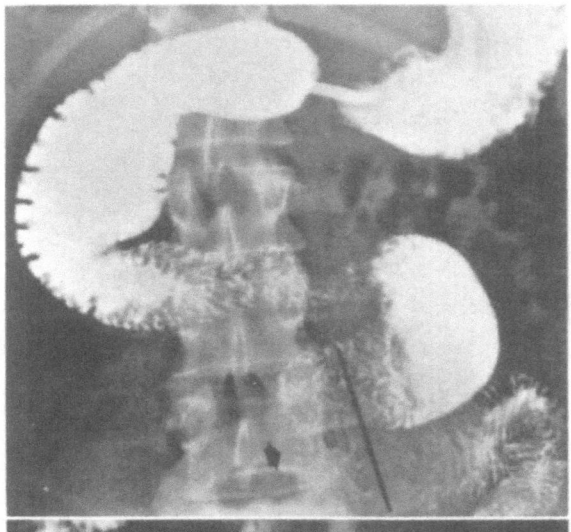
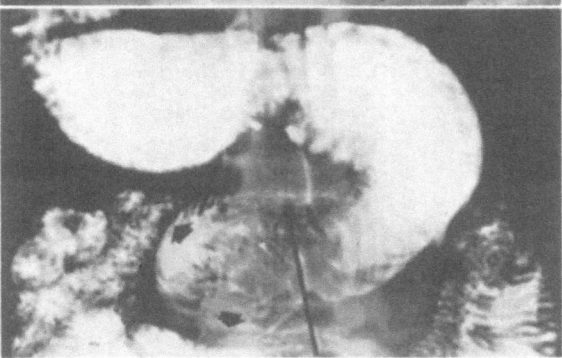
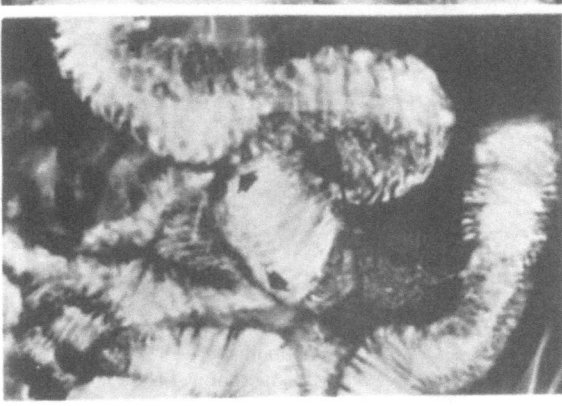

Fig. IV.23. Herniation of a segment of the proximal jejunal loop through a small defect in the mesentery (straight black line) that developed after surgical removal of a mesenteric cyst. Proximal to the herniation is a prestenotic dilatation. On the distal side is local, pronounced hyperperistalsis that caused the colic-like attacks of abdominal pain.

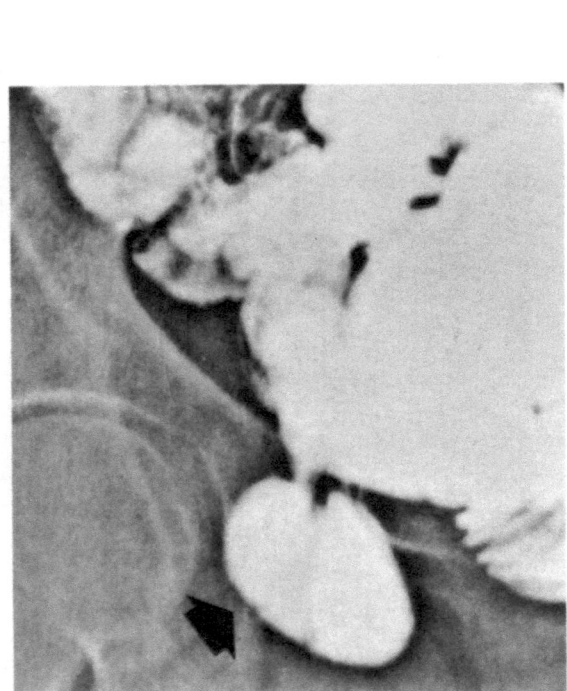

Fig. IV.24A. Right inguinal hernia.

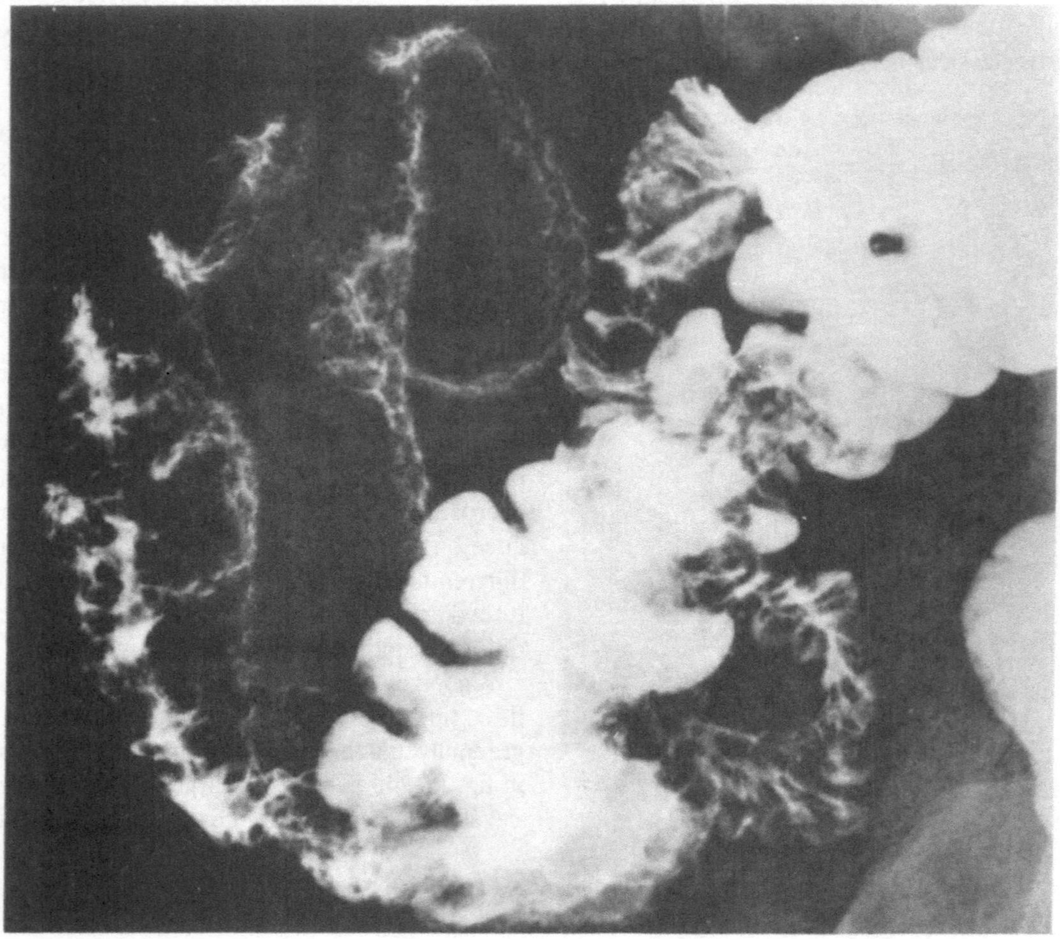

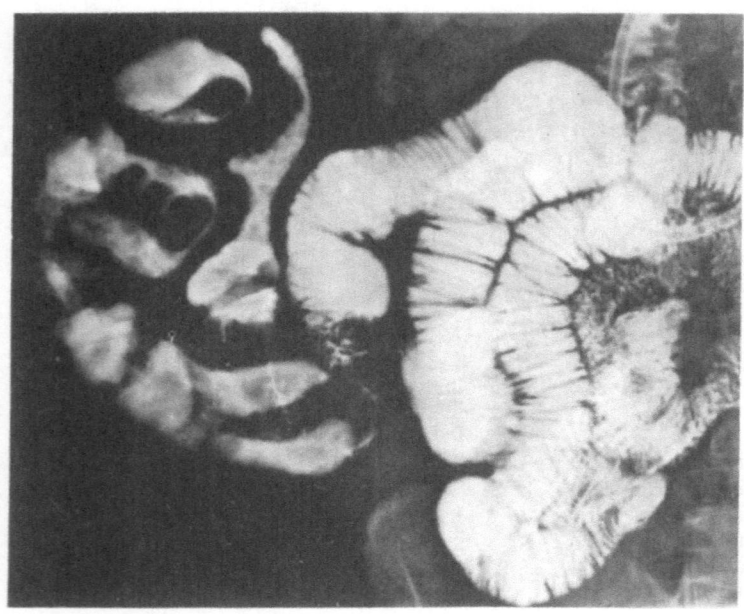

Fig. IV.24B. Lateral hernia through the abdominal wall after previous kidney operation. The hernial sac contains part ot the ascending colon and a mass of jejunal loops that show the results of a disturbed venous flow. The abnormalities, consisting of multiple longitudinal ulcerations, asymmetric and circular shrinkage, markedly thickened intestinal wall and frequent spasms cannot be differentiated from those in Crohn's disease or radiation enteritis.

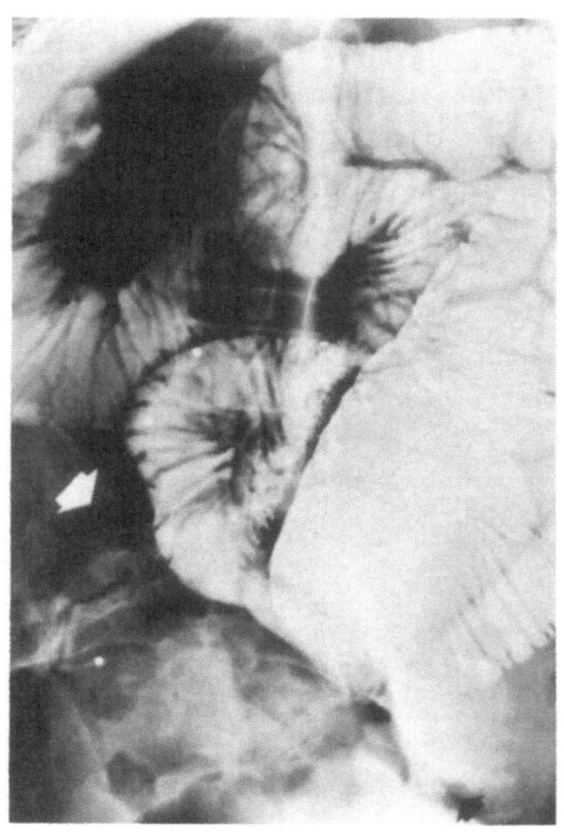

kidney operation. The patient could in fact only report that the hernial sac was much smaller in the beginning and that it was not until later that he was able to push the intestinal loops in the sac back through the hernial opening into the abdominal cavity. It is interesting that the very rigid and stiff intestinal loops were easily palpable through the thin flabby wall of the hernial sac and that it could be established that the most lateral loops were fused with the wall of the hernial sac.

Because of their constricting nature, bands sometimes cause a volvulus of the intestine. On the röntgenogram the point of torsion of the volvulus can often be identified by concentric rings of mucosal folds in the dilated intestinal loop which decrease in size towards the centre (fig. IV.25).

Volvulus of a mass of intestinal loops can be caused by a particularly long mesentery or when fixation of the mesentery to the posterior abdominal wall is too short or inadequate. A good example of the latter is shown in fig. IV.26, it can be seen that the mass of intestinal loops changes position very easily which may result in intermittent complaints. When in a patient with unexplained colic-like abdominal pain a positional anomaly is demonstrated, the possibility of a volvulus should always be considered. In volvulus the circulation is often seriously disturbed in the involved intestinal segment. There may be signs of mucosal swelling due to the elevated venous pressure as well as hyperperistalsis from anoxia of the intestine (fig.IV.27).

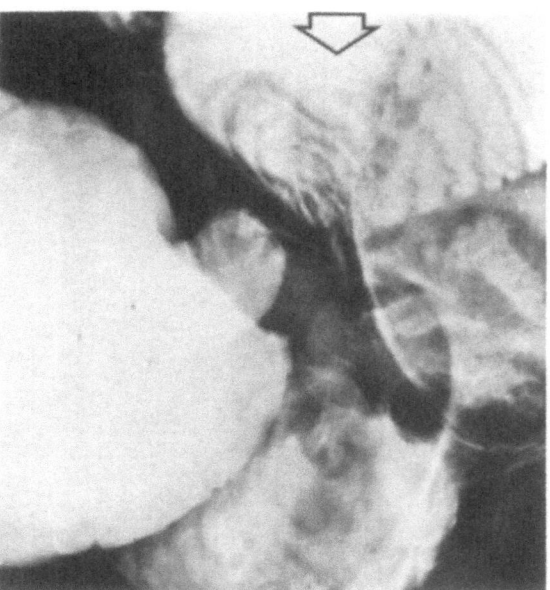

Fig. IV.25. Almost total obstruction of the small intestine from a crossing band, running from the upper right to the lower left quadrant (solid arrows) in a patient with a 'short bowel' (Crohn's disease). This band constricted one loop completely and another quite markedly, thus causing a volvulus. Upper: Survey film after administration of 1200 ml contrast fluid. Lower:Subsequently the site of obstruction was approached from the distal side by filling of the colon. The point of torsion can be recognized on this röntgenogram by the mucosal folds that form concentric rings (open arrow).

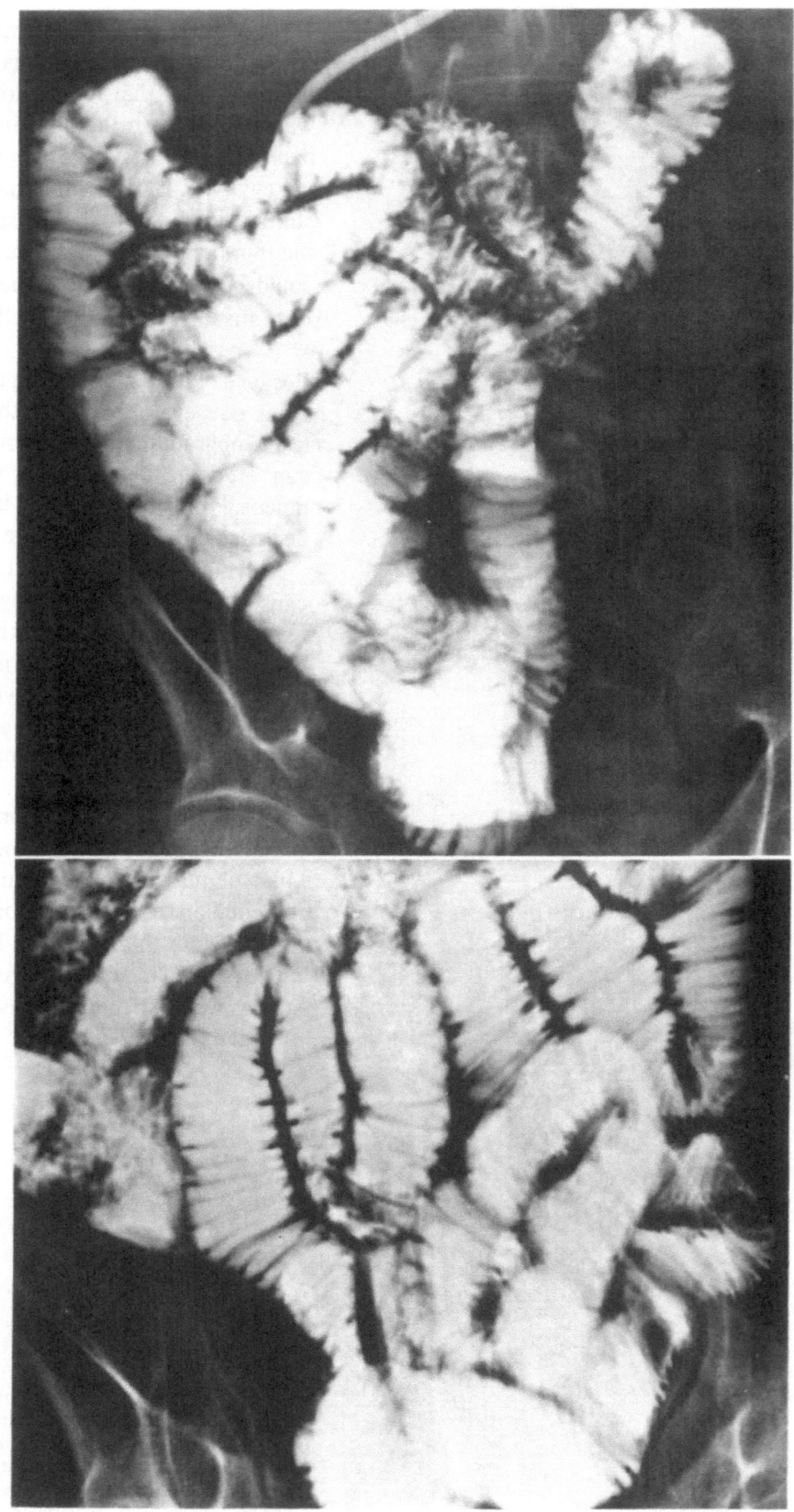

Fig. IV.26.

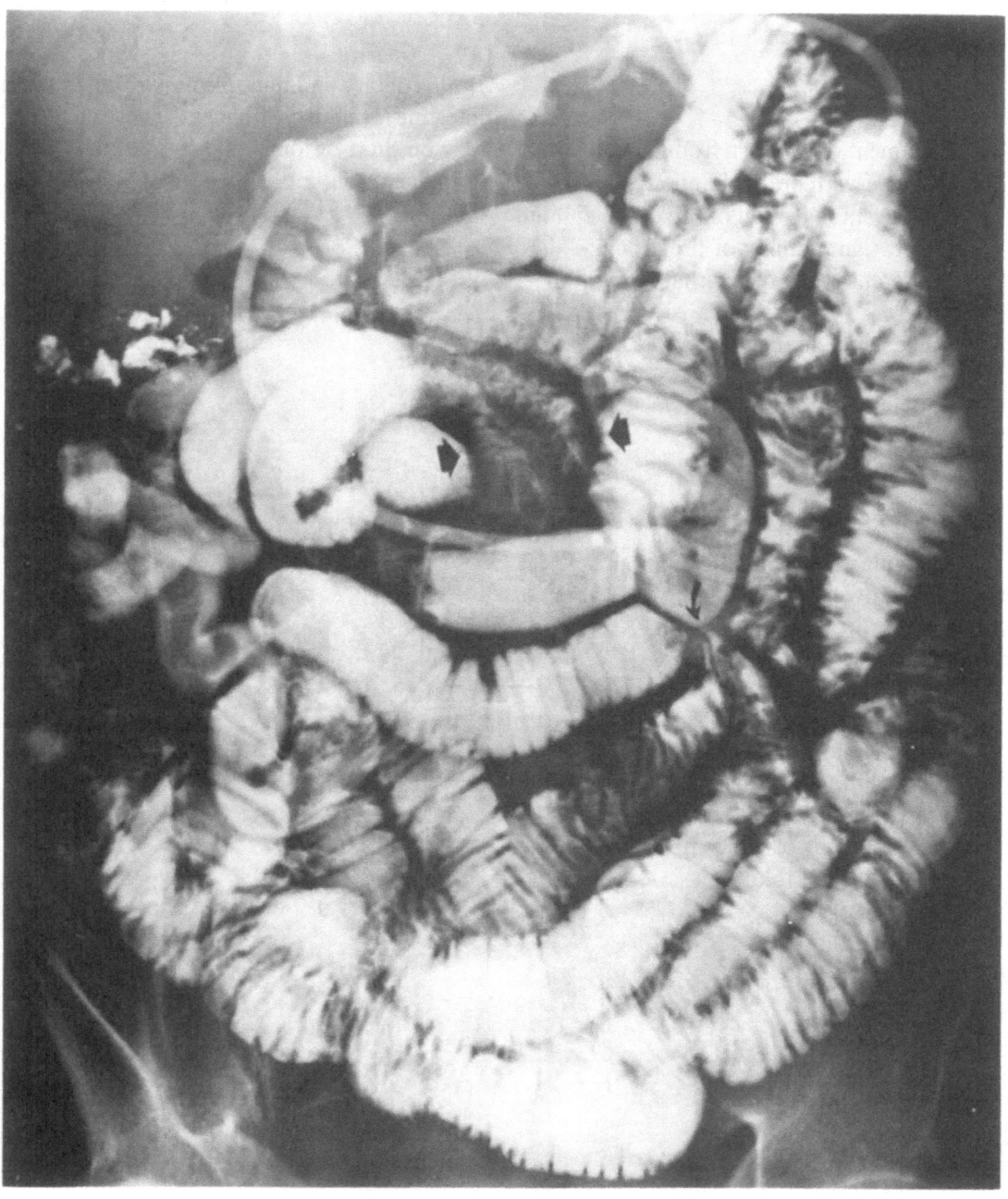

Fig. IV.26. Volvulus of the small intestine because the attachment of the mesentery was too short. An attack could be provoked by having the patient bend over as far as possible. The jejunum is in the upper right quadrant, the ileum in the lower left. The moderately dilated ileal loops show multiple indentations and the mucosal folds are stretched perpendicular to the axis of the intestine (left page). During periods without complaints the jejunum lay in the lower left quadrant and the ileum in the upper right. The mass of intestinal loops is therefore rotated through a 45° angle with respect to the normal position. To the left of the navel is an elongated intestinal loop with a pointed bulge (thin arrow) probably caused by a band.

Local hypermotility with mucosal folds stretched perpendicularly above the navel (thick arrows on right page).

3. Summarised positional anomalies

Involving more or less the whole small intestine.
    congenital:
        transpositions
Partial transpositions.
    congenital:
        ligament of Treitz in front or to the right
            of vertebral column
        recurrent inversion of proximal jejunum
        excessive mobility of the cecum
        different types of internal herniation
    acquired:
        defects in the mesentery
        traumatic
        inflammatory process
        surgery
        external hernias
            inguinal
            in the abdominal wall
        volvulus from band formation
Increasing chance of volvulus in case of long
mesentery or short mesenteric base.
Clinical picture:
        colic-like abdominal pain
        hypermotility of small intestine
        fixed position of several loops
            with fluid levels and air
        vascular abnormalities (edema)
        development of concentric tapering of
            mucosal folds

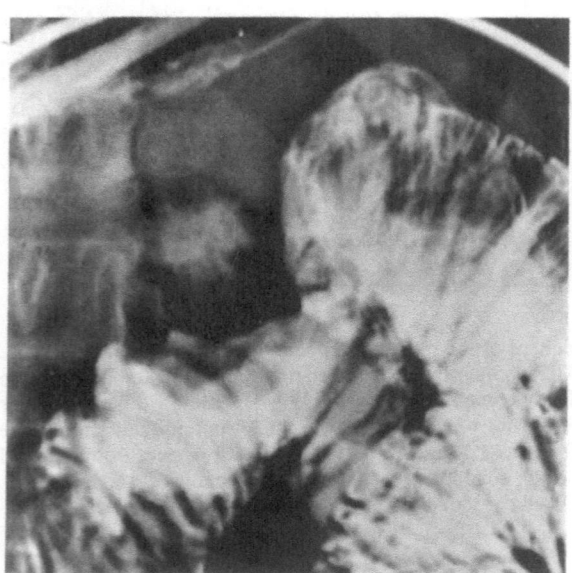

C. Alteration in intestinal diameter

1. Locally restricted narrowing

1.1. General

Both, solitary and multiple narrowing of the small intestine is relatively frequent. These constrictions may be short or long, mild or marked, smooth or irregular in outline, as well as circular or asym-

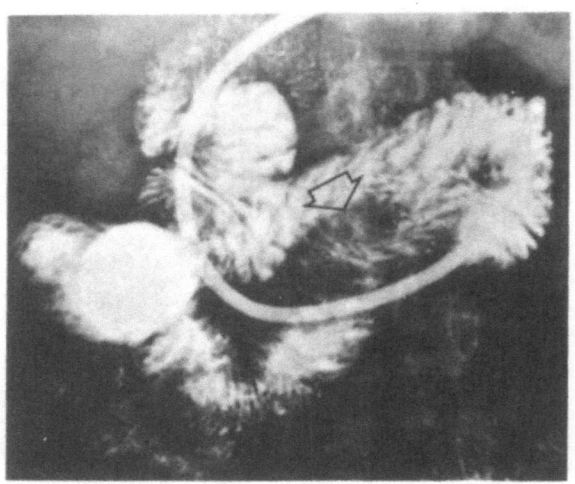

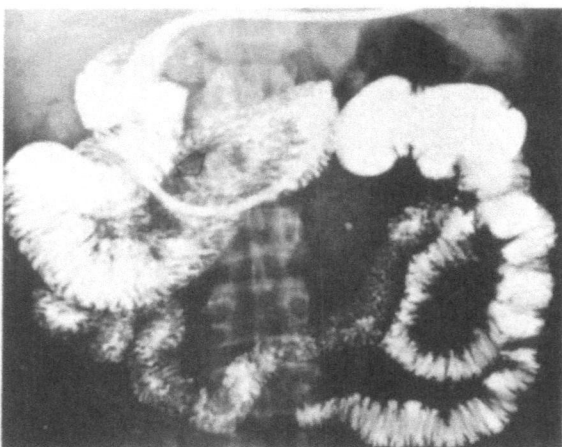

Fig. IV.27. Intermittent moderately severe attacks of abdominal pain presumably connected with slight torsion of several proximal jejunal loops in the right upper quadrant. Locally there was quite pronounced hypermotility (arrows) so that it was not possible to visualize this segment of the intestine in a well-filled state.

Fig. IV.28. Leiomyoma of the jejunum with centrally located calcifications. *(Courtesy of prof. A. de Schepper – Antwerp.)*

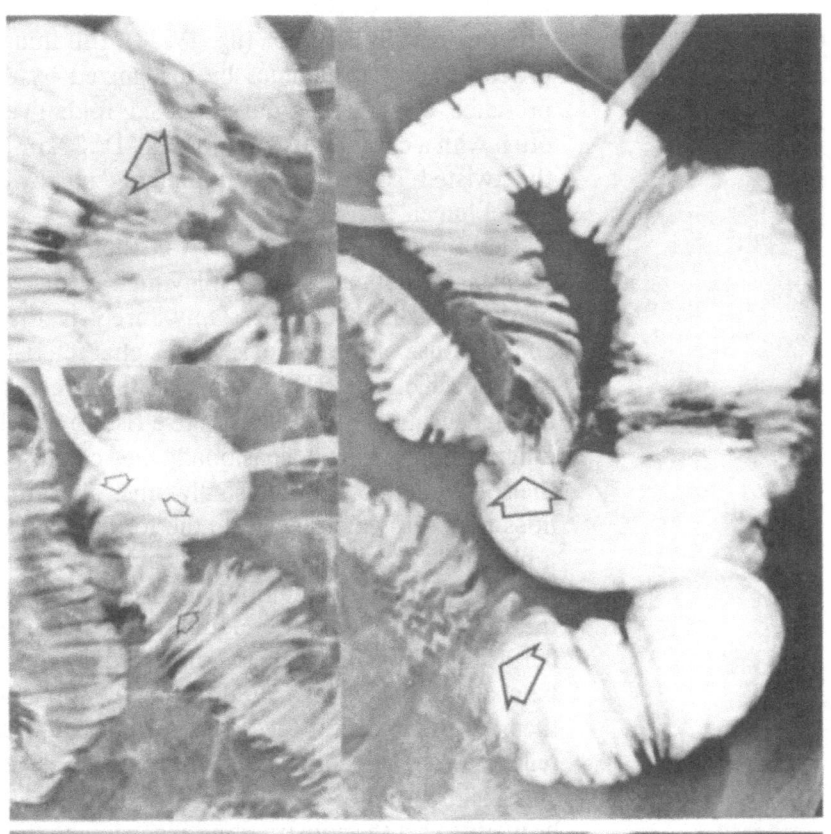

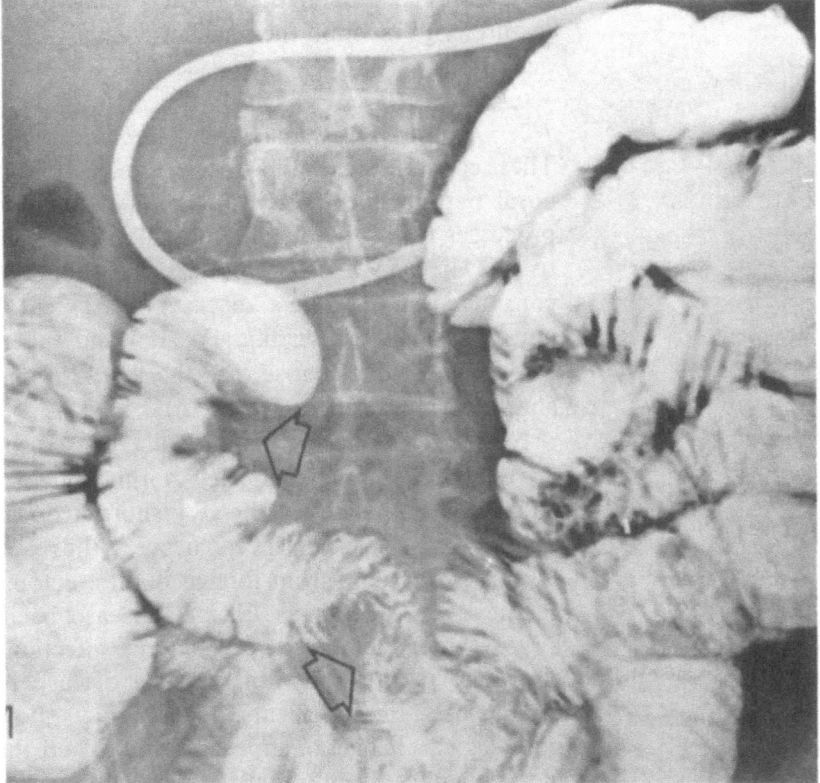

Fig. IV.29. Reticulum cell sar-coma with predominantly extra-mural growth and therefore com-pression-like patterns and stretched mucosal folds at the sites of the lesions. The mucosal relief in the proximal jejunum in the upper left quadrant resembles that of the ileum (above) and be-comes strikingly smooth as filling of the lumen increases (below). The presence of celiac disease is highly suspected.

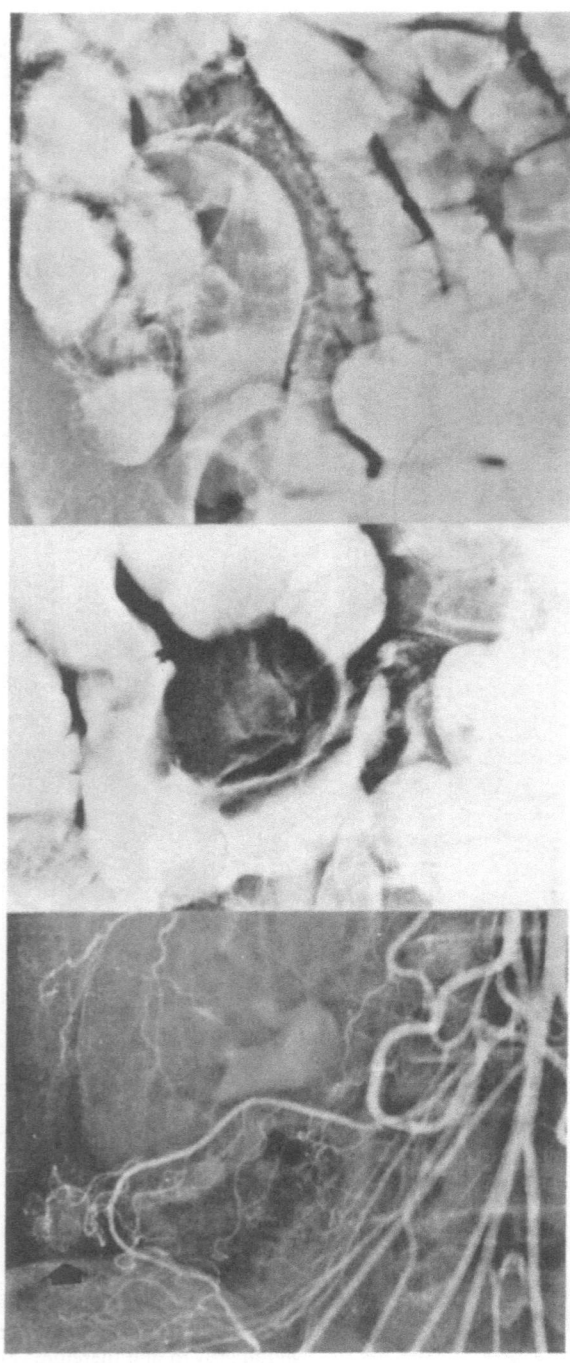

Fig. IV.30. Carcinoid in Bauhin's valve with stretched distal ileum, almost invisible on the plain film (upper), but easily seen on the compression spot film (middle). An angiogram (lower) revealed not only the carcinoid but also metastases in the liver.

metric. An asymmetric stenosis can be the result of fibrous contracture or an intramural growth process, usually a tumor (fig. IV.28). Intramural processes may sometimes be recognized by the presence of stretched-out mucosal folds, very often with a circular distribution (fig. IV.29) or by the twisted course of the remaining narrowed bowel lumen (fig. IV.30).

The conditions responsible for such appearances are legion and may display their own scala of distinguishing features. Only rarely is there some feature of the stenosis that is characteristic for a specific cause. Depending on their severity and localisation, stenoses can give rise to widely differing complaints. Occasionally they constitute the sole finding but more usually other abnormalities are seen which facilitate the formulation of a probability diagnosis.

In the presence of multiple stenoses and where the contrast medium is not administered with sufficient rapidity, often only the more proximal can be visualised. This leads, unfortunately now and then, to the necessity of a second operation to relieve recurring complaints. Although a strict classification is not very feasible, an attempt wil be made to list the constrictions according to their features and mention their salient ancillary characteristics.

1.2. Narrowing with smooth-walled borders

These constrictures mainly result from loss of mucosal pattern due to ischemia or inflammatory processes with subsequent contraction of fibrous tissue. The *inflammatory processes* that should be considered are Crohn's disease (fig. IV.31M), non-specific ulceration (fig. IV.31K) and tuberculosis where the stenoses are short ($1/2$-$2^1/2$ cm) and often multiple (figs. IV.55AB).

Non-specific ulcers, occasionally caused by KCL tablets, show a completely normal mucosal pattern on both sides of the very short stenosis. Solitary non-specific ulcers can occur as the result of mucosal trauma from foreign bodies, ectopic gastric mucosa, Zollinger-Ellison's disease, bacillary dysentery and systemic bacterial infections elsewhere in the body. In Crohn's disease or tuberculosis the adjacent mucosa may show pathological changes or appear normal. Where the ulcer has not been circular, markedly asym-

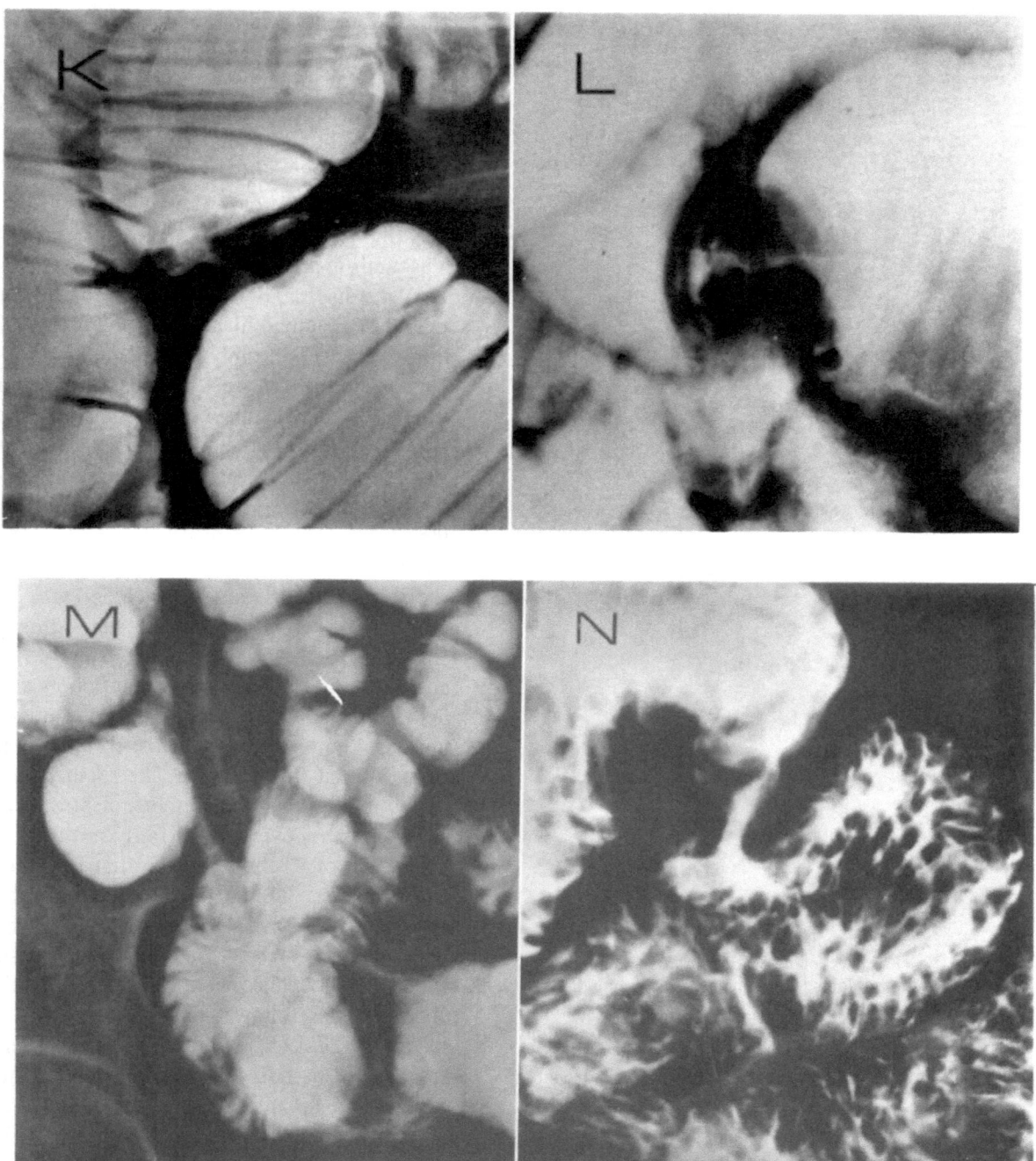

Fig. IV.31. Stenoses in the small intestine, 0.5-1.0 cm long, as a result of non-specific ulceration (K) and carcinoid (L). In both cases fibrosis is pronounced. Stenoses in the small bowel more than 1 cm long due to skip lesions in Crohn's disease (M) and an adenocarcinoma (N).

metrical contracture leads to the formation of the so-called 'shell sign' (fig. IV.32).

Stenosis of *ischemic* origin are generally in excess of 2 cm, frequently circular and do not always show marked narrowing. They can arise by:

1) Fairly acute occlusion of the superior mesenteric artery from arteriosclerosis. Where these occlusive processes have developed more

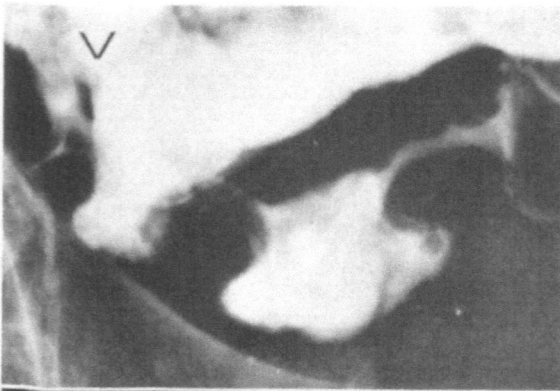

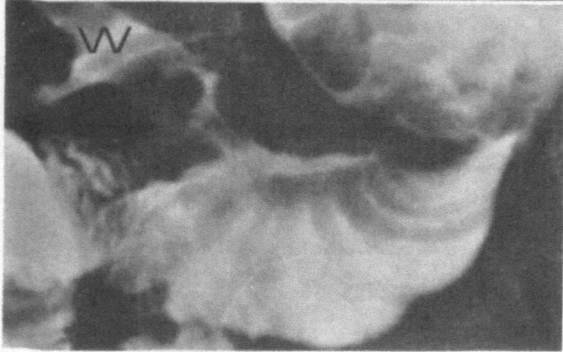

Fig. IV.32. Emblem of the Shell Oil Company (above). Asymmetric shrinkage of ulceration in the intestinal wall causes the mucosal folds to assume a radial course directed towards the ulcer; this pattern closely resembles the emblem of the Shell Oil Company (the Shell sign). Differentiation between old ulcers in Crohn's disease, ischemia and tuberculosis is impossible: (v) ischemia; (w) Crohn's disease after 14 years remission.

gradually and collateral circulation from the celiac trunk, inferior mesenteric artery or vessels of the abdominal wall has been established, they do not necessarily lead to complaints (fig. IV.33).

2) Mechanical obstruction of the intestine from adhesions or bands, volvulus or internal hernia is usually accompanied by obvious impairment of the arterial and venous circulation.

3) After surgery, involving the major vessels in the abdomen, there may be a temporary decrease in the blood flow through the superior and inferior mesenteric arteries.

4) Microemboli, occuring in polycythemia vera or as a result of valvular disease, atrial fibrillation or a myocardial infarction, can cause sudden occlusion of the relatively small vessels (fig. IV.34).

5) Vasculitis in arteries or small veins, as seen in Burger's disease, Schönlein-Henoch disease, diabetes, rheumatoid arthritis or mesenteric fibrosis causes thrombosis and multiple occlusions in these vessels. This can also occur in many collagen diseases associated with abnormal skin conditions, such as periarteritis nodosa (fig. IV.35), lupus erythematosus or dermatomyositis. The relatively long (often measured in decimetres) moderately severe constrictions associated with radiation enteritis can be included in this group. The appearances are here mostly smooth-walled but folding can still be recognized (fig. IV.36A). Short radiation stenoses are also found resulting from ischemic fibrosis, tumor recurrence or compression from without (fig. IV.36B). The slightly narrowed smooth-walled stretches of bowel resulting post recovery in the fairly rare superficial form of Crohn's disease that is somewhat reminiscent of an ulcerative colitis of the small intestine, have also their origin in extensive loss of mucosal folding from diffuse widespread occlusion of the smallest peripheral arteries, followed by mild diffuse fibrosis (fig. IV.37MNO). A similar picture is seen in graft-versus-host disease following bone marrow transplantations, but here the appearances are somewhat more irregular with more spindle-shaped areas of widening arising from prestenotic dilatations (fig. IV.38).

6. Vasoconstrictors, ergotamine preparations for example, can also cause a temporary reduction in the blood supply of the intestinal wall.

Smooth-walled constrictions can also be caused by *tumor growth*. The better known are the short stenoses of adenocarcinoma (fig. IV.31N) or car-

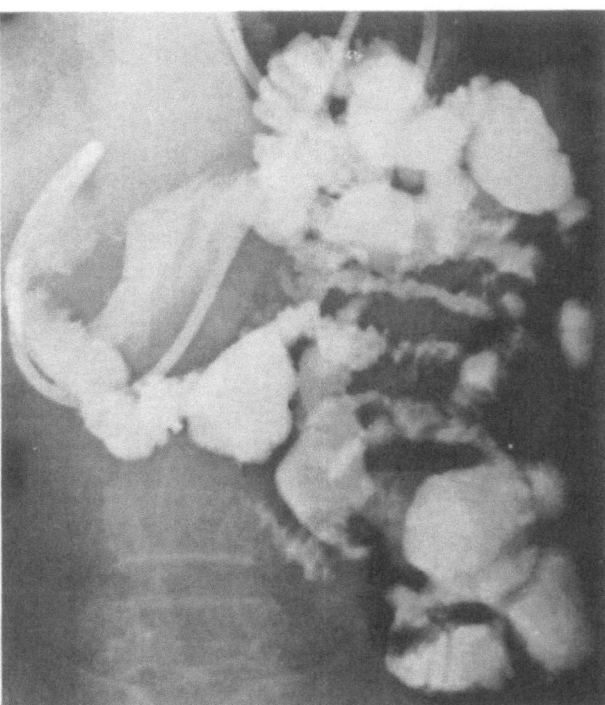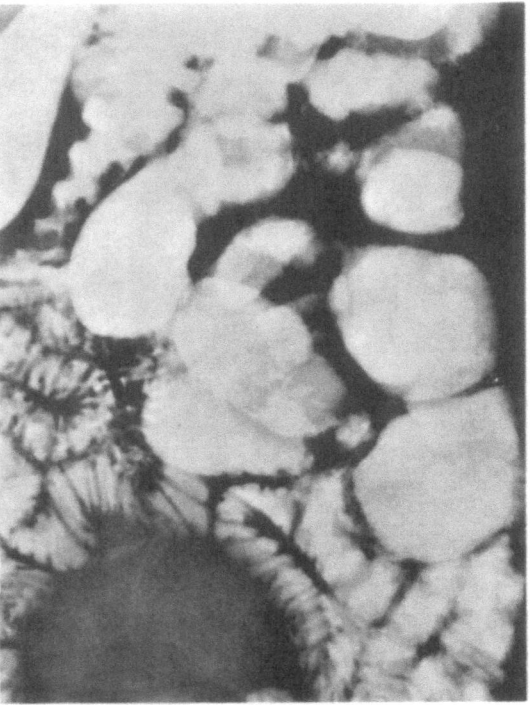

Fig. IV.33. Elderly male with multiple ischemic stenoses several centimetres in length in the jejunum. The mucosal pattern has disappeared in the intestinal segments between the stenoses. An angiographic examination revealed a vascular insufficiency in this part of the small bowel and the appearance of the vessels indicated contracture of the mesentery. Impression of large prostate in lower abdomen.

cinoid focus (fig. IV.31L) and the mainly longer stenoses of less marked severity associated with intra-mucosal or intra-mural lympho-reticular malignancies (fig. IV.40) or scirrhus metastases (fig.IV.41). Less frequently seen are the short but severe stenoses from metastases (fig. IV.39). Adenocarcinoma is found chiefly in the duodenum or proximal jejunum and carcinoid or lympho-reticular malignancy more frequently distal in the ileum, but all can occur anywhere in the small intestine. In cases of lympho-reticular malignancy where destruction of intestinal wall is sometimes limited, longer segments of constriction may be caused by external pressure from massive mesenteric lymph-gland involvement that leads to bizarre combinations of very numerous, short, in themselves smooth-walled constrictions (fig. IV.42).

A continuous smooth-walled mildly constricted segment, by definition beginning in the duodenum and not extending further than to the ileum, may be based on a *celiac syndrome* with additional edema of the bowel wall from superimposed infection (fig. IV.43B1).

1.3. Constricted segments arising from swelling of intact mucosa

The appearances here involve short to very limited segments constricted by local but very pronounced swelling of the mucosa that can originate in congestion of blood or lymph or result from an interstitial inflammatory process. A classical instance is the recurrence of Crohn's disease proximal to the anastomosis, which regularly appears after resection, most frequently from the ileocecal region (fig. IV.44).

Sometimes a collateral inflammation of the distal ileum, associated with infiltration of the appendix or cecum can show well marked swelling of the mucosal folds (see fig. IV.107). After reduction of an invagination, sometimes successful in small children, a very marked mucosal edema accompanied by a somewhat reduced tran-

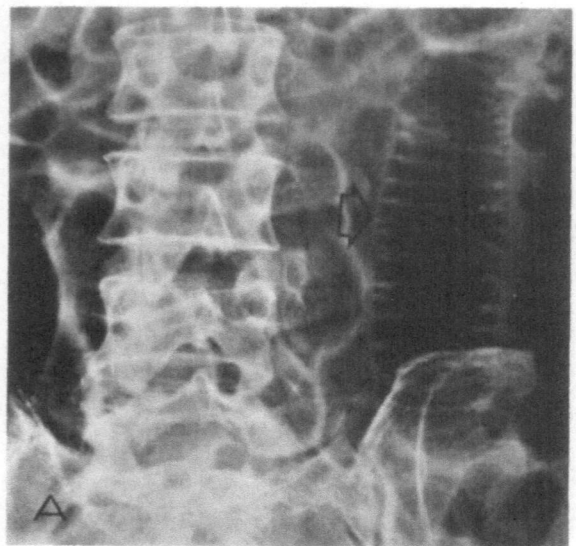

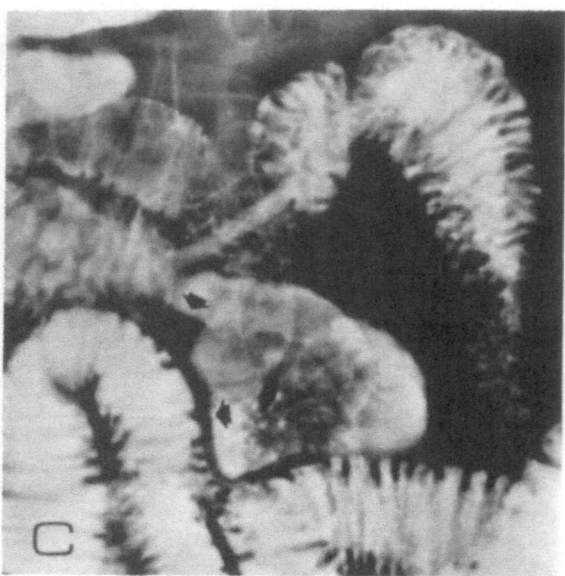

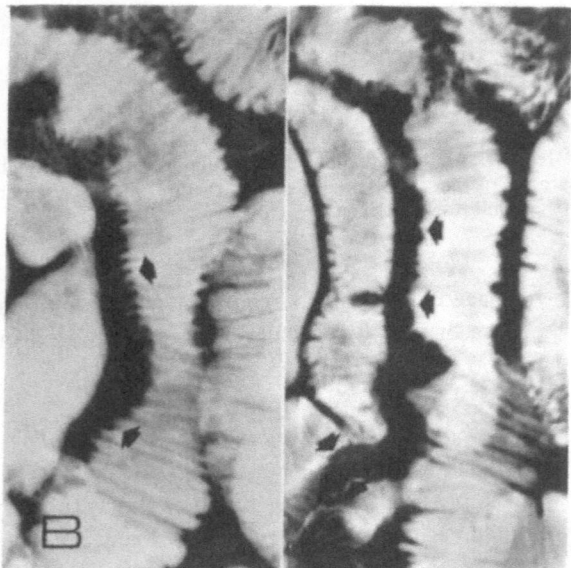

Fig. IV.34. Vascular accident in the small bowel of a patient with atrial fibrillation. (A) There were definite signs of an ileus, both radiologically and clinically. (B) In the distal jejunum, one loop contains highly edematous swollen mucosal folds; this is called 'thumbprinting'. The bowel wall is obviously thicker. No peristaltic movements could be seen in this region. (C) Several weeks later a definite clinical recovery was apparent. The röntgenograms now showed complete obliteration of the mucosal relief in the involved segment. The intestinal lumen is slightly narrower, thickening of the wall is reduced and signs of peristalsis could be seen during fluoroscopy.

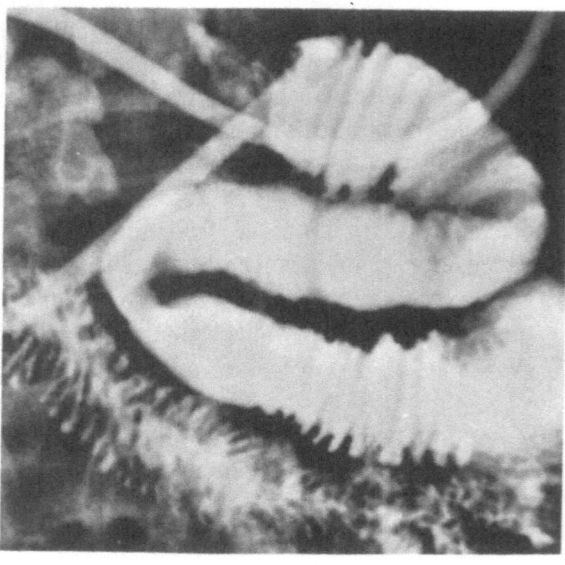

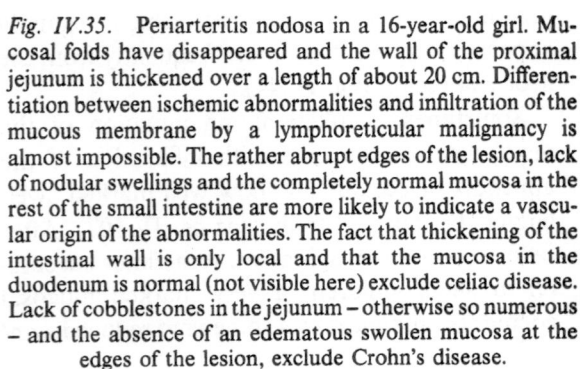

Fig. IV.35. Periarteritis nodosa in a 16-year-old girl. Mucosal folds have disappeared and the wall of the proximal jejunum is thickened over a length of about 20 cm. Differentiation between ischemic abnormalities and infiltration of the mucous membrane by a lymphoreticular malignancy is almost impossible. The rather abrupt edges of the lesion, lack of nodular swellings and the completely normal mucosa in the rest of the small intestine are more likely to indicate a vascular origin of the abnormalities. The fact that thickening of the intestinal wall is only local and that the mucosa in the duodenum is normal (not visible here) exclude celiac disease. Lack of cobblestones in the jejunum – otherwise so numerous – and the absence of an edematous swollen mucosa at the edges of the lesion, exclude Crohn's disease.

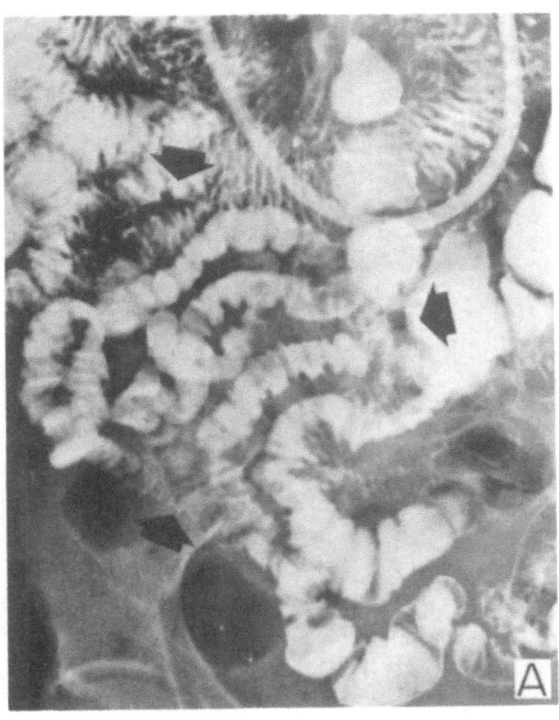

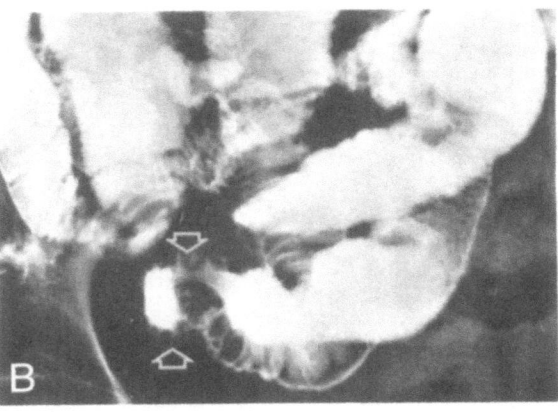

Fig. IV.36B. Stenotic area in the intestine due to fibrosis in radiation enteritis.

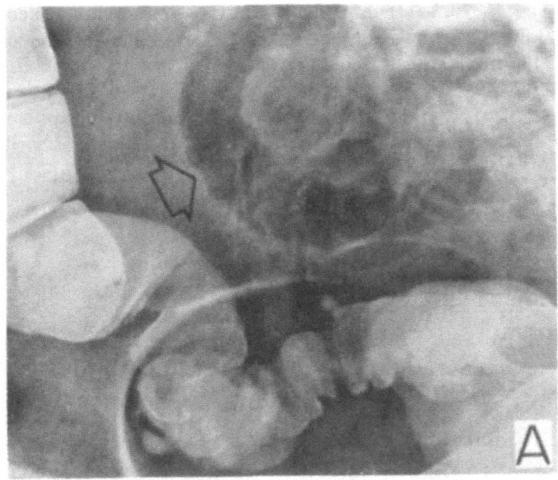

Fig. IV.36A. A tube-like air-filled small intestinal loop was noted on radiogram taken during a colon examination from elsewhere (below). On enteroclysis examination (above) the proximal ileum appeared affected by radiation enteritis. The calibre is decreased and the intestinal wall is thickened. There is a loss of mucosal folds with thickening of those remaining.

sit can persist for up to day (fig. IV.45). Obvious mucosal swelling is in a number of cases associated with the regularly observed spasms resulting from vasculitis, radiation enteritis and crossing bands (figs. IV.46 and IV.47).

1.4. Constriction with irregularly defined wall
Fundamentally, narrowed segments with irregular border can be caused by tumors, inflammatory processes or vascular abnormalities including the various forms of vasculitis and spasm.

1.4.1. Tumors are the wildest in appearance and as a result of necrosis can show local widening in a constricted segment and are often surrounded by a considerable space occupying mass (figs. IV.48WXYZ). The wild mucosal appearances found in the duodenum where it crosses the aorta can very deceptively resemble a tumor. Absence of a surrounding tumor infiltrate betrays its illusory nature (fig. III.8). An exception to this general picture is formed by malignant lymphomas growing in the superficial layers of the mucosa, which do not give rise to stenoses or only in

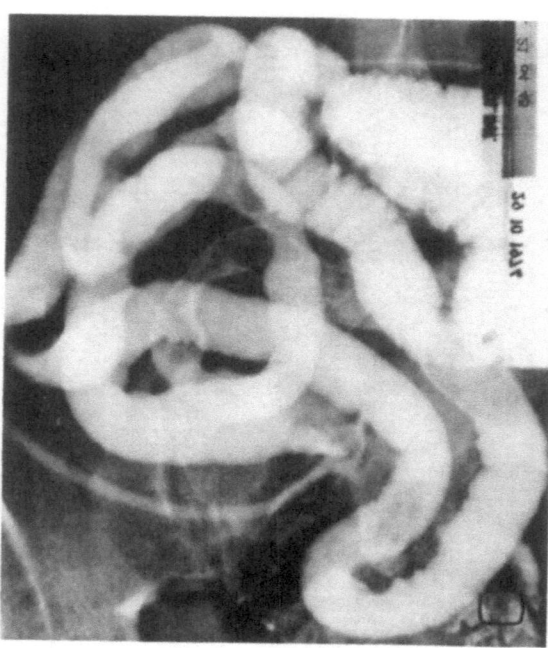

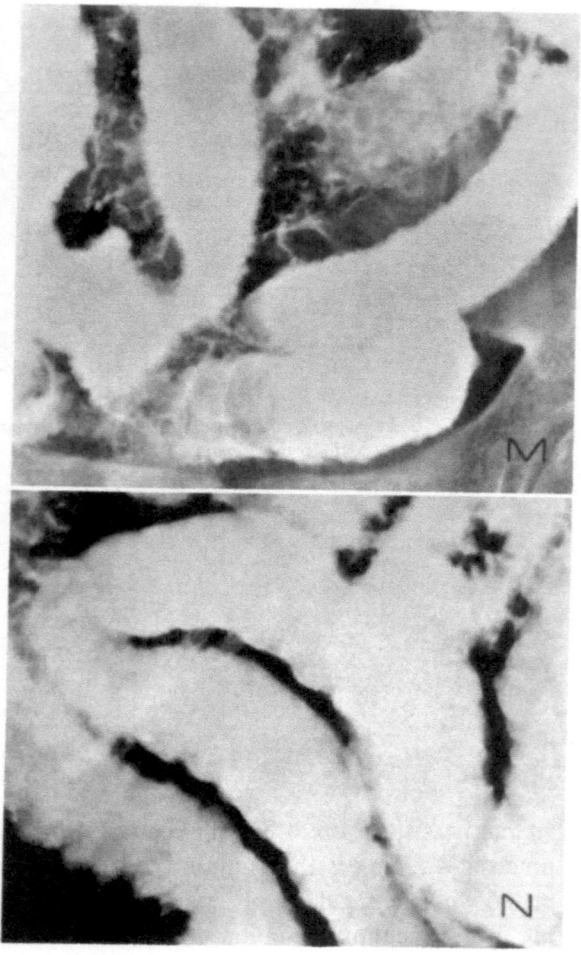

Fig. IV.37. (M) Superficial, more or less merging ulcerations in Crohn's disease, slightly resembling the mucosal abnormalities in the colon in a case of ulcerative colitis. There are only a few cobblestones, no skip lesions and no healthy segments.(N) One year later the ulcerations have disappeared and the intestinal wall is more or less smooth with no visible mucosal relief. (O) After two years.

a later stadium and are typified by thick, flat, stiff mucosal folds that can easily smooth out, in particular in the ileum. With the bowel moderately filled they form only a gross longitudinal folding (figs. IV.49 and IV.109) that clearly differs from the subtle longitudinal folds found in a 'burned-out' Crohn's disease with a supple, fairly thin intestinal wall (figs. IV.50 and III.21B). Tumors can occur throughout the small intestine with a slight preference for the distal ileum and proximal jejunum. The length of the affected segment varies between 3-13 cm with an average of 5 to 6 cm.

1.4.2. *Inflammatory* processes can produce constriction of the intestinal calibre and here the most important is Crohn's disease. These constrictions can have a length from circa 1 to 10-15 cm, are often multiple and are partly the result of powerful spasm of the intestinal wall muscle that has become hypertrophic. Their borders may be slightly or more grossly irregular from more or less superficial ulceration sites or roughly uneven (cushion-like) from the cobblestone appearance of the swollen mucosa (fig. IV.51). A recent recurrence shows intact mucosal folds which are, however, markedly thickened (fig. IV.44). Where the mucosa has been replaced by the growth of fibrous tissue the outline may be fairly smooth (fig. IV.52).

The often quite abrupt transition from so-called 'skip lesions' to apparently normal mucosal pattern is remarkable. Short skip lesions in Crohn's disease (fig. IV.53) cannot be distinguished from similar non-specific ulcerations (fig. IV.54) and the scala of abnormalities resulting from tuberculous infections identical with that of Crohn's disease (fig. IV.55).

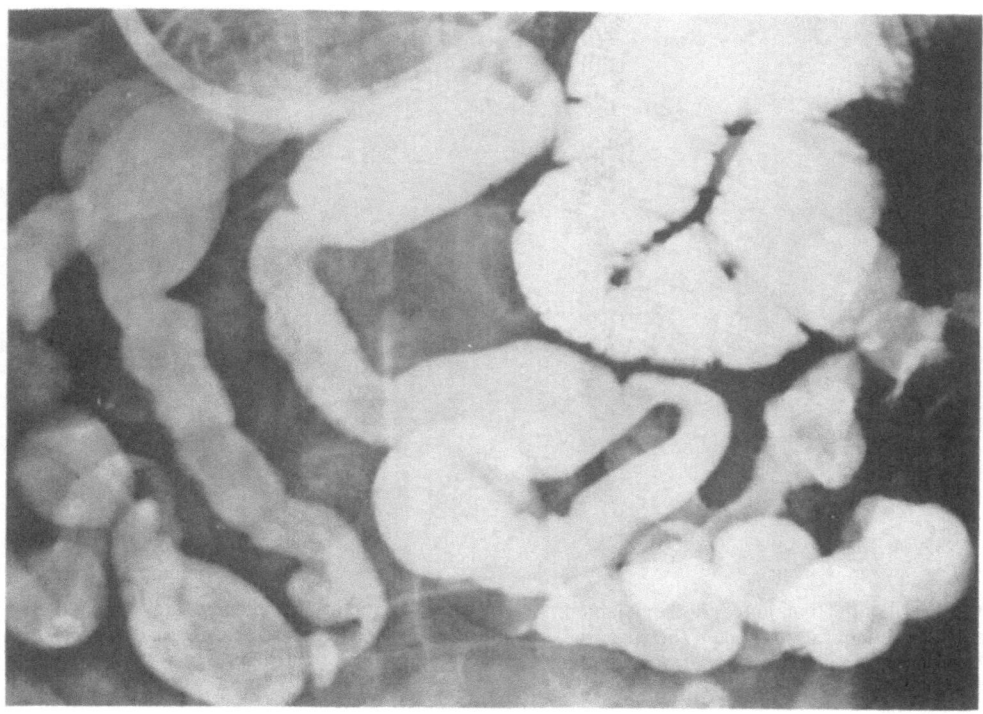

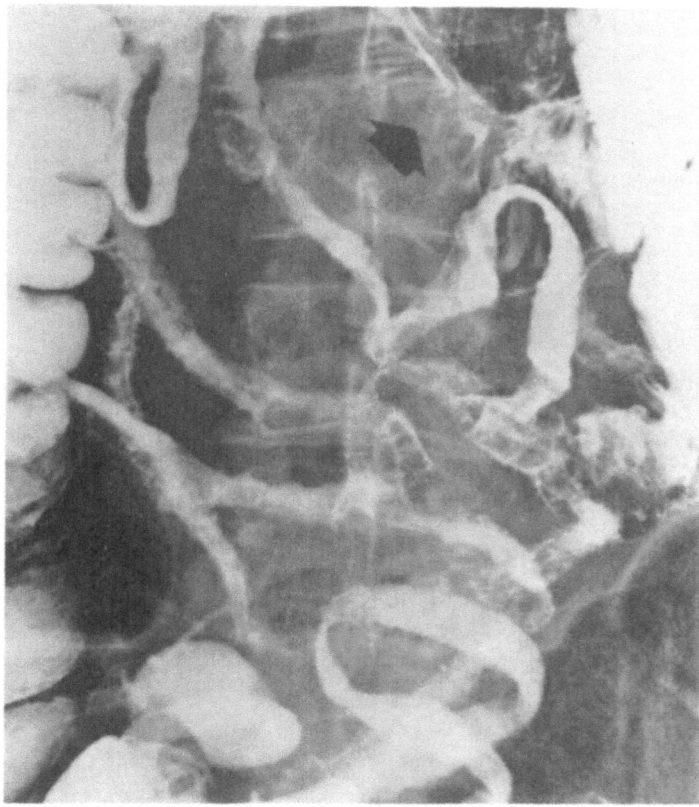

Fig. IV.38. Extensive ischemic abnormalities, predominantly in the ileum, after bone marrow transplantation: the so-called 'graft versus host' disease. There are multiple stenoses and longitudinal ulcers with pseudo diverticula-like contractures (arrows). The abnormalities do not differ so much from those seen in fig. IV.33. However, no abnormalities were revealed on angiography, thus indicating that the vascular occlusions were predominantly peripheral.

84

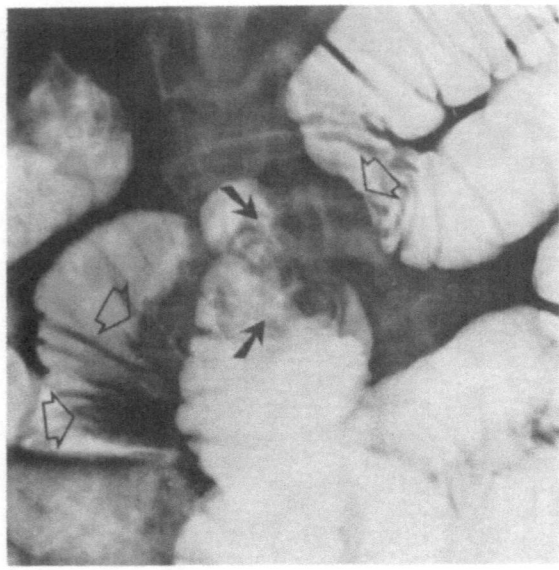

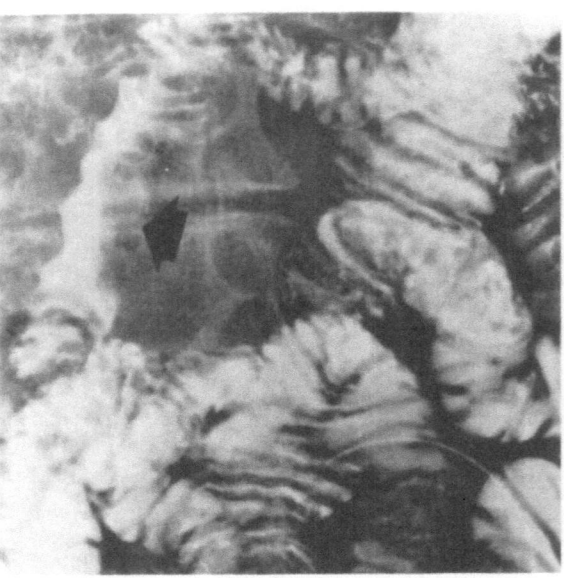

Fig. IV.39. Stenosis, about 3 cm long, in the jejunum caused by metastasis of a tumor in the cecum (between the solid arrows). At the stenosis the tumor has invaded the mesentery (open arrows).

Fig. IV.40. A solitary lymphosarcoma is encountered less frequently. It presented here as an extended stenosis in the jejunum.

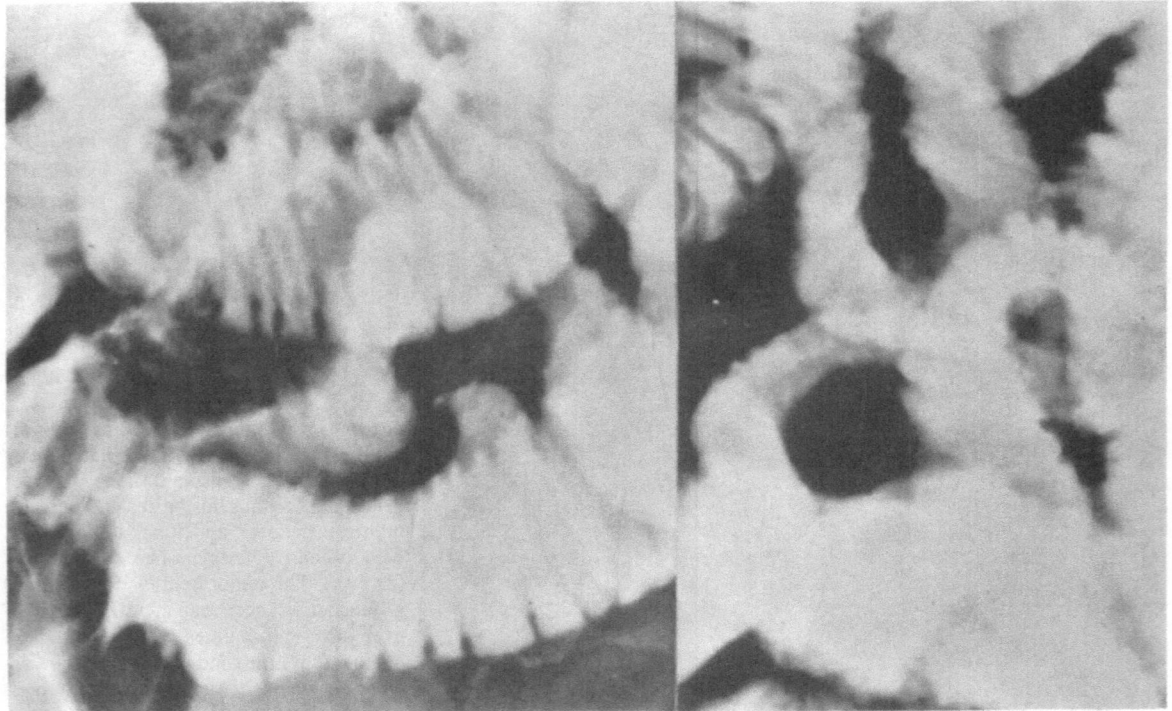

Fig. IV.41. Innumerable plaques with contracture and loss of mucosal relief throughout the entire digestive tract. These abnormalities could be attributed to metastasis of linitis plastica.

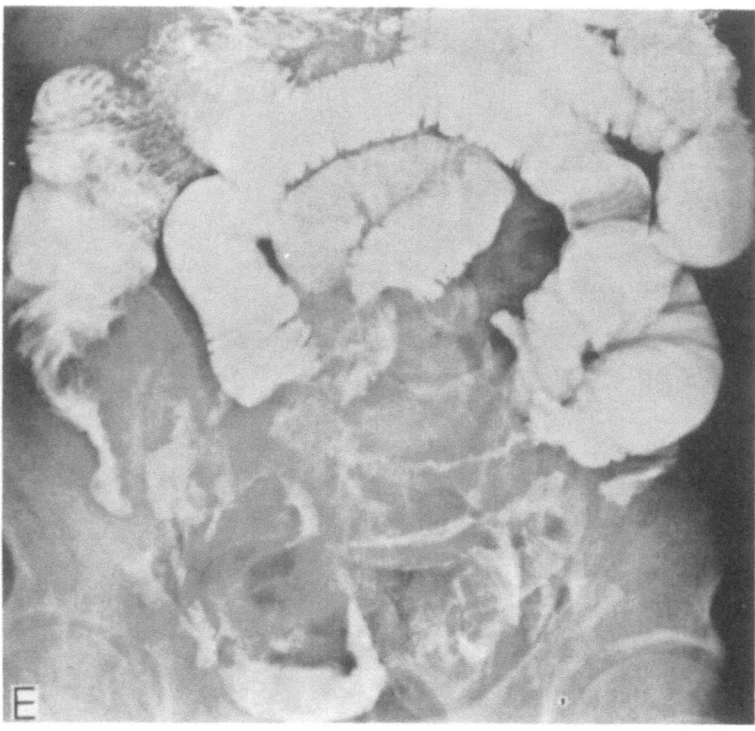

Fig. IV.42. Hodgkin's disease with pronounced involvement of the mesentery leading to erratic stenoses of the intestinal loops in the middle of large 'empty' spaces in the lower abdomen.

1.4.3. *Vascular* causes of limited constrictions are best represented by hematomata of the intestinal wall (fig. IV.56B). When intramural accumulations of gas are visible, then the central lumen filled with contrast fluid has become so narrow and its wall so irregular, that no suggestion of a clearly definable border remains (fig. IV.56A). This appearance of gas, associated with a fatal outcome, must be expressly distinguished from that of intestinal pneumatosis in which the mucosal pattern and wall thickness are normal.

1.5. Constrictions without significant mucosal changes

These are mainly based on local adhesions which for no obvious reason give rise to hypermotility and narrowing of the ileum. The bowel often shows multiple pointed projections marking the sites of local adhesions (fig. IV.57). Provided the vascularisation remains normal, further mucosal abnormalities are absent. Contact adhesions are by far most common in the lower abdomen and are but seldom seen in the upper. The affected segment can vary in length from 10 or 20 cm to as much as 2 or 3 metres (fig. IV.58).

1.6. Crossing bands, spasm and fake patterns

These occupy a place apart in the study of stenotic appearances. In these cases the picture consists of short, apparently very narrow segments where the concomitant transit delay of these appearances is scarcely present and certainly not if prestenotic dilatation is absent. A crossing band may present as a markedly asymmetric indentation (fig. IV.59) or as a narrow track impression crossing the bowel more or less at right-angles (fig. IV.60) and often passing over a number of loops (fig. III.17B). A similar picture but with a broader impression is seen in fake patterns where the bowel is crossed by vessels or other structures with higher tonus (fig. III.9). At the site of a kink in the intestine the double kinking in the wall of the inner bend can cause a similar impression on the lumen (fig. IV.61). This latter condition is as with spasm merely transient. Spasms present in celiac disease (fig. IV.62) and in all situations where the blood

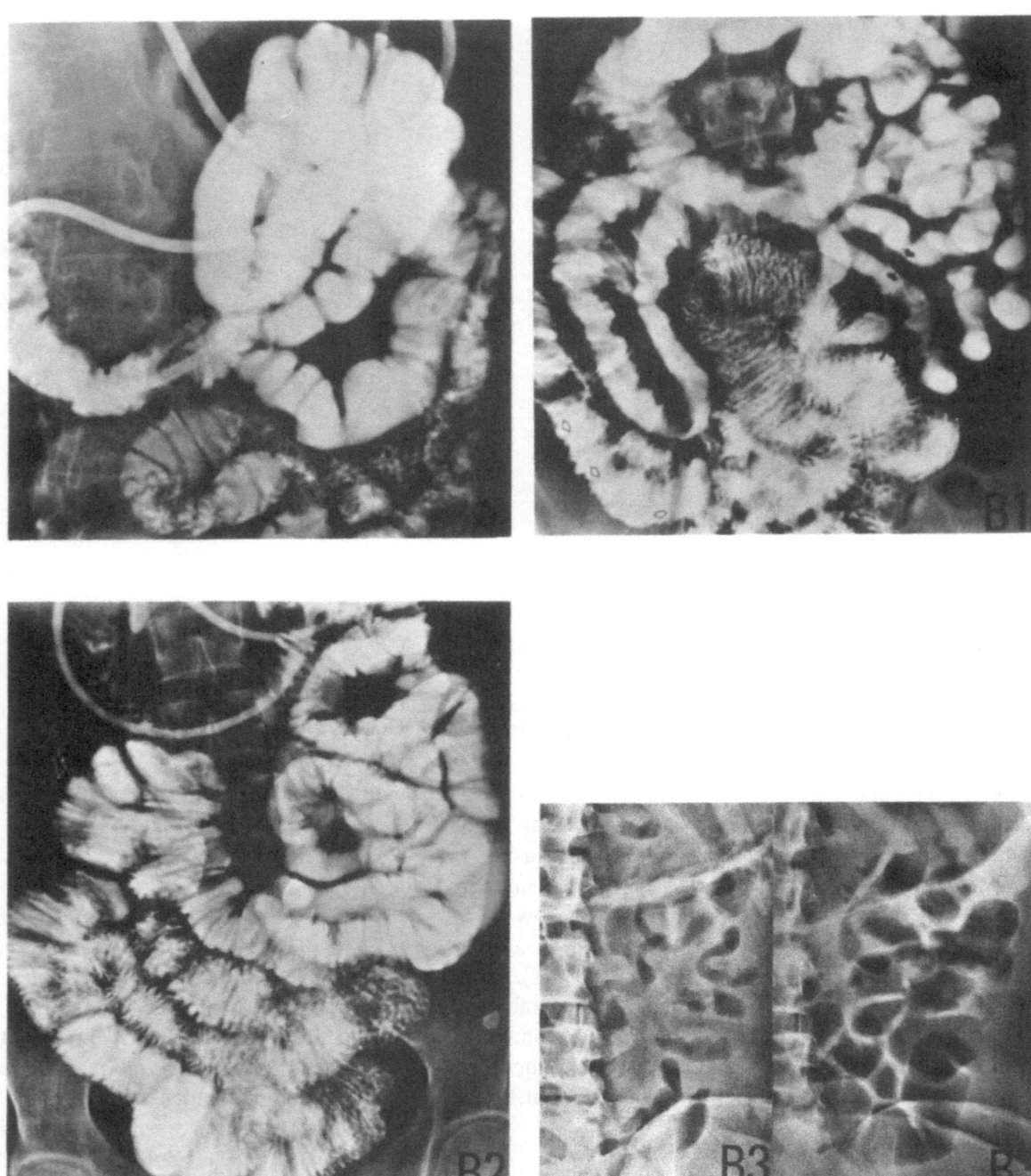

Fig. IV.43. Patient B (see fig. B1) Symptomless celiac disease (patient unaware of condition). Hypoalbuminemia present; possibly in part from a secondary infection acquired while on a camping trip. It is obvious that the walls of the jejunum are markedly thickened (solid arrows) and that the more distally situated mucosal folds are greatly broadened (open arrows). After treatment of the hypoalbuminemia, the thickness of both the intestinal wall and the mucosal folds was again normal. The pattern of an uncomplicated celiac disease remained (B2). It is interesting that the improvement could be seen on the abdominal survey film (B3). Right: after treatment. Left: intestinal gas pattern upon admission to the hospital. However, six years later the patient retorhed with a malign antlymphoma.

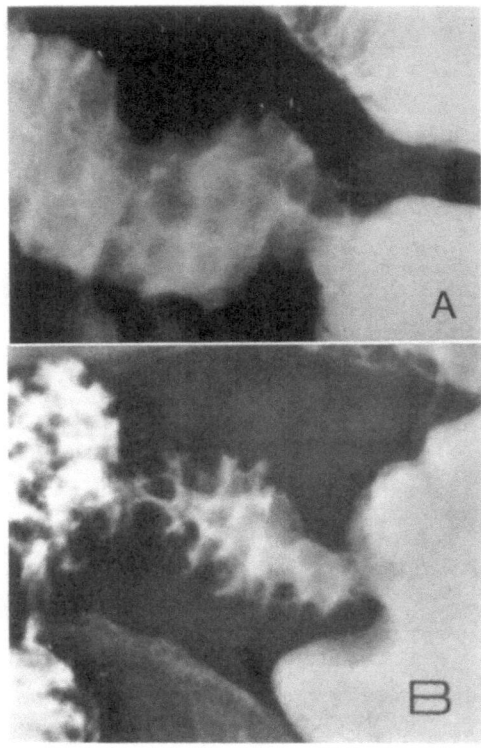

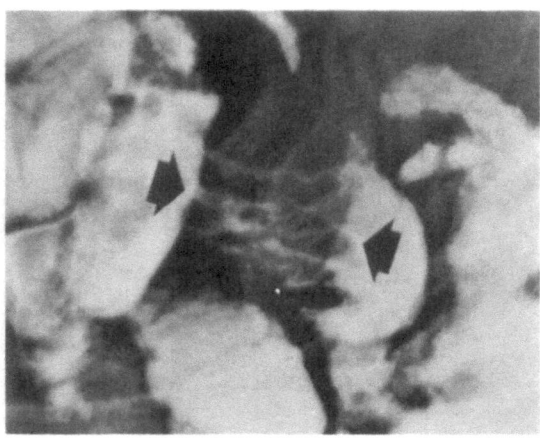

Fig. IV.46. Coblestone pattern in the distal ileum as a result of periarteritis nodosa.

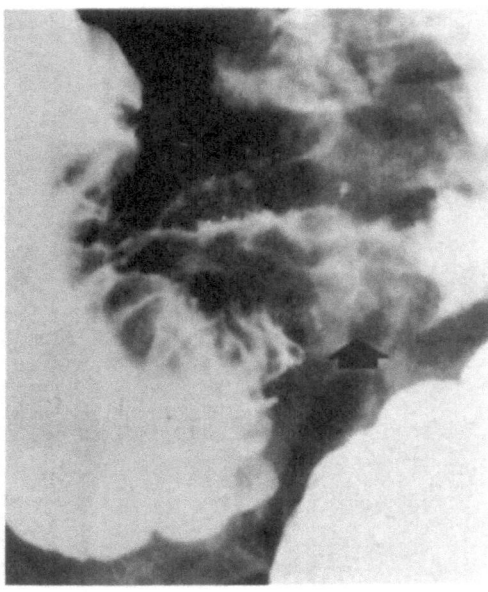

Fig. IV.44. Local edema due to a reccurence of Crohn's disease in two patients with a short bowel.

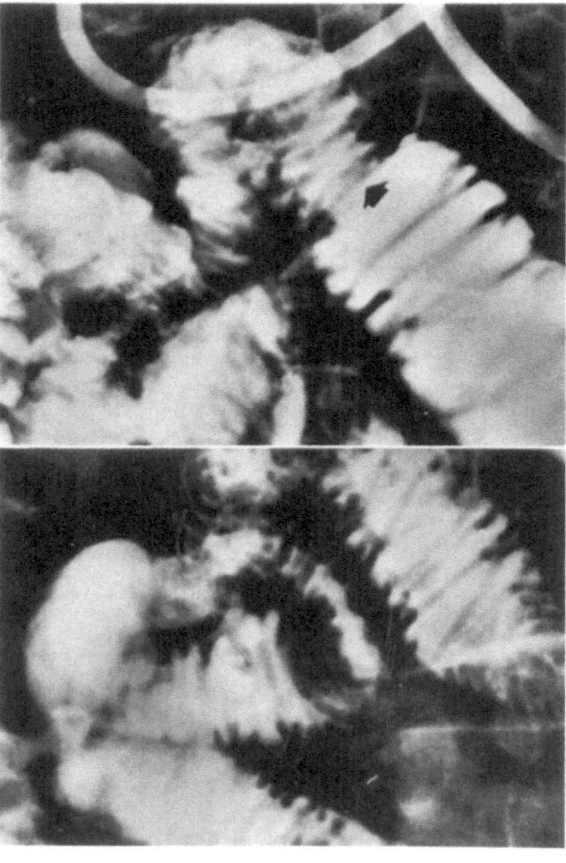

Fig. IV.45. Cobblestone relief in the distal ileum and edematous swollen Bauhin's valve after repositioning of an ileo-colic intussusception.

Fig. IV.47. Radiation enteritis with edematous mucosa. Between the highly swollen mucosal folds are narrow spaces filled with barium that resemble a coarsely toothed saw. The transition to the normal intestinal segments is very abrupt (arrow).

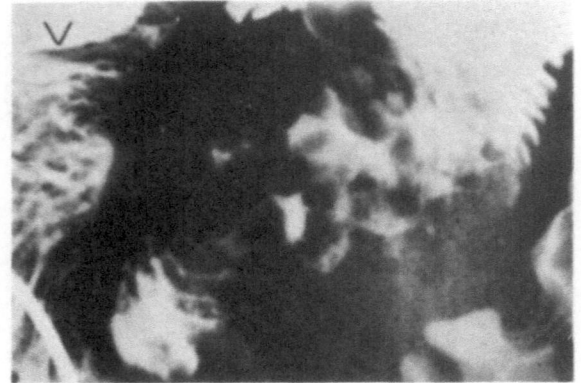

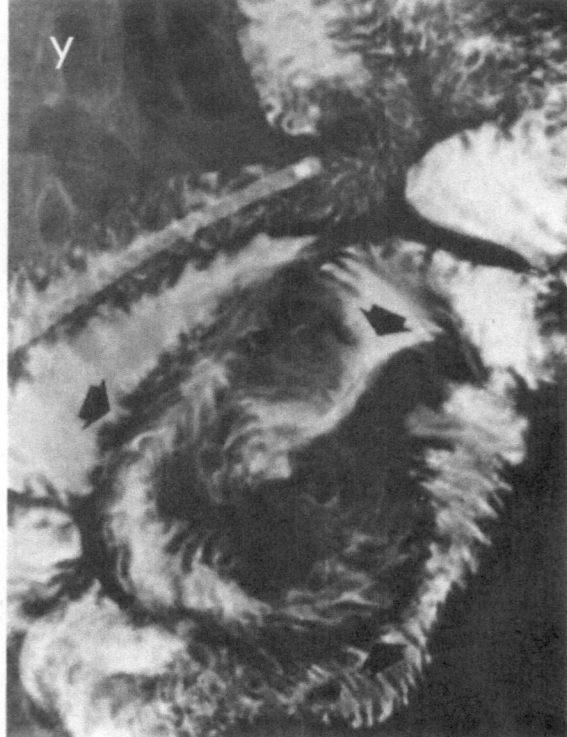

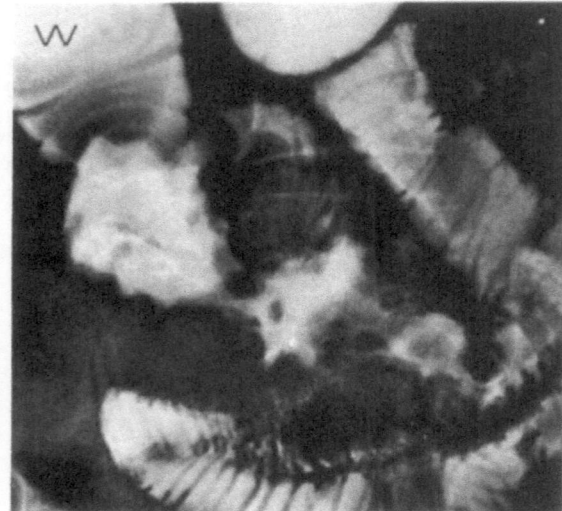

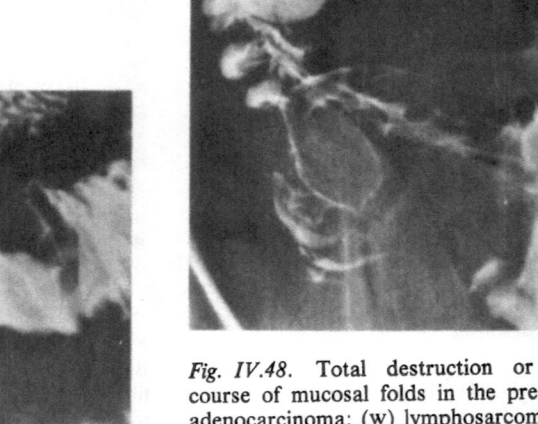

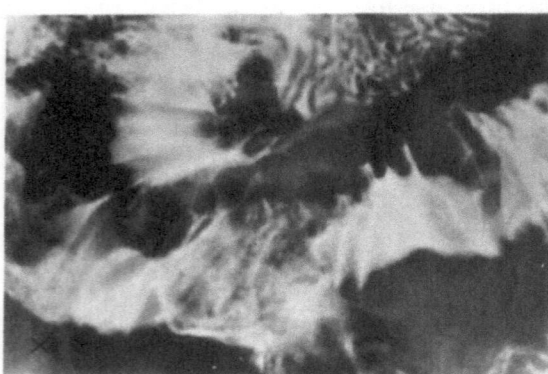

Fig. IV.48. Total destruction or completely irregular course of mucosal folds in the presence of a tumor: (v) adenocarcinoma; (w) lymphosarcoma; (x) malignant lymphoma; (y) leiomyosarcoma; (z) reticulum cell sarcoma.

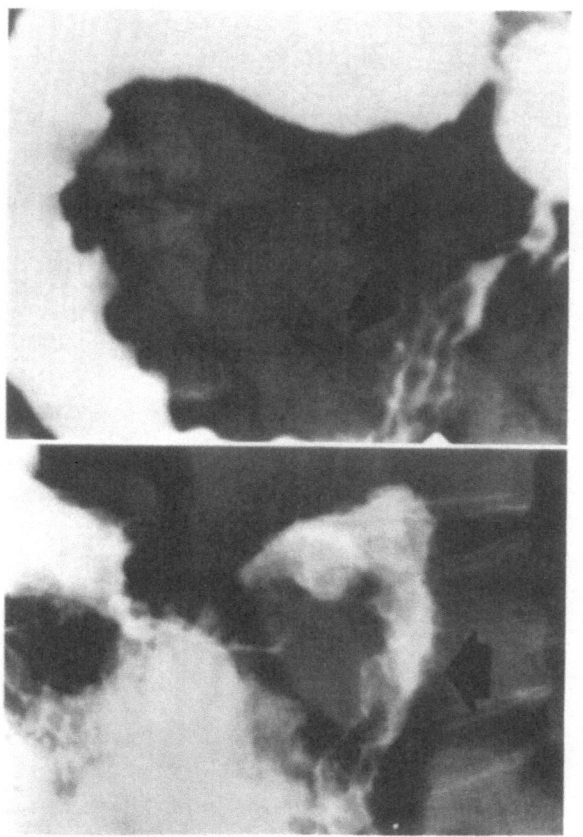

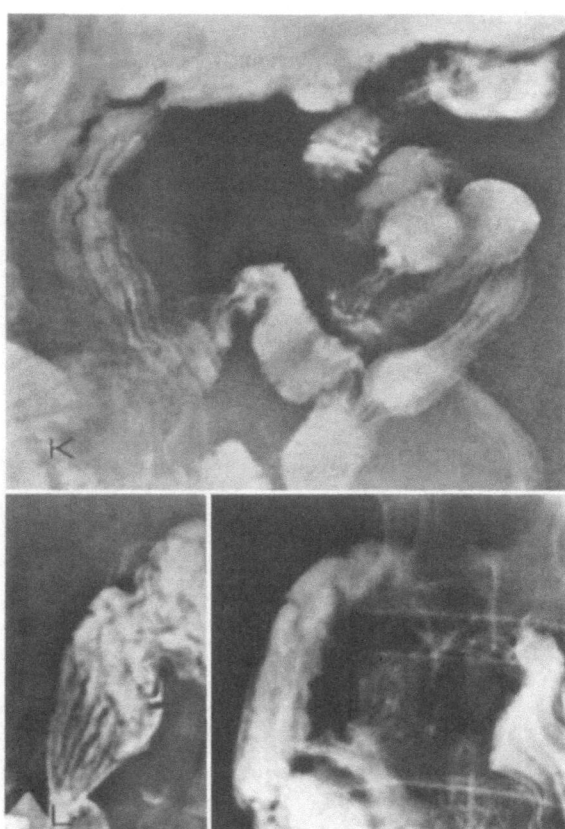

Fig. IV.49. Two patients with cobblestones in the duodenum due to lymphosarcoma.

Fig. IV.50. Examples of atrophied mucosa after Crohn's disease with longitudinal folds when the intestine is inadequately filled: the so-called 'bike tire' phenomenon; (ĸ) proximal jejunum, (ʟ) duodenum.

flow to a short segment suffers hindrance, as with crossing bands (fig. IV.63) and extensive adhesions.

Local hypermotility with reduced intestinal calibre is also seen in the immediate vicinity of carcinoid lesions (fig. IV.64), probably the result of their local adrenaline production. If additionally in this area a compression effect on the lumen, the 'kinking sign' or an indentation from a fibrous band is visible, the diagnosis is highly improbable (fig. IV.65). It is also possible that in collagen diseases a local hypermotility with reduced intestinal calibre can occur, the degree of vasculitis should be considered as not universally uniform (fig. IV.66).

Finally, the slight but constantly present constriction of a suture line, only visualised with a sufficiently rapid flow of contrast medium, can give the impression of a stenosis (fig. IV.4). There is here no suggestion of stenosis under normal conditions and functionally no difference from a normal contraction.

2. Narrowing of the small intestine in its entire length

When the whole small intestine has chronically lapsed into disuse, for example after one or two years parenteral feeding, its calibre gradually reduces but returns to normal when eating is recommenced. Further, reduction in calibre throughout the entire length of the small intestine is seen only in combination with *marked hypermotility* as found in massive adhesions, carcinoid and in particular in nearly all collagen diseases.

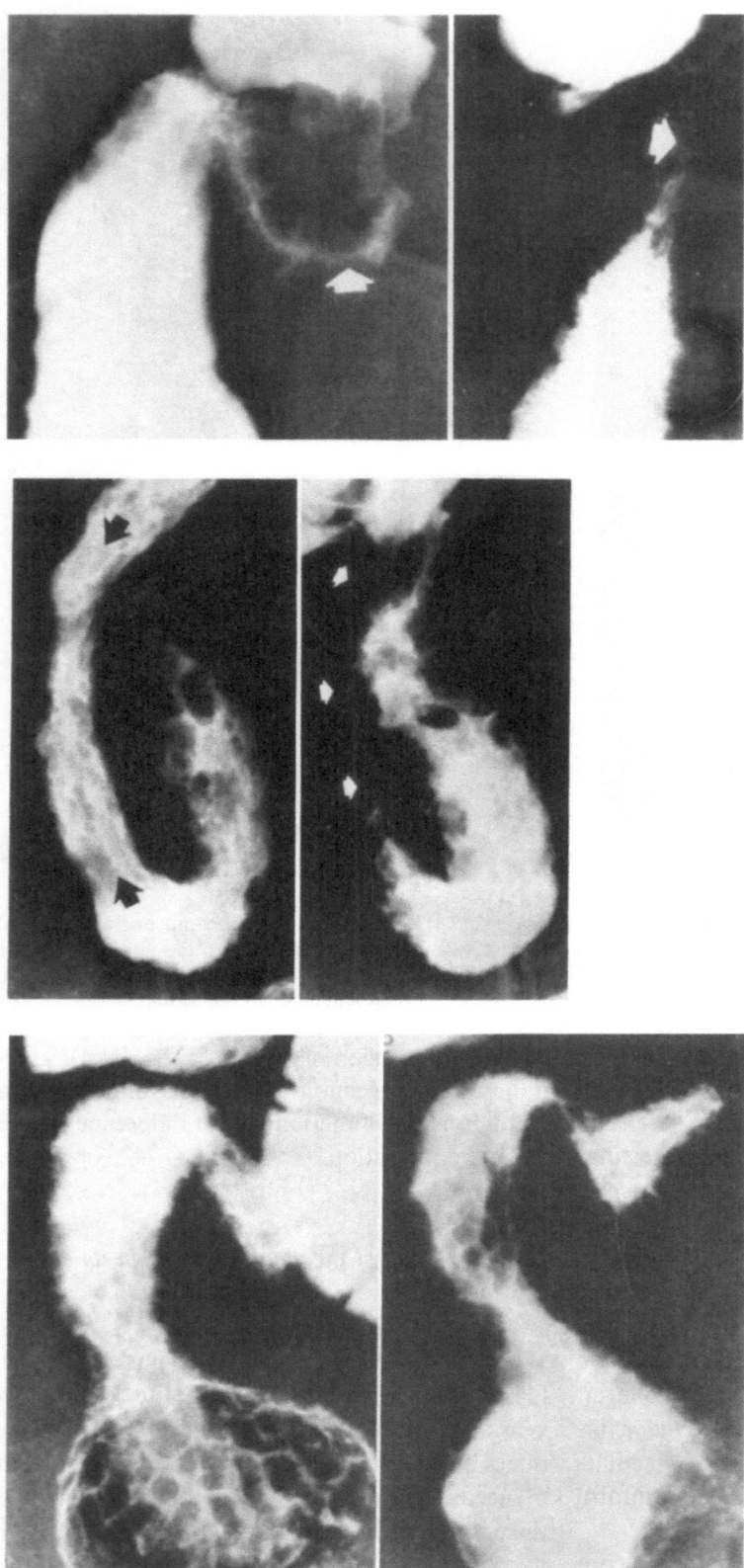

Fig. IV.51. Several examples of the so-called string sign in Crohn's disease caused by spasms due to a marked hypertrophy of the muscular layers. There is no indication of either a stenosis or a prestenotic dilatation. Superficial ulcerations (upper), coarse ulcerative surface (middle) and cobblestones (lower).

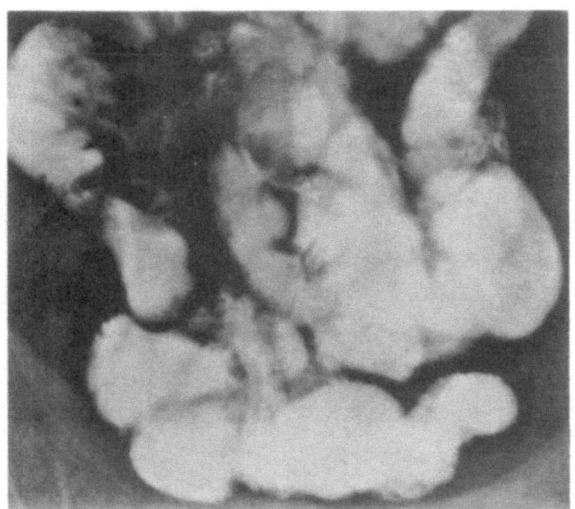

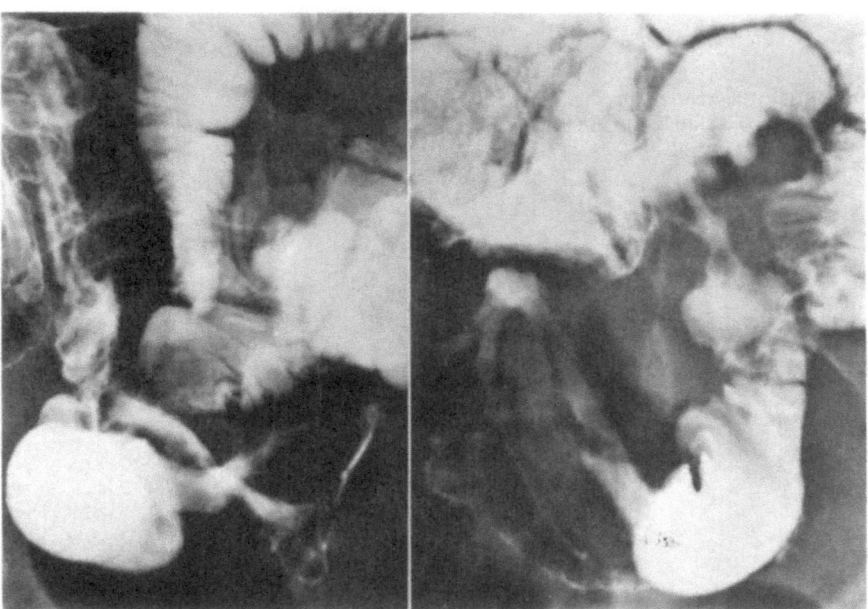

Fig. IV.52. Patient with Crohn's disease. Multiple stenoses as a result of ulcers that have healed with fibrosis. The abnormalities could be seen only on the spot films taken under compression!

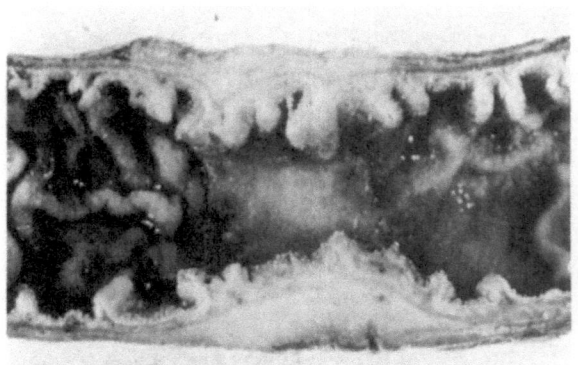

Fig. IV.53. Skip lesions in Crohn's disease; fairly normal mucosa on both sides of the lesion.

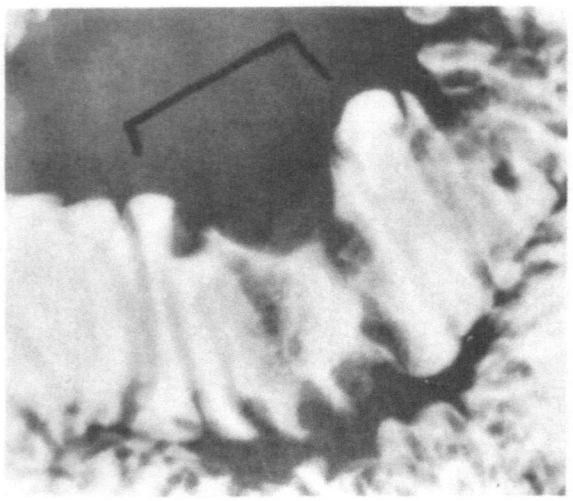

Fig. IV.54. Non-specific ulceration in the jejunum; the ulceration closely resembles a skip lesion in Crohn's disease or tumor growth.

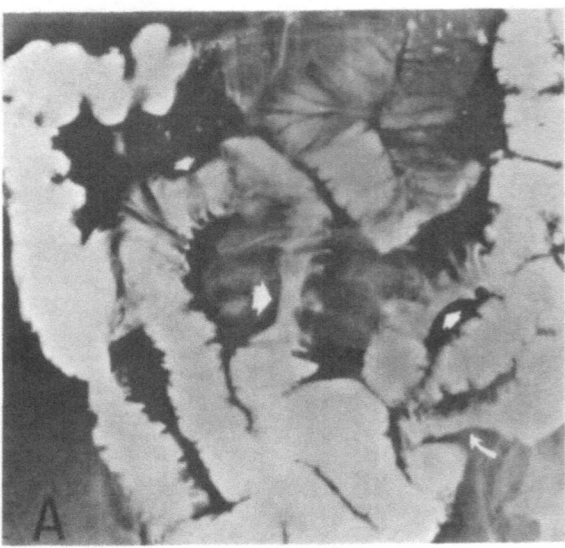

Fig. IV.55A. Shrinkage processes due to tuberculosis with pseudo-diverticula, undifferentiable from those seen in Crohn's disease. In ischemia, the abnormalities generally merge.

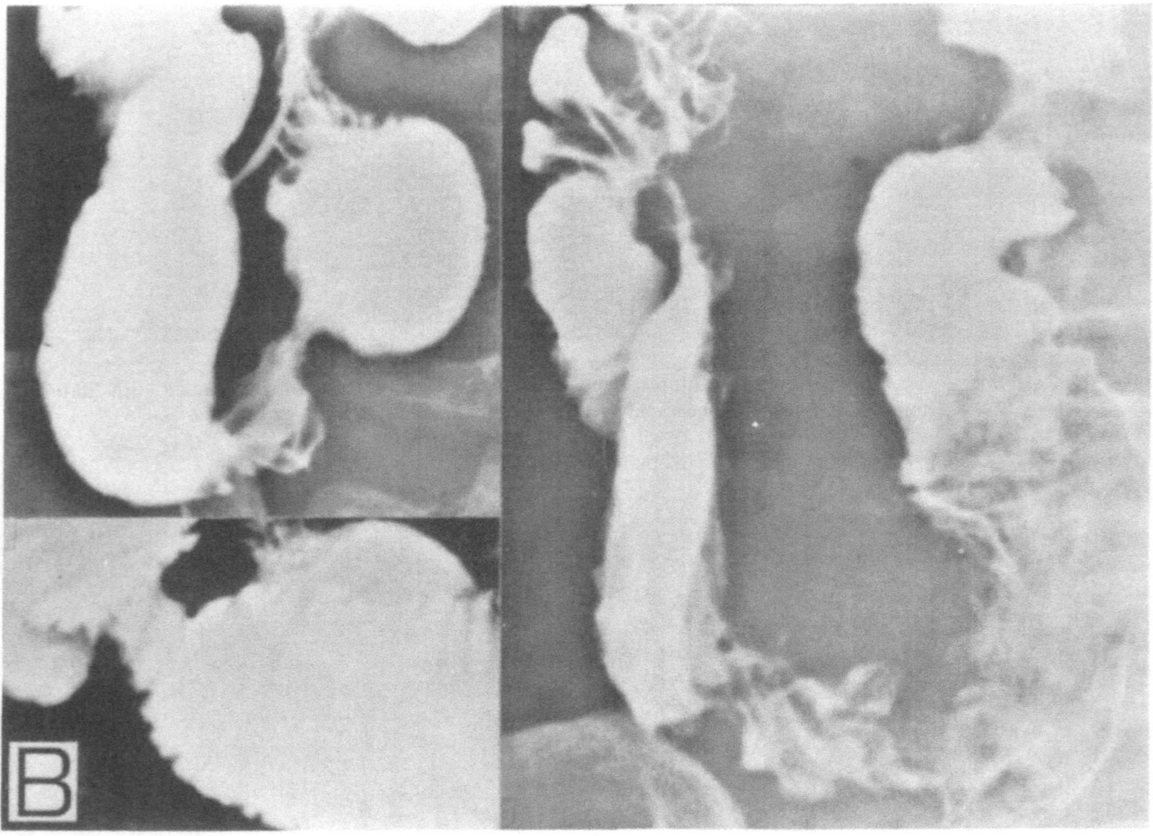

Fig. IV.55B. These X-rays, showing multiple stenoses with prestenotic dilatations, were taken after an intestinal resection, necessitated by a traffic accident. It appeared, however, that the stenoses were due not to vascular abnormalities but to tuberculosis.

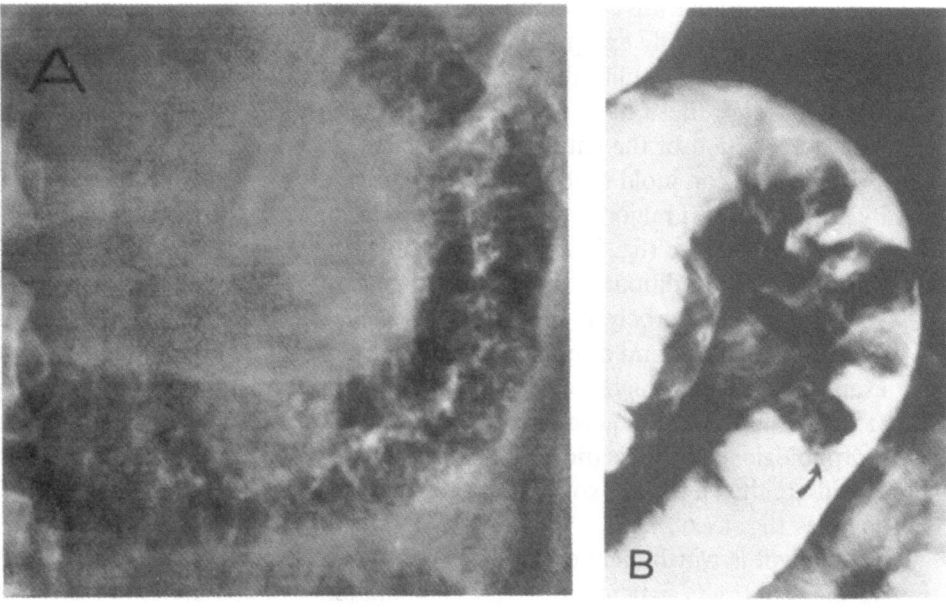

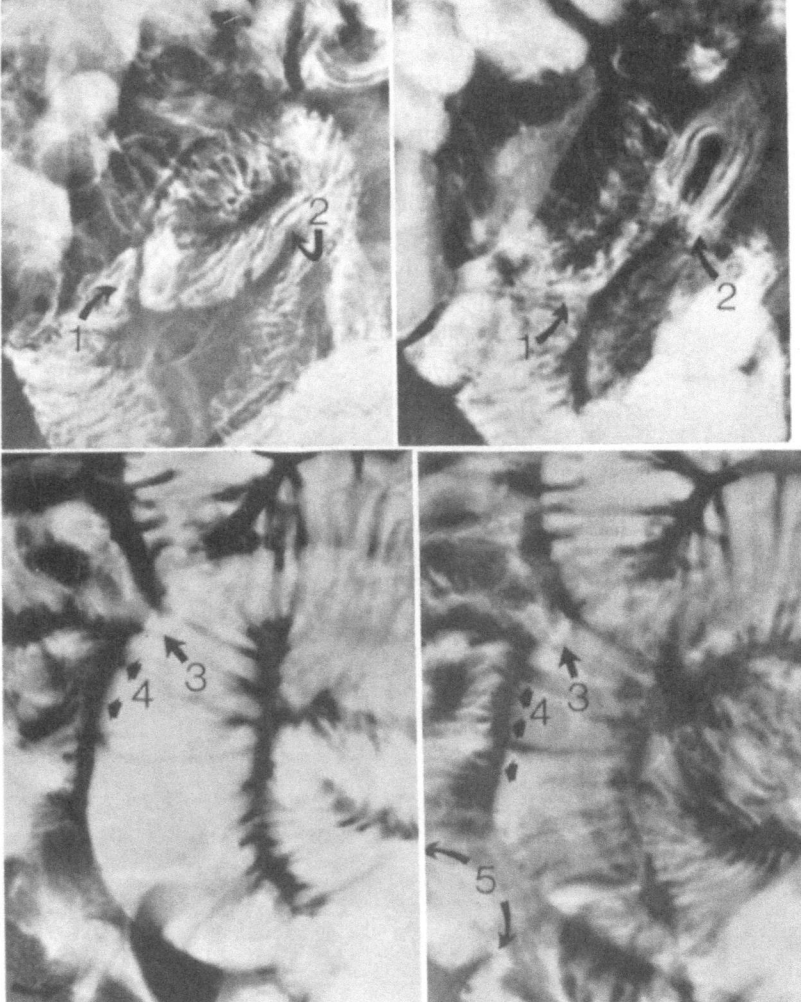

Fig. IV.56. Erratic intramural gas accumulations (A) and large pseudotumors bulging out into the intestinal lumen (B) as a result of submucosal hematomata in a patient with mesenteric thrombosis.

Fig. IV.57. Stretched mucosal folds extending along the length of the intestine (2) and local adhesion of two intestinal loops (1). Pointed bulges on elongated intestinal loops (3) due to fusion. Also visible are several indentations (5) as well as slight elongation of the somewhat thorn-like spaces between mucosal folds (4).

Since adhesions are rare in the upper abdomen and the jejunum only exceptionally influenced by the marked hypermotility that can be caused by this condition, these have practically no rôle in calibre reduction of the entire small intestine.

In practice carcinoid is comparatively rare and by far the greatest majority of cases are the result of collagen disease (fig. IV.67). Hypermotility in this group of conditions can be so marked that with orthodox enteroclysis the cecum is reached with a mere 200 ml and a supplementary phase of examination with a higher rate of administration (150-200 ml/min) is required for the purposes of morphological diagnosis (fig. II.3B). Cases of carcinoid are thus a regular source of surprising discoveries (fig. IV.68).

Finally it is worth mentioning that in case of a normal contraction percentage, an examination carried out with a too low flow rate of 50 ml/min or less, can produce a definite suggestion of calibre reduction (fig. II.20), thus *a fake pattern*.

3. *Summary of bowel constrictions*

Limited in length
  smooth walled
    ischemia plus fibrous contracture
      arteriosclerosis
      bands – volvulus – hernia
      post-operative
      micro emboli
      vasculitis
      vasoconstrictors
    inflammatory process with fibrous contracture
      Crohn's disease

      tuberculosis
      non-specific ulceration
    tumor growth
      adenocarcinoma (mainly jejunum)
      carcinoid
      lympho-reticular malignancy
      scirrhus
      metastases
    celiac disease plus infection (mainly jejunum)
  From mucosal edema
    lymph or vascular congestion
    inflammatory process after reduction of invagination
    bands
    marked spasm
    vasculitis
    Crohn's disease
    appendicular infiltrate
  Irregular wall
    tumors
    inflammatory processes
    vascular (mainly hematomata)
  No significant alteration in the mucosa
    mild degree of band formations with spasm
    local spasm associated with collagenoses
    suture line
    fake patterns.
Involving more or less the entire length of the small intestine.
  marked hypermotility
    collagen disease
    carcinoid lesions
    extensive adhesions
  infusion rate less than 50 ml/min.

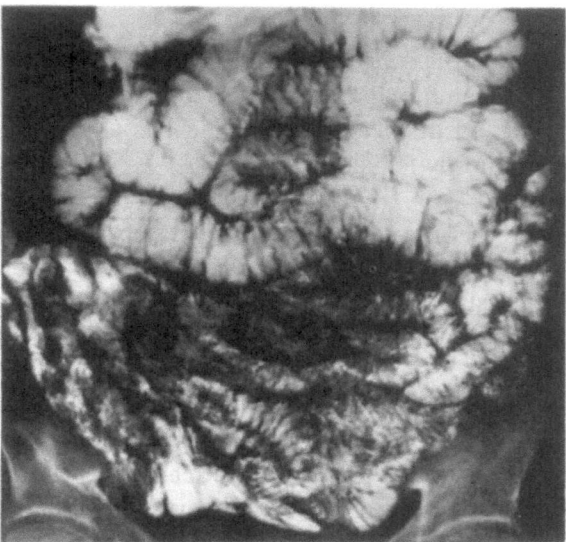

Fig. IV.58. Pronounced hypermotility of the entire ileum with some stagnation of the contrast fluid in the jejunum as a result of numerous fusions and adhesions in the distal half of the small bowel. Compression showed that all ileal loops were totally fused. The patient complained of considerable rumbling in the stomach and attacks of pain, especially when he assumed certain positions. Occasionally a subileus developed with numerous fluid levels.

4. Short or limited segment with dilated lumen

4.1. General

Local dilatations, which may be isolated or multiple, must in the majority of cases be regarded as pre-stenotic in relation to the immediately distal constriction. Since these stenoses form a serious hindrance to the flow of contrast medium, the most distally situated are as a rule not revealed. It is therefore advisable in these cases to conduct a supplementary retrograde small bowel enema examination (figs. IV.69 and II.14). Multiple stenosis with pre-stenotic dilatation are to be expected in Crohn's disease, tuberculosis, non-specific ulceration, radiation enteritis, metastases, peritoneal carcinomatosis, mesenteric fibrosis, carcinoid lesions, scleroderma and bands. In scleroderma, naturally, stenoses are not the causative factor since the dilatations result from a disturbed tonus in the bowel wall. All these conditions can also produce solitary dilatations and this is typically true of superior mesenteric artery syndrome, primary tumor, internal hernia, invagination, local

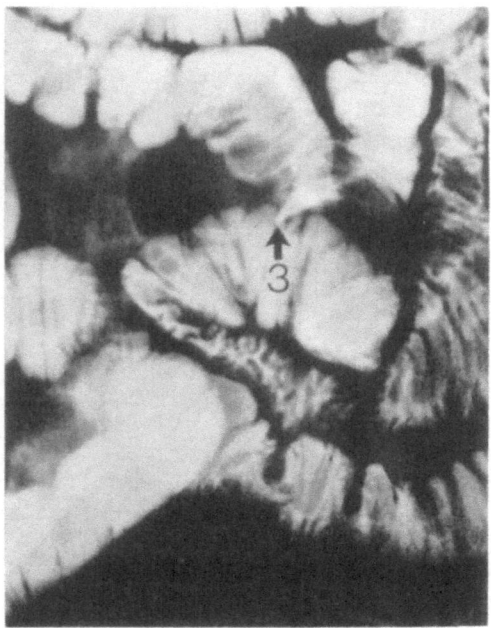

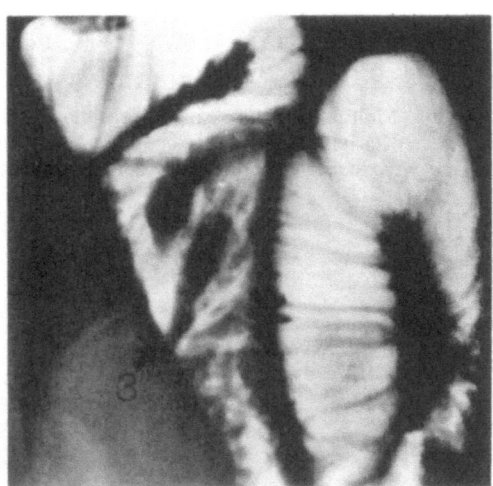

Fig. IV.59. The upper photo shows two asymmetrical constrictions with rounded edges caused by traversing ligamentous adhesions. In the case of contact adhesions (lower photo) this cleft is narrower and the edges are sharp.

ischemia, obstructing polyp or foreign body. When judging a local dilatation, it is important to study the nature of the associated distal constriction and check whether similar mucosal changes are present elsewhere in the small intestine. A number of possibilities in the differential diagnosis should be considered in accordance with these observations.

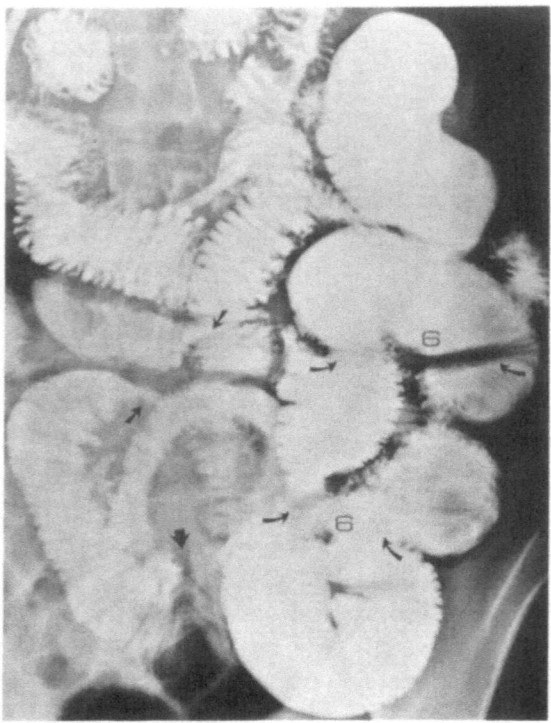

Fig. IV.60. Multiple bands crossing several intestinal loops in a patient who had never undergone abdominal surgery. The bands were livid blue and possibly congenital in origin.

4.2. *Mucosal changes absent*

4.2.1. *Superior mesenteric artery syndrome:* Duodenum only affected due to compression of aorta on duodenum. The patient is always thin and mostly female.

4.2.2. *Crossing band:* Where the obstruction is but slight, mucosal abnormalities from venous congestion can be completely absent and the prestenotic dilatation show a varying degree of severity.

4.2.3. *Extraluminal carcinoid lesions:* The mucosal folds are unaffected but can none the less show a stretched or bizarre course due to underlying fibrous contracture in the bowel wall. Obstruction is usually but slight and hypermotility is present.

4.2.4. *Mesenteric fibrosis or retractile mesenteritis:* Frequently multiple dilatations from local fibrous contracture in the bowel wall and above all in the mesentery, without abnormality in the mucosal folds themselves. As a result of operative resections the intestine is as a rule short and despite a central void, lies fairly well central in the abdomen thanks to contracture of the mesentery (fig. IV.5).

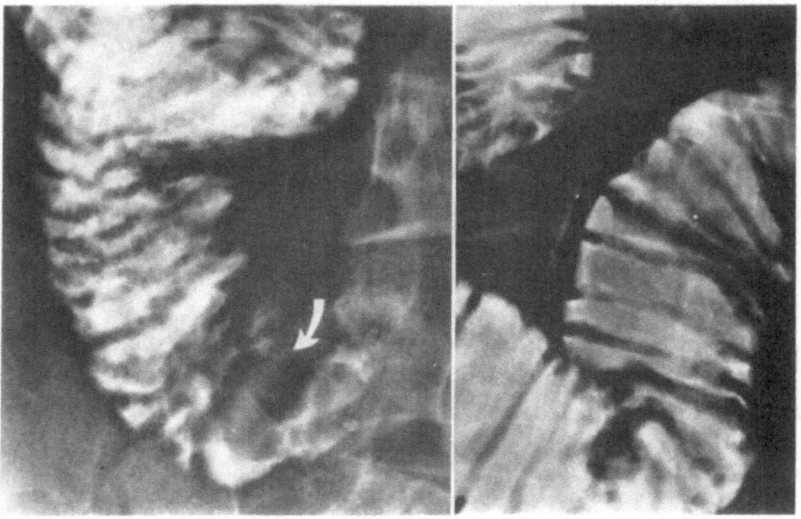

Fig. IV.61. Impression on a jejunal loop, here caused by a sharp curve in this loop.

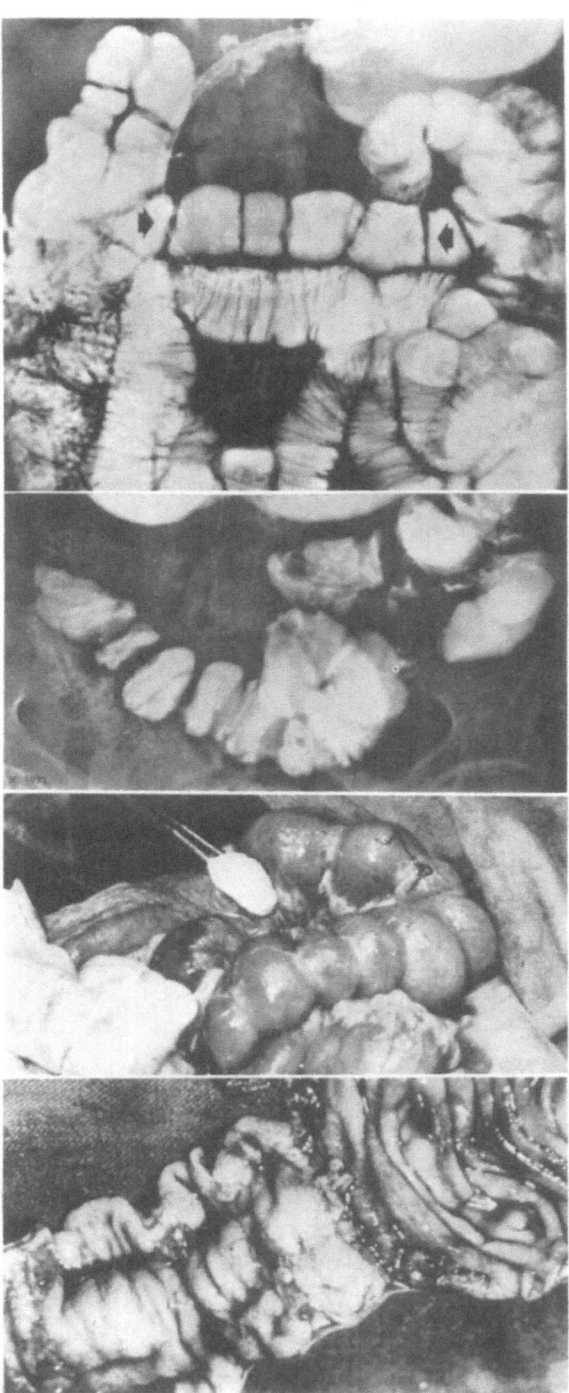

Fig. IV.62. Colon-like haustration in the jejunum. The abnormalities resemble ischemic abnormalities. During surgery they appeared to be caused by spasms and cicatrization at the site of circular ulcerations. These stenotic ulcerations in this patient possibly resulted from atrophy of the vascular system. On the surgical photographs, the colonization pattern is clearly visible and also in the open intestine, the atrophied mucosal relief in the jejunum.

4.2.5. Adhesions: In contrast to bands the majority of adhesions cause no obstruction but passive dilatations caused by the contraction of neighbouring adherent loops. Characteristic is a considerable diameter of empty bowel which on cross-section has been pulled flat (fig. IV.70AB).

4.2.6. Scleroderma: This can often present with asymmetric sac-like dilatations resulting from reduced tonus in the intestinal wall and in no sense related to distally situated obstructions (fig. IV.71).

4.2.7. Internal hernias: Internal hernia is characterised by the presence of a hernia orifice through which a herniated loop can enter and return (fig. IV.19). At the level of this more or less narrow orifice the involved loop can show a concentric fold pattern resulting from tapering of the bowel calibre. Pre-stenotic dilatation is generally but slight. Vascularisation of the loops contained in the hernial sac may be so disturbed that motility ceases and constantly present fluid levels under accumulations of gas are seen.

4.3. Thickening of mucosal folds

4.3.1. Crohn's disease: After ileocecal resection marked edema frequently appears in the region of the suture as a result of recurrence. Since the ability to dilate is in this suture area moreover limited, a slight prestenotic dilatation occurs. Inflammatory edema of such intensity that it gives rise to pre-stonic dilatation is further unknown except in the distal ileum in the presence of an adjacent appendicular infiltrate.

4.3.2. After bowel resection: Although it is rare, disturbed vascularisation can lead to a postresection edema of such intensity that transient ileus or subileus results.

4.3.3. Disturbance of circulation: A vascular accident in combination with local edema and clinical ileus or subileus, is certainly the most frequent cause of a generally transient local dilatation of a loop. There is no suggestion of stenosis. The edema can be seen both in the dilated and more distal segment. Moreover the intestinal wall is obviously thickened, motility in this area has ceased and in erect posture local fluid levels are

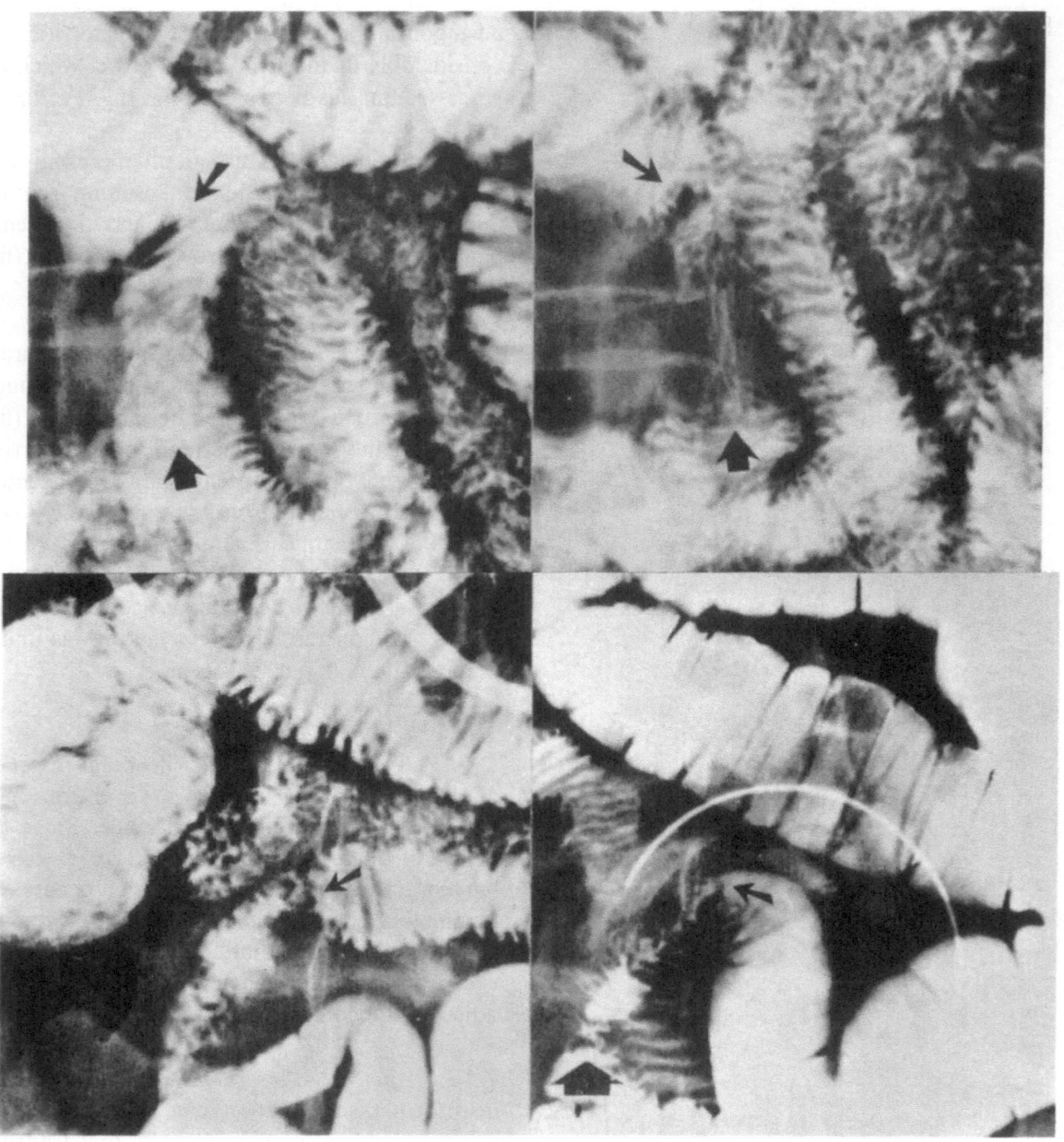

Fig. IV.63. Local hypermotility in two patients, in a segment several centimetres long, caused by a band crossing the intestinal wall (thin arrow).

seen. The majority of vascular accidents heal spontaneously and, if venous in origin, without residual lesion. In cases of ischemia a local loss of mucosal pattern sometimes persists (fig. IV.34).

4.3.4. Crossing bands etc.: Where compression by crossing bands or a stenosis of an hernial orifice is severe, obviously thickened folds can arise, resulting from disturbed vascularisation which at first is venous but later also arterial. If a clinical policy of 'wait-and-see' is adopted it is of importance to study the thickness of the mucosal folds and bowel wall on the consecutive abdominal exposures (with *vertical* beam) with the

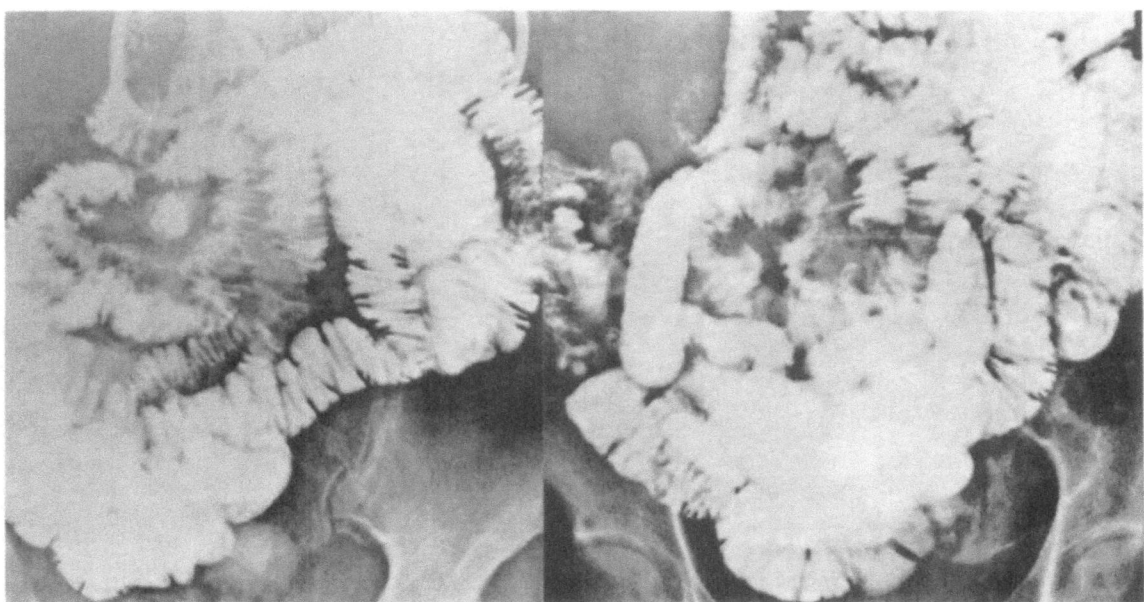

Fig. IV.64. Local hypermotility in a patient with carcinoids and metastases in the liver. The translucent spaces in the middle of the convolution of intestinal loops are probably caused by a combination of mesenteric contracture and the carcinoid foci themselves.

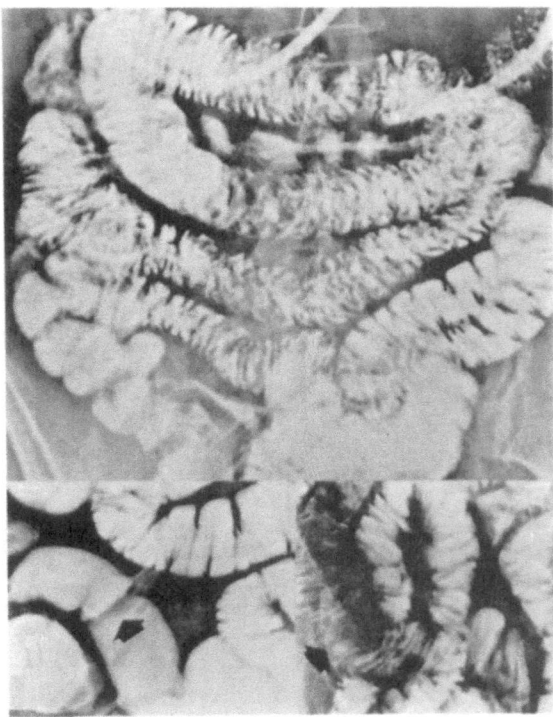

Fig. IV.65. Patient with hypermotility of the small bowel. Moreover, a very subtle lesion in the distal ileum consisting of an intramural defect in the intestinal wall during the empty phase of the examination (lower right) and a constriction when the intestine was well filled (lower left). At operation the suspected carcinoid was found.

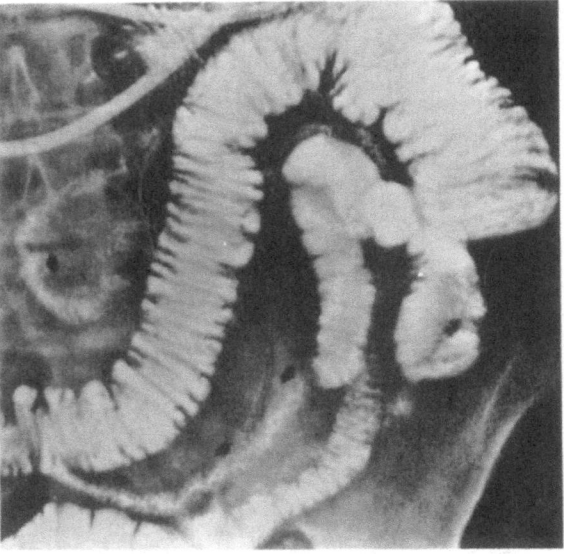

Fig. IV.66. Spasms of an entire intestinal segment are rare in the jejunum. No abnormalities of the mucosa or intestinal wall could be seen in this patient. Etiology unknown, suspected collagen disease.

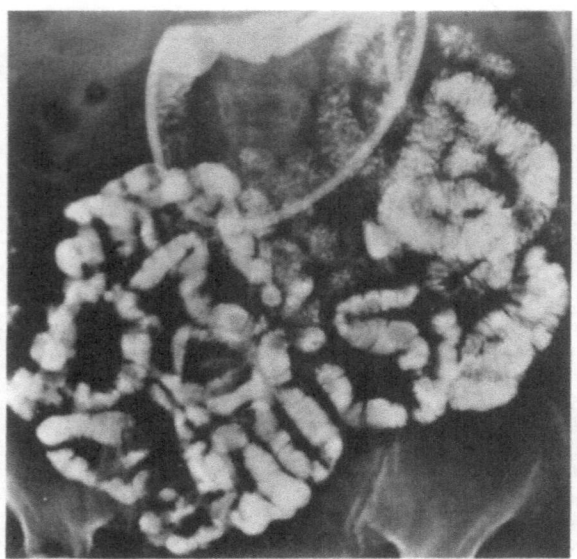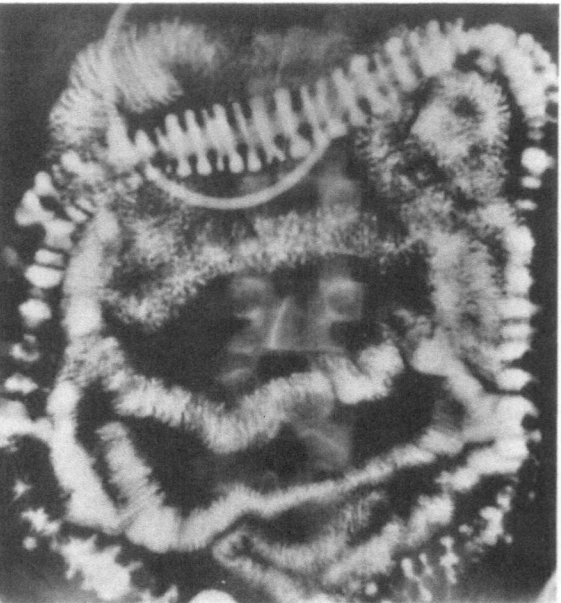

Fig.IV.67. Two patients with chronic abdominal cramps as a result of SLE. The loops of the small bowel show a pronounced hypermotility, but no ischemic mucosal lesions can be found. Many of the loops are in the contraction phase and the lumen of the intestine is obviously smaller than normal. Since the colon can also be quite spastic, it is sometimes possible in these cases to fill both the large and the small intestine with only 400 ml barium suspension.

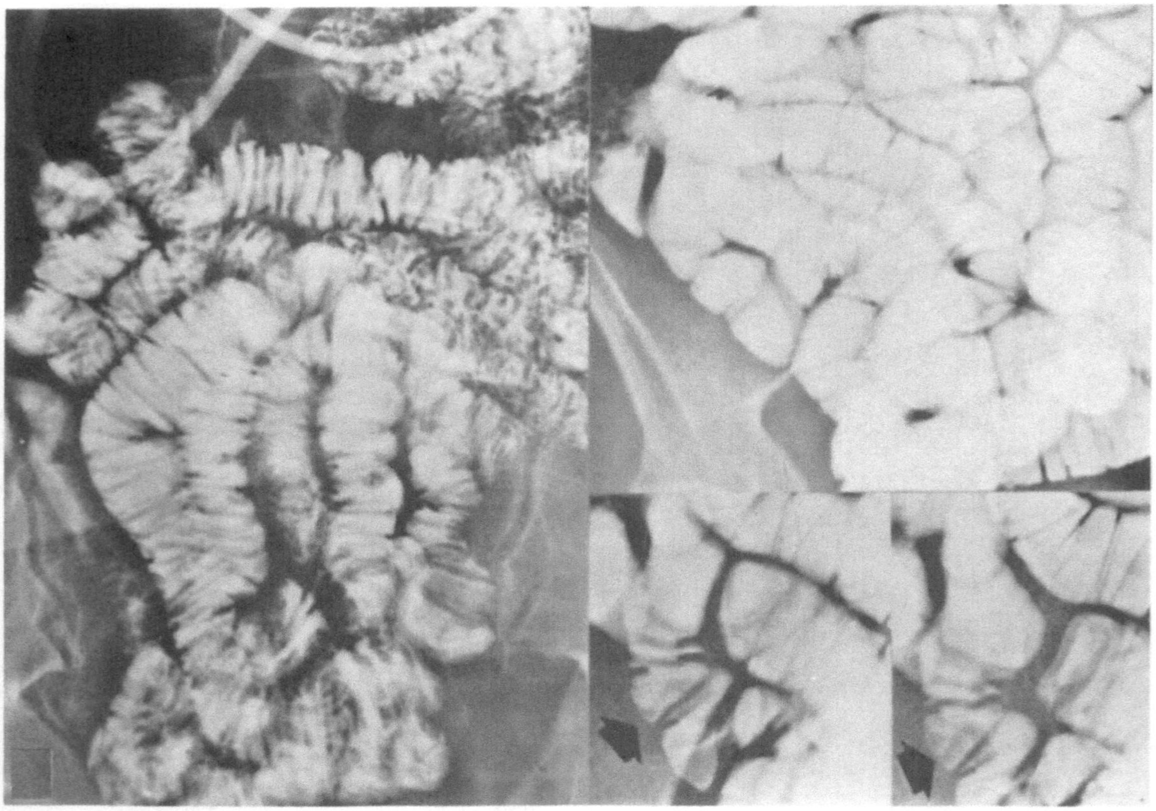

Fig. IV.68. Generalized hypermotility of the intestine. At a rate of flow of 75 ml/min, less than 400 ml contrast medium were needed to reach the cecum – instead of the statistical average of almost 700 ml. Since carcinoids were suspected and such a moderate filling of the intestine prevents proper evaluation of the mucosa, the examination was then continued by increasing the rate of flow to 150 ml/min. This detail of the plain film thus obtained shows that even in the case of hypermotility such a high rate of flow causes paralysis of the intestine. Intramural carcinoids were not found during this phase of the examination; however, the 'kinking sign' in the distal ileum (arrow) can be regarded as a secondary indication of carcinoids. This diagnosis was surgically confirmed.

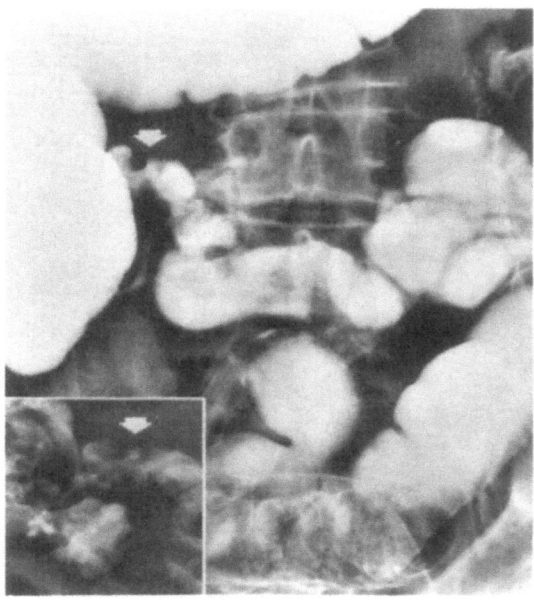

Fig. IV.69. With the enteroclysis technique, this smaller tumor in the distal ileum was not reached although 2500 ml contrast fluid and water were administered and the examination was continued for 1 hour. The tumor was quickly visualized via filling of the colon. The patient had a history of five previous admissions for rectal bleeding.

greatest possible care. Surgical intervention is necessary when these show an increase.

4.3.5. Radiation 'enteritis': Hyperemia and edema preceded by spasm can arise in the mucosa under the influence of radiation therapy. This is seen on the X-rays as a clear broadening of the mucosal folds with very thin, fairly pointed interspaces ('spikes'). As a result of the thicker intestinal wall, the distance between adjacent intestinal loops is obviously increased. These abnormalities are probably due to a local anoxia of the intestinal wall and are partly similar to those seen in some cases of hypermotility. The edema seems to develop only when the anoxia is irreversible. An enteroclysis examination may reveal a moderate degree of prestenotic dilatation, probably not present (fig. IV.47) under physiological circumstances.

4.4. Disappearance of mucosal fold pattern
Where a local dilatation of the bowel results from a more distally situated smooth-walled stenosis the following possibilities may be considered:

4.4.1. Crohn's disease or tuberculosis: Other abnormalities frequently found in association with these conditions render the diagnosis relatively simple (figs. IV.119 and IV.55B).

4.4.2. Tumor growth: An adenocarcinoma may be smooth-walled and appear as a solitary abnormality (fig. IV.31N). In Hodgkin's disease or scirrhus metastases, multiple, more or less connected and slightly constricted segments are involved, which give rise to almost negligible dilatations (fig. IV.41).

4.4.3. Vascular abnormalities: A short smooth-walled stenosis can remain as end result of local ischemia. This condition is mainly caused by small emboli originating from the mitral valves. Where more or less adjacent constrictions of varying severity, chiefly in the ileum are involved, arteriosclerosis or radiation enteritis is the probable cause. Distinction between these two conditions should never give rise to difficulties when the numerous other signs and information are considered. On the other hand, the differential diagnosis of Crohn's disease and arteriosclerosis in the older patient may give rise to great difficulties (fig. IV.32). In systemic lupus erythematosis smooth-walled constrictions may occur of some centimetres long which are hardly ever severe enough to give rise to dilatations. The ischemia associated with this condition is too superficial and thereby has also clinically a too imperceptible course for the formation of deeply structured fibrosis. A celiac syndrome with loss of mucosal pattern in the jejunum can produce multiple smooth-walled spasmodic constrictions which cause no or only very transient dilatations (fig. IV.62).

4.5. Irregular mucosal pattern
Where a dilatation is the consequence of a constriction that shows an irregular mucosal pattern then the folds or their remnants are still recognizable, while in contrast, this is no longer the case with a destructive lesion. Such irregular mucosal appearances are to be found in:

4.5.1. Crohn's disease or tuberculosis: Here the folds can have a bizarre course and ill-defined

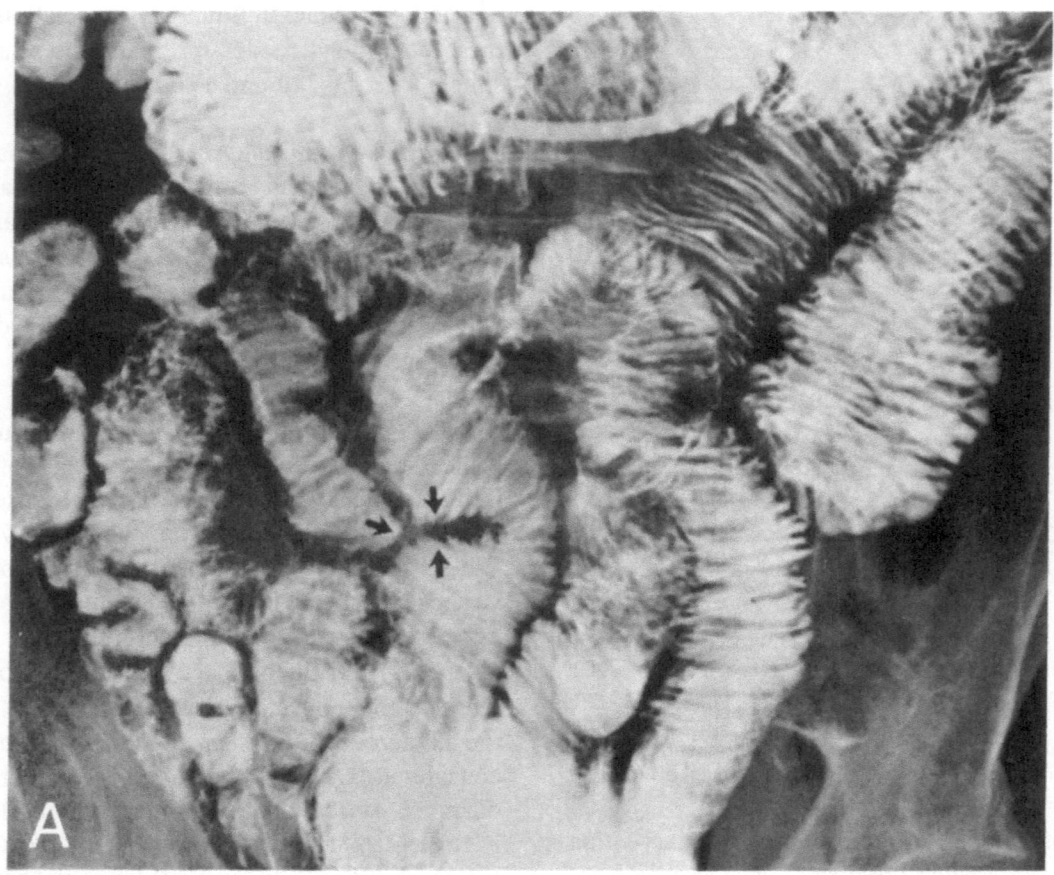

Fig. IV.70AB. Extensive fusion between the loops of the ileum and the distal jejunum. Enteroclysis examination several weeks after the patient had suffered from severe abdominal pain and a state of subileus following a copious dinner (A). Presumably this is a case of temporary ischemia (severe intestinal angina) resulting in a coat of fibrin on the intestine. A follow-up examination 4 months later showed that the fusions had entirely disappeared and that the calibre of the intestine was again normal (B). (lower X-ray on page 103)

borders (fig. IV.72) while the dilated areas may show abnormalities such as radial arrangement (fig. IV.73), cobblestones or mucosal islands (fig. IV.74). Severe spasm of long duration can play a role in the appearance of transient dilatations with Crohn's disease. These appearances result from the pronounced hypertrophy of the muscular layers in the intestinal wall which so often accompany Chrohn's disease. Spasm of these thickened walls can further give rise to a threadlike configuration of the contrast medium, known as 'string sign' (fig. IV.51).

4.5.2. Radiation 'enteritis': Here too the mucosal pattern can still be recognizable in a stenotic area resulting from severe local edema or from fibrous contracture. Where caused by edema the constriction and thus also the dilatation is indeed less pronounced (fig. IV.75).

4.5.3. Tumor growth: Mild constriction of the lumen with prestonic dilatation can occur where tumor growth is slow or but little destructive. Good examples of still easily recognizable but abnormally situated mucosal folds are shown in figs. IV.29 and IV.76. In the second radiograph a tumor with intramucosal infiltration has not yet resulted in obstruction but this is only a matter of time.

4.5.4. Carcinoid lesions: Fibrosis in the bowel wall can here lead to a very bizarre arrangement

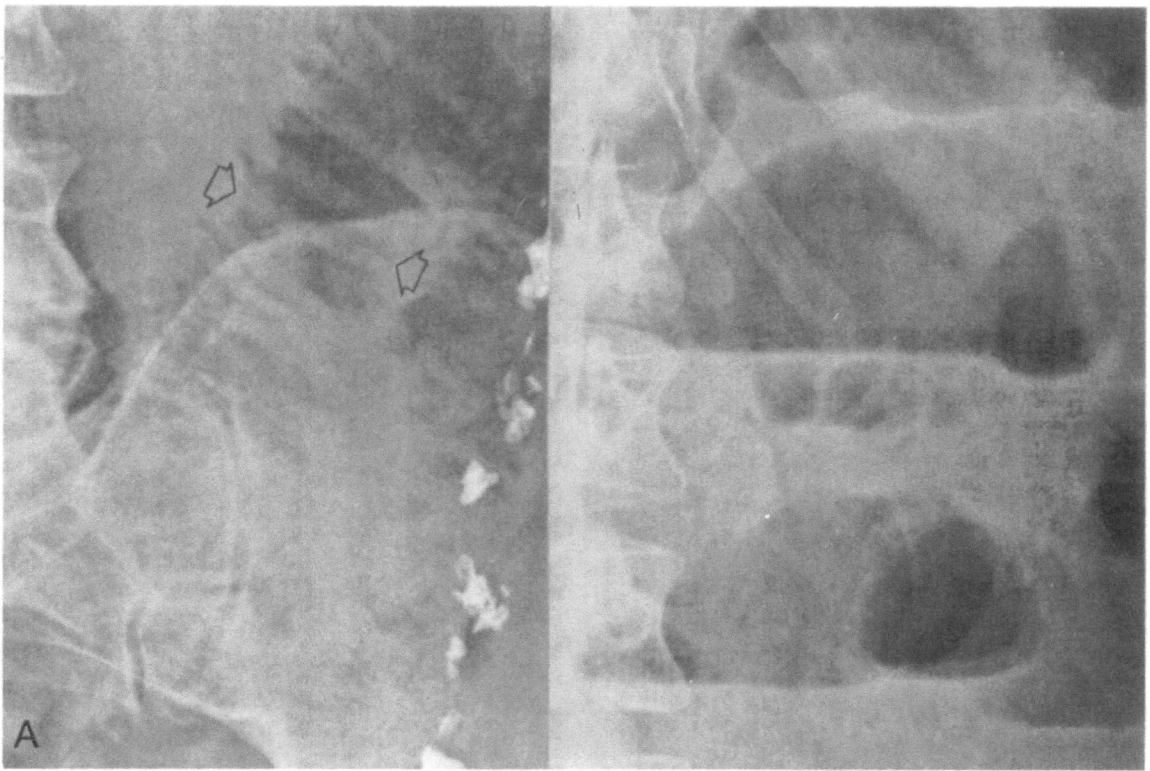

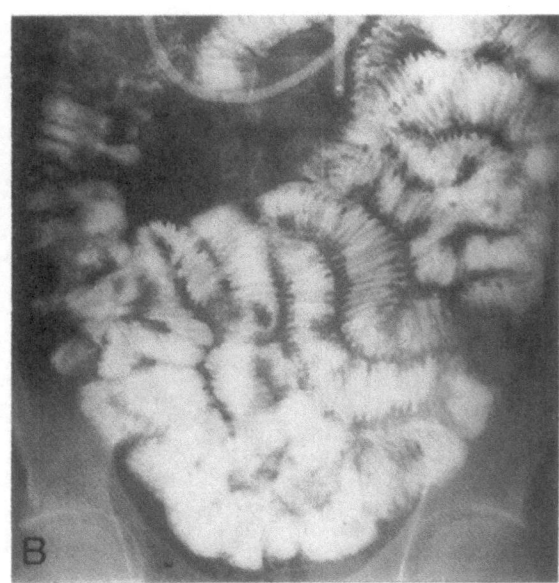

Fig. IV.70AB.

of individually intact mucosal folds and to severe constrictions and dilatations that are further enhanced by the hypermotility that may accompany carcinoid foci (fig. IV.77).

4.6. Destruction of mucosa

Where a very irregularly defined wall bordering is found at the site of a constriction, it can originate in one of the following conditions:

4.6.1. A malignant tumor:
All malignant tumors can lead to severe destruction of mucosa and the whole bowel wall; the most frequently occurring in the gut are:

    lympho-reticular malignancies;
    adenocarcinomata and all sarcomata (fig. IV.48).

In the case of extensive necrotic destruction wide spaces may arise, in which absolutely no trace of normal bowel wall bordering can be found (fig. IV.78).

4.6.2. Non-specific ulcerations:
These can manifest as solitary or multiple lesions, are very short (1-2 cm), penetrate to deep within the bowel wall and cause severe constrictions from active fibrosis (fig. IV.79) with prestenotic dilatation.

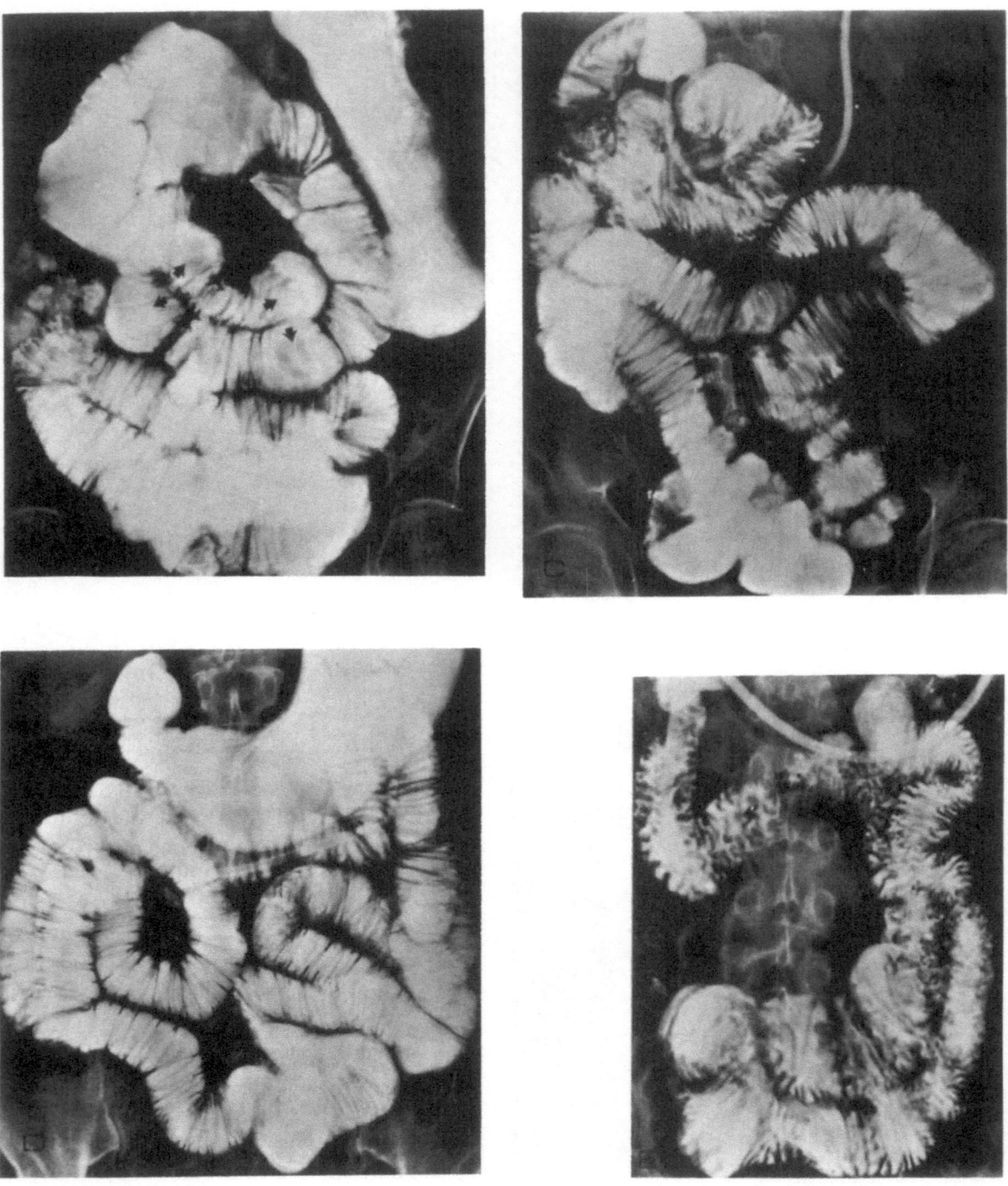

Fig. IV.71. Four patients with scleroderma and the resulting abnormalities encountered in the small intestine. (A) Very large stomach with pronounced dilatation of the descending limb of the duodenum. The jejunum that is also dilated shows several local sacculations (arrows) but there are also contractions in the right upper quadrant. This patient also had abnormalities of the skin and esophagus. (C) Unequal dilatations in the jejunum but also many contracted loops (in contrast to a drug-induced atony, where this is not seen). In this patient there were also abnormalities of the hands and esophagus. (D) Abundant reflux into a normal-sized stomach. Dilatation of the duodenum and jejunum without sacculations or contracted intestinal segments. This patient also had abnormalities of the esophagus. Differentiation from a drug-induced atony of the small bowel is not possible. (E) Sacculations in the jejunum. Motility was initially normal but became obviously disturbed within several minutes. In this patient, abnormalities of the skin, hands and esophagus were also seen.

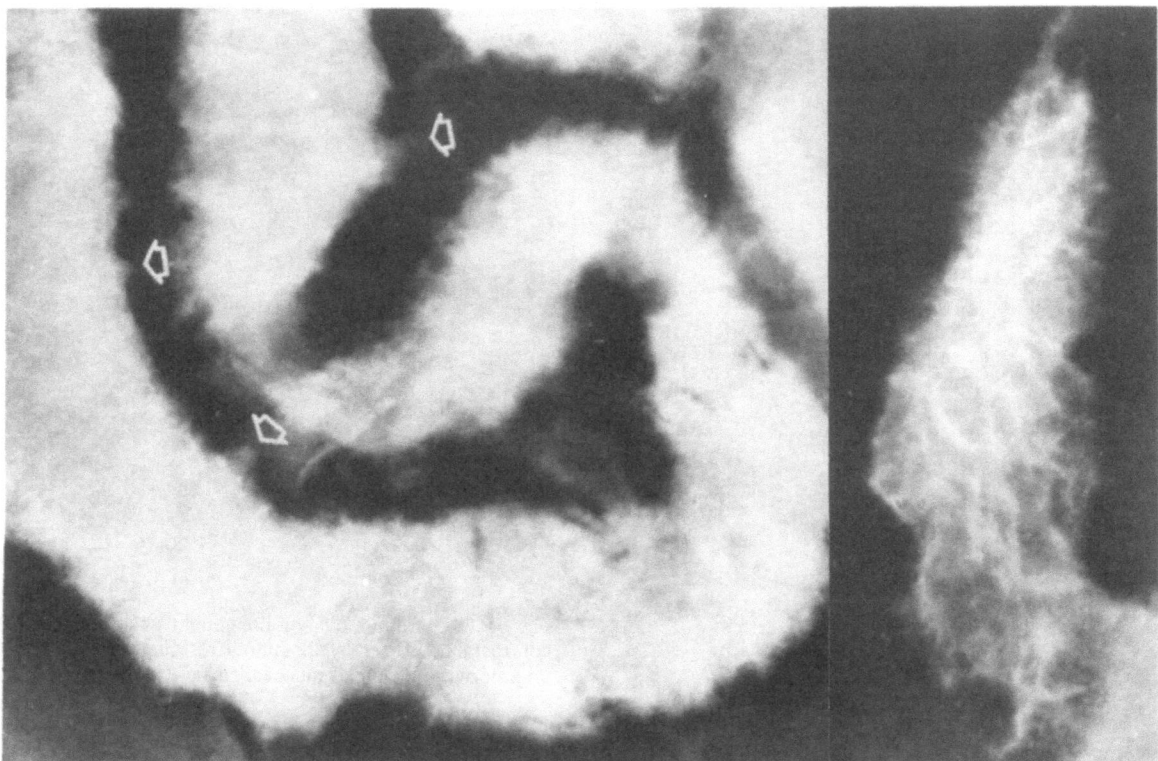

Fig. IV.72. Locally stiff and thickened wall of the intestine. A very long section of the contrast column has ragged margins, irregularly striped in the distal ileum. Deep ulcerations are observed most easily along the margin of the intestine (arrows). If the film density is too high, they can no longer be seen because of overexposure. Vaguely defined intestinal wall is due to purulent secretion on an ulcerated mucosal surface.

4.6.3. Skip lesions in Crohn's disease: Similar abnormalities to those described in subsection (2) may also arise with the more frequently encountered Crohn's disease. These abnormalities, called 'skip lesions' can be somewhat longer than those of non-specific ulceration and generally lead to a less severe stenosis and dilatation. Differential diagnosis of these two conditions gives usually no problem since Crohn's disease is accompanied by numerous other abnormalities and has a completely different complement of clinical findings and progress. An exception to this rule is provided by fig. IV.80.

4.7 Extraluminal mechanical obstruction
In principle a distinction can be made between compression by structures lying outside the bowel and the sort of auto-compression exercised by intramural foci. The latter naturally exert a more marked effect on the transit in the bowel lumen.

4.7.1. Extramural causes: Hindrance of transit by compression of the bowel lumen from without is seldom of serious nature unless a longer segment is involved in extensive lymph gland infiltration or tumor masses (fig. IV.42).

4.7.2. In the presence of *serious hypomotility* from prolonged use of sedatives, antispasmodics, tranquillizers etc. compression from other organs may well cause some dilatation and transit hindrance. This is particularly so for the effect on the ileum of transversing vessels or a well-filled rectosigmoid and for that of the aorta on the duodenum (figs. IV.81 and IV.87B). More severe compression can be exercised by large abdominal cysts or tumors.

4.7.3. Intramural lesions: Only benign or very mildly malignant tumors can attain sufficient size in the bowel wall without destroying it and con-

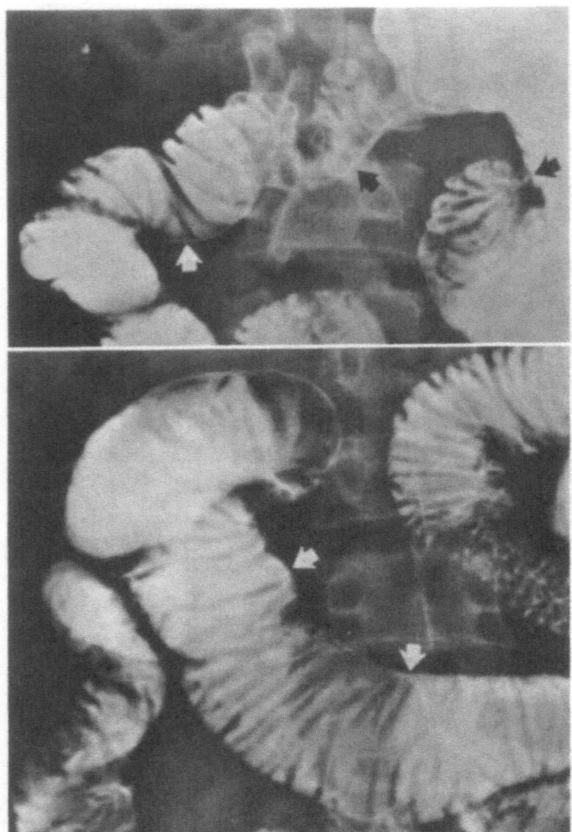

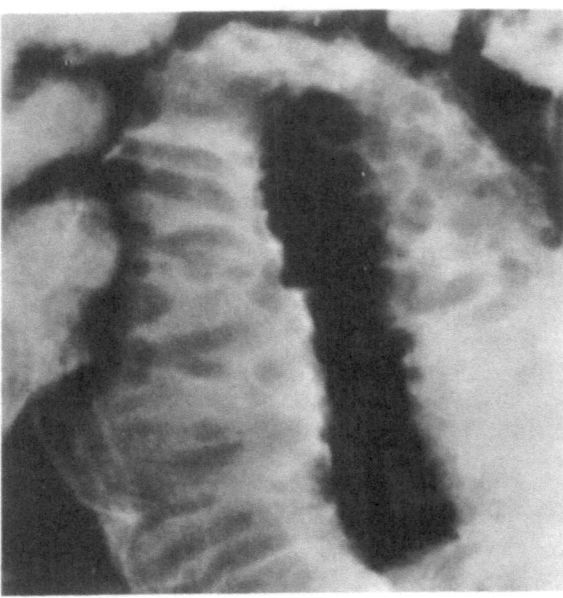

Fig. IV.74. Round, oval or elongated translucencies in the contrast fluid caused by edematous residual mucosal folds in an otherwise atrophied mucosal surface in Crohn's disease.

Fig. IV.73. Ulcerations due to Crohn's disease that have healed with fibrotic contracture. On one side of the intestine the mucosal pattern has completely disappeared.

tinue their growth in the lumen. In practice this is illustrated by carcinoid foci (fig. IV.30), leiomyomata (fig. IV.28) and hematomata of the intestinal wall (fig. IV.82).

4.8 Intraluminal mechanical obstruction
It is selfevident that intraluminal obstacles can exercise a greater influence on transit with earlier development of mild dilatation of a limited segment proximal to their site, than the conditions listed in subsection (g). The following list is given in order of frequency and probability:

4.8.1. Food residue in the distal ileum in case of pronounced hypomotility from chronic use of medicaments listed in subsection 'g 2' (fig. IV.83).

4.8.2. A gallstone that has perforated into the intestine. Hypomotility resulting from peritoneal irritation is here also an associated factor.

4.8.3. A large solitary polyp or multiple polyps may cause a, usually, moderate degree of obstruction and dilatation (fig. IV.110). Sometimes an invagination can occur (fig. IV.85).

4.8.4. A large solitarity polyp or multiple polyps may cause a, usually, moderate degree of obstruction and dilatation (fig. IV.110). Sometimes an invagination can occur (fig. IV.85).

4.9. Spasm
Spasm may occasionally be so severe and enduring that dilatation with hindrance of transit arises proximal to the site of action. This can be seen in Crohn's disease (fig. IV.86) (massive hypertrophy of the muscle wall), collagen diseases and crossing bands or very extensive adhesions (fig. IV.58). In these last three conditions the dilatations and hindrance of transit are most probably the result of local ischemia.

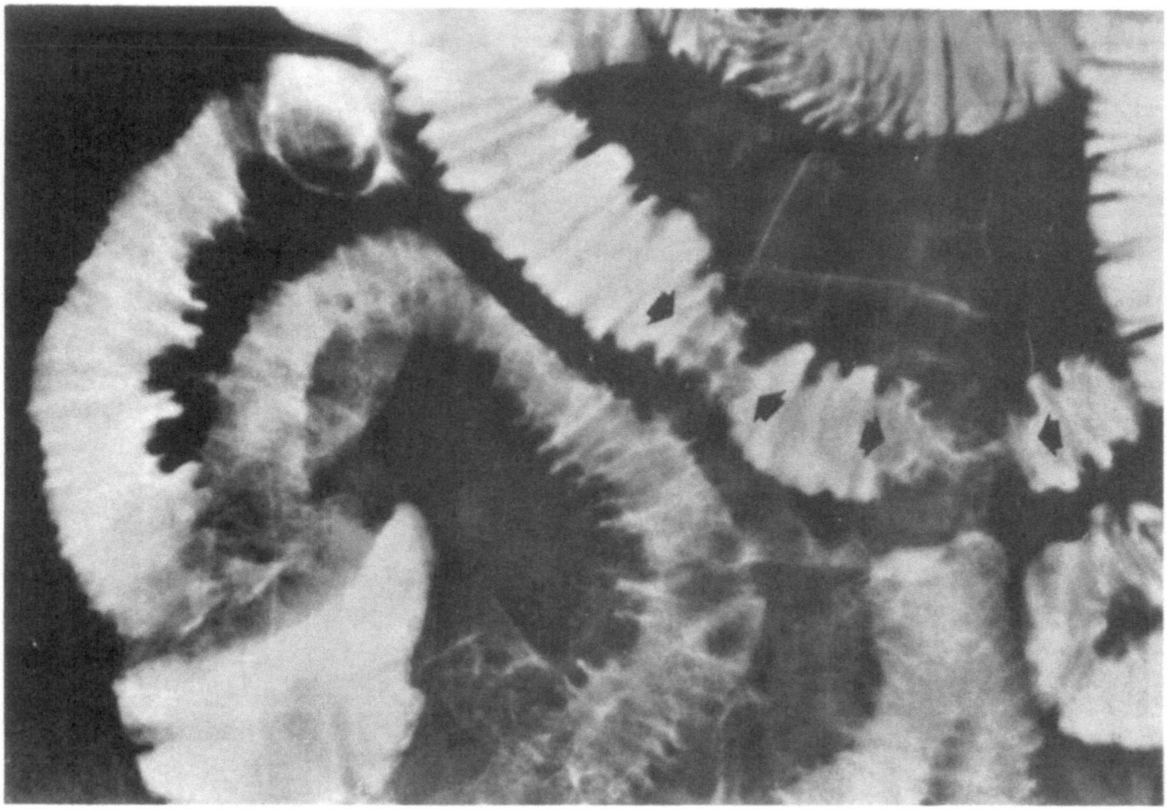

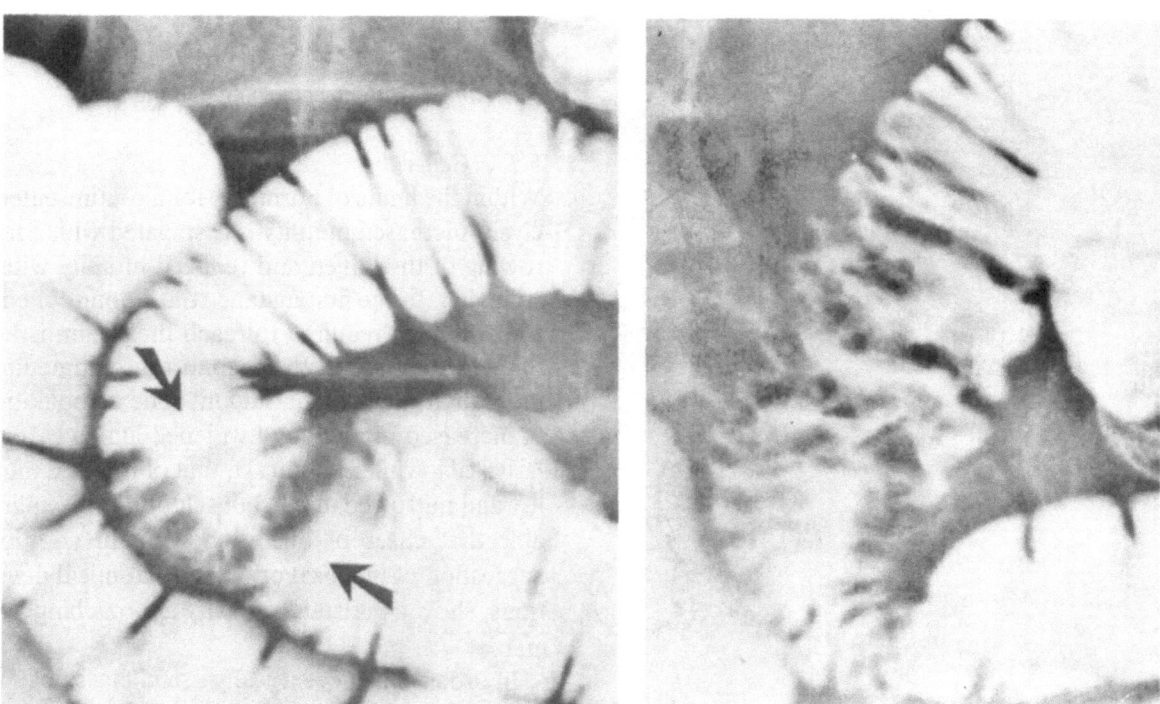

Fig. IV.75. Adhesion of intestinal loops in radiation enteritis; irregular mucosal surface and multiple small ulcerations. Thickened intestinal wall is due mainly to fibrosis rather than edema. Areas resembling skip lesions are indicated by arrows.

Fig. IV.76. In a 40-year-old woman, an accidental finding consisting of five iregularly thickened folds on the compression spot films; a conglomeration of lymph follicles is clearly visualized in this region. The distance between the relevant barium column and that of the adjacent loop has not increased so that the intestinal wall itself cannot be thickened. In spite of the radiological report of a suspected very small lymphoreticular malignancy, growing within the mucosa, the surgeon was exceedingly reluctant to perform laparotomy. Eventually the suspected diagnosis was confirmed by the pathologist.

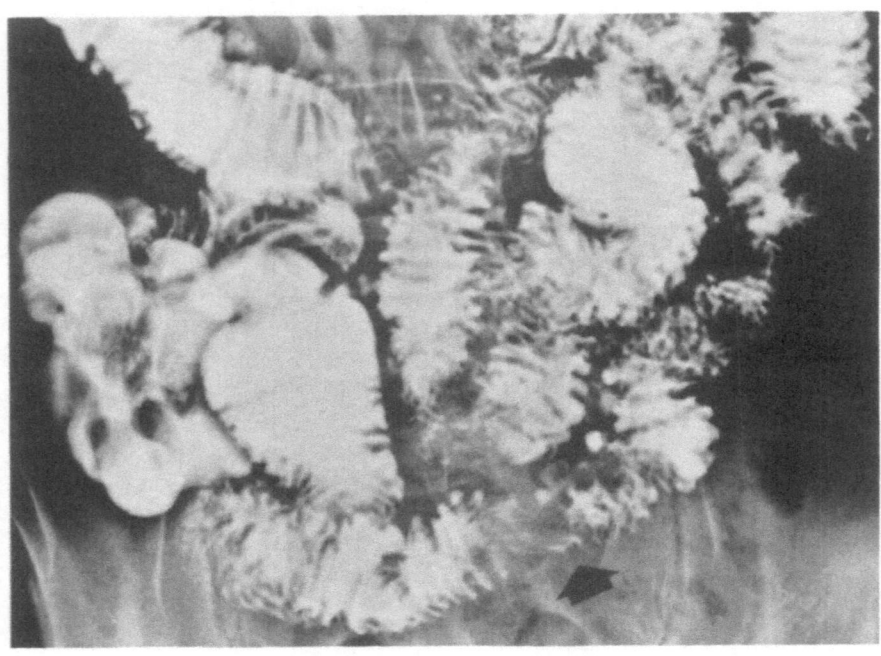

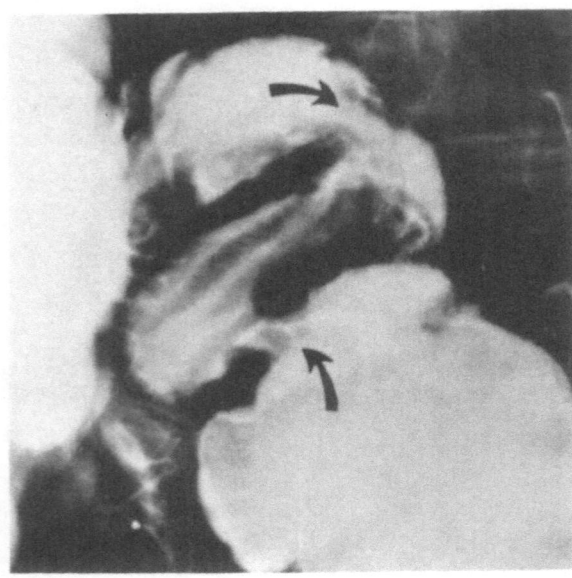

Fig. IV.77. Hypermotility with formation of diverticula in the ileum (upper) and abrupt changes in the course of the intestine (kinking) caused by local contracture of the mesentery due to a carcinoid (below)

5. Long segment with dilated lumen

5.1. General

Within the limits of normality for a routine entero-clysis, increased motility is associated with a narrowing of the lumen and reduced motility with a widening. In the first instance the amount of contrast medium required to reach the cecum is less than 700 ml and in the second up to sometimes more than double that amount. The combination of increased motility and widened lumen is regularly seen, while in contrast, that of reduced motility and narrowed lumen but seldom. It is remarkable that cases of dilatation with, in addition, suggestion of mucosal or other anatomical deviations, show a peristaltic activity approaching normal.

In order to achieve a really useful classification scheme for critical interpretation of examinations revealing increased calibre of a long segment or full length of the intestine, the conditions that must be considered in the differential diagnosis have been arranged as follows:

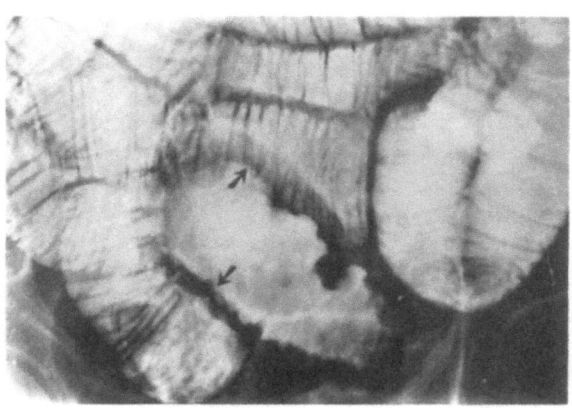

Fig. IV.78. Plaque-like carcinoids are rare; they are diffi-cult to differentiate from a local intramural lymphosarcoma. The lumen of the intestine is dilated locally and the intestinal wall is thickened. Local absence of mucosal fold relief. There was metastasis in the liver.

5.2. *Dilatation with reduced motility*

5.2.1. *Rate of infusion too high (more than 100 ml/min).* It is characteristic for this frequently occurring technical error in enteroclysis that mo-tility is initially completely normal but disappears in the course of the examination. This normal period, in practice a half minute, becomes shorter in proportion to the excess of infusion rate. Dila-tation is more marked in the jejunum than in the ileum as is shown in subsection 2. It is important that taking radiograms early in the examination be adopted as standard procedure.

5.2.2. *Atony resulting from medication.* In case of prolongued medication with antispasmodics, hypnotics and sedatives the intestine is dilated in

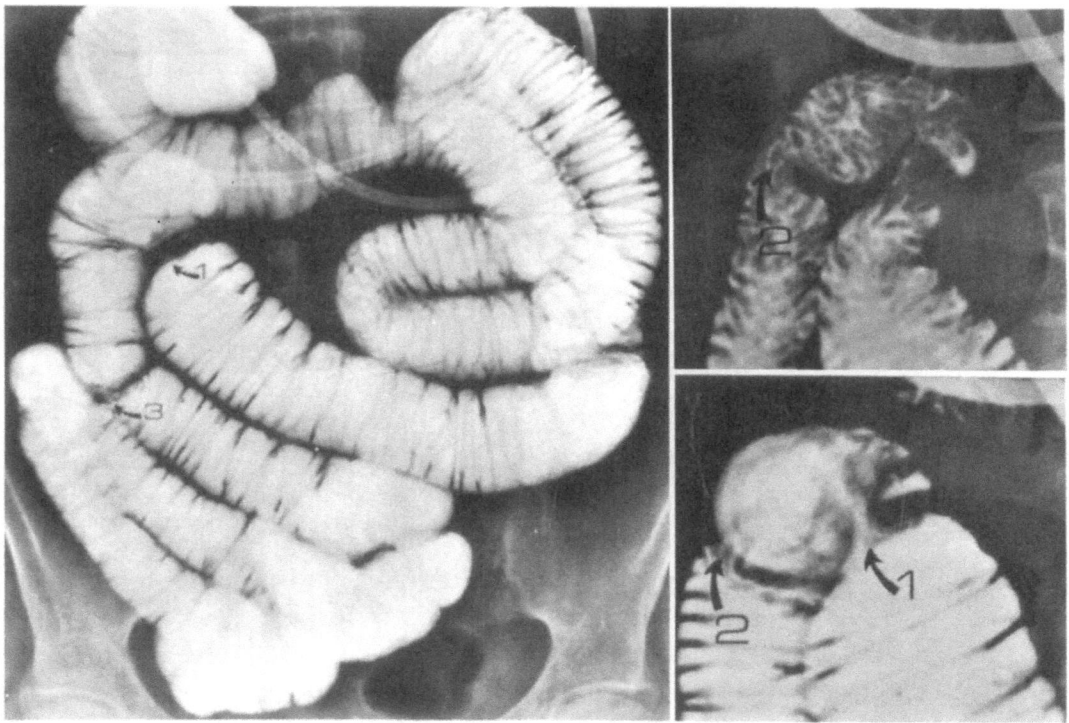

Fig. IV.79. Survey films of a patient who had complained of colic-like pain in the abdomen for years. Dilated intestinal loops with two short annular strictures (1 and 3). The spot films revealed, however, that there were in fact three stenoses that were clearly visible only when the loops were well filled. The dilatation of the loops on the distal side of the third stenosis suggested that further constriction existed distally; this was confirmed at surgery. None of the conventional examinations had ever revealed any abnormalities. This patient had been considered un unconfirmed Crohn's disease case for 20 years and was scheduled for an ileocecal resection. It is obvious that Crohn's disease is unlikely.

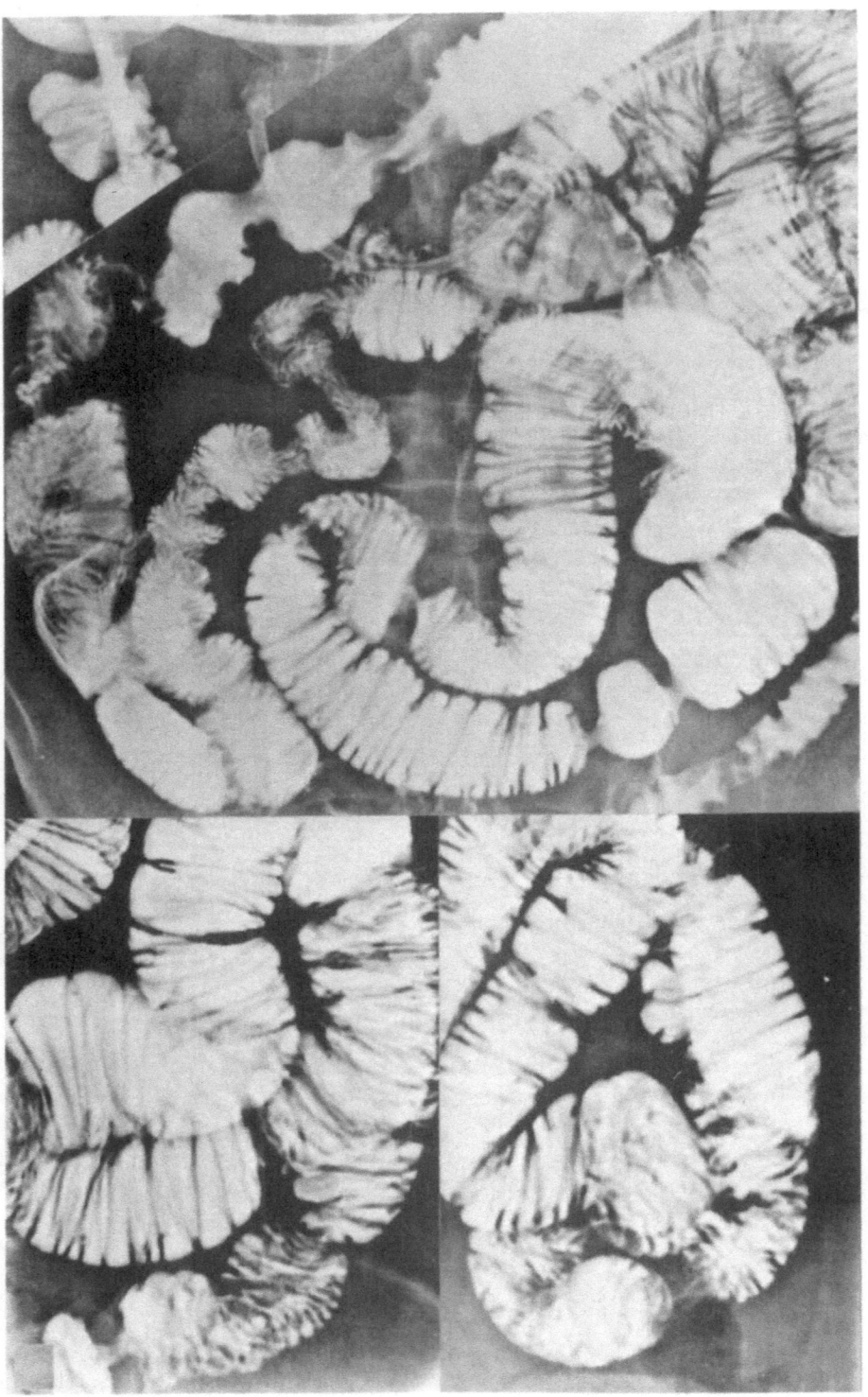

Fig. IV.80. Multiple very short strictures, mainly in the duodenum and jejunum, without further abnormalities of the mucosa. Although quite unusual in Crohn's disease, pathological examination indicated that these abnormalities were indeed attributable to this illness.

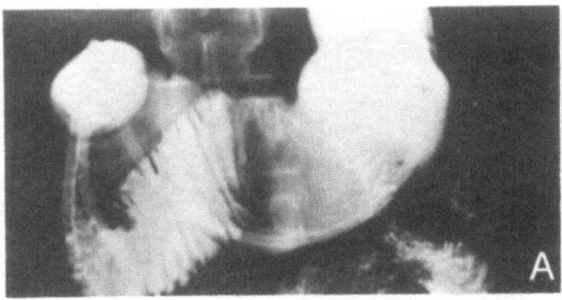

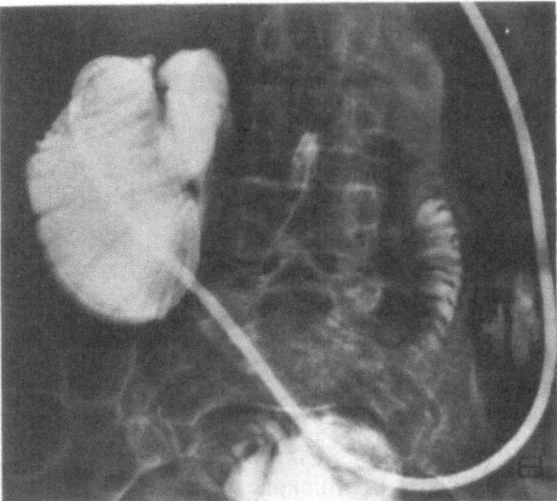

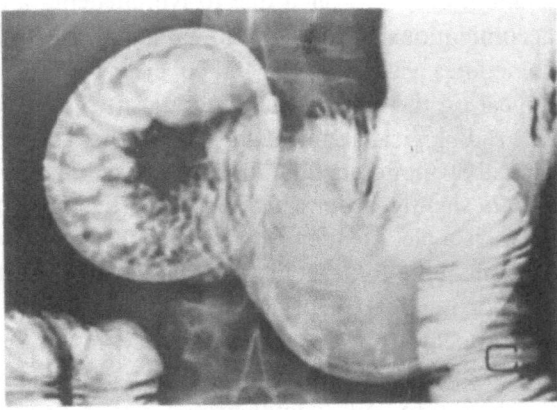

Fig. IV.81(A). The tube turns back in a prestenotic sacculation in the duodenum that has developed as a result of a
mesenteric artery syndrome. The tip of the tube is in the
duodenal bulb and is therefore close to the pylorus so that a
large quantity of contrast fluid flows back into the stomach.
(B) The tube is coiled in the descending limb of the
duodenum, which is greatly dilated as a result of scleroderma.
(C) it is not always possible, especially in those patients who
use drugs for atony, to pass the spinal column or the aorta
with the tube. The chance of reflux to the stomach is then
considerably greater and decreasing the rate of flow of the
contrast fluid to 50 ml/min and administering metoclopramide to the contrast fluid is to be recommended.

its entire length and peristalsis is very characteris-
tically, in even the very earliest phase of the
examination reduced or absent, depending on the
degree and duration of the medication. The contraction percentage shown on a general view is
from less than 50% to near enough absent (figs.
IV.87AB and IV.88). In some cases differentiation
from amyloidosis may be very troublesome but
the peristaltic disturbance in the proximal jejunum, so characteristic for drug atony, is consistently absent in amyloidosis (fig. IV.89).

5.2.3. Paralytic or obstructive ileus. The causes of
obstructive ileus are diverse and include bands,
adhesions, tumors, Crohn's disease or the result
of radiation therapy. Motility and intestinal
calibre are typically completely normal in the most
proximal portion of the small intestine but become
increasingly more disturbed distally as the site of
obstruction is approached; in contrast to what
has been described in subsections 1 and 2 (figs.
IV.90 and IV.91).

In paralytic ileus, often caused by ischemia or
thrombosis, motility in the proximal segment may
also be disturbed. Some increase in calibre is
present up to the site of the vascular accident but
is here not so marked as in the case of obstruction.
Paralytic ileus or sub-ileus frequently undergoes
spontaneous recovery which, depending on the
causitive factor, is unusual in the obstructive type.

5.3. Dilatation with increased motility
5.3.1. Whipple's disease. This is a fairly rare
disease, which is sometimes hereditary. The
complaints ot these patients, predominantly
middle-aged men, include abdominal pain, steatorrhea, weight loss and recurrent shifting pain in
the joints. Physical examination shows a generalized lymphadenopathy, enlarged liver and spleen
and polyserositis. The skin is often pigmented as
in Addison's disease. Hematological determina-
tions reveal a low Hb and decreased protein and
calcium concentrations; in addition, the resorption of various food components is obviously
disturbed. The lymph nodes and the lamina pro-
pria of the thickened intestinal wall are filled with
deposits of fat and fatty acids containing large
foamy macrophages. During the active phase of
the disease, bacteria conglomerate in the macro-

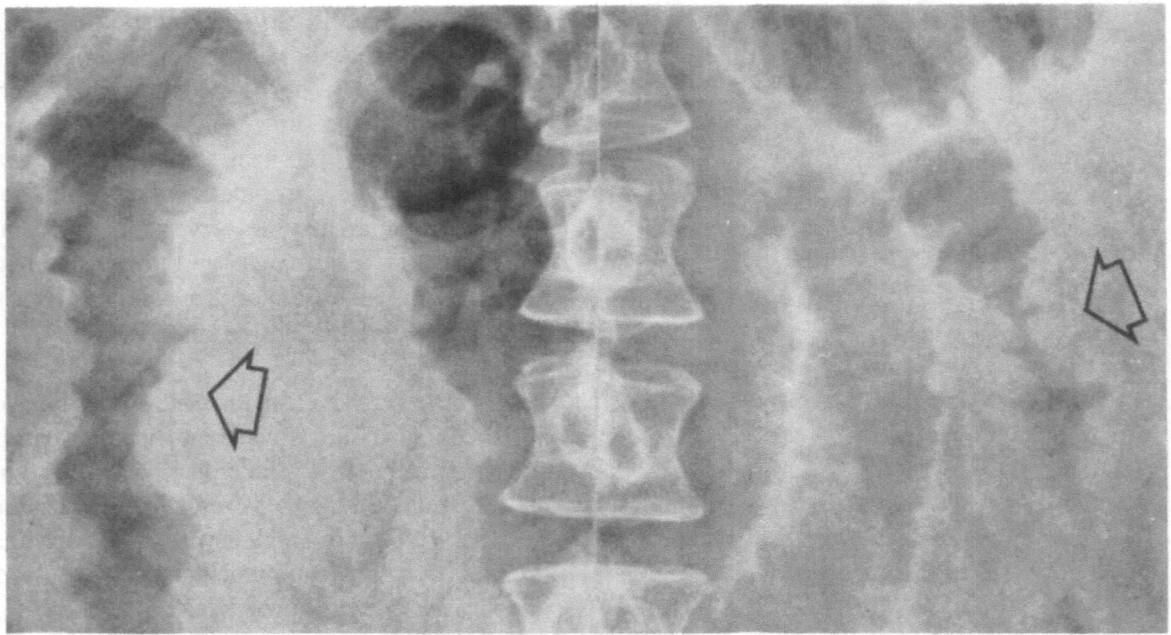

Fig. IV.82. Persistent gas in several dilated intestinal loops. The irregular appearance, the so-called 'thumbprinting' sign, is from hemorrhage in the intestinal wall. Patient hemophilic.

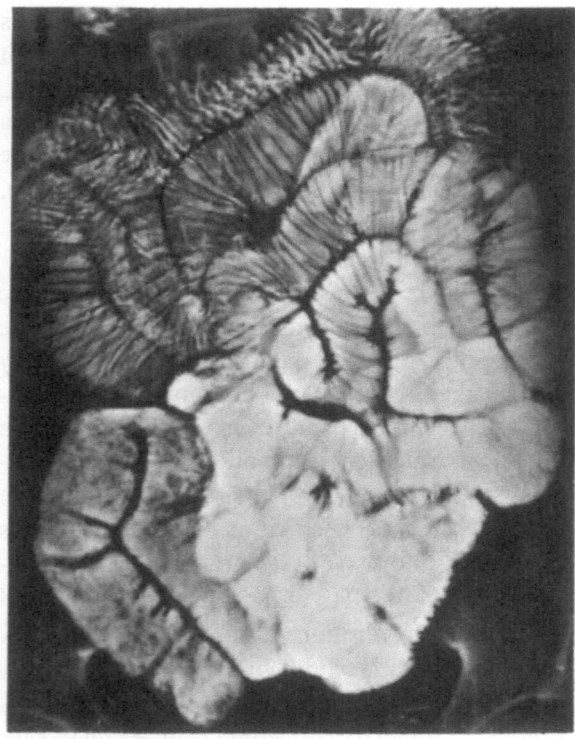

Fig. IV.83. Drug-induced atony of the intestine. Food residue from the previous day acts as additional mechanical obstruction in the distal ileum.

phages but disappear after prolonged treatment with antibiotics.

The villi on the thickened mucosal folds in the jejunum are so swollen due to lymphedema and accumulations of lipogranulomata that they are sometimes visible to the naked eye. They then appear on the films as small nodules (fig. IV.92). The radiological abnormalities are further characterized by moderate dilatation of the jejunal loops and a slightly accelerated passage (fig. IV.93). There is a clear tendency towards flocculation or dilution of the contrast fluid so that the time available for making useful films is rather short.

It appears that the marked coarsening of the mucosa in the jejunum, consistently mentioned in the literature and demonstrated on röntgenograms, can be attributed to a large extent to disintegration of the contrast fluid; it is less pronounced than is generally assumed.

5.3.2. *Celiac disease.* This disease, which can occur both in small children and adults, is characterized by abdominal pain, fatigue, loss of weight and diarrhea. Usually the stools are pulpy and voluminous but some cases present with obstipation. The patient, having learned to live with his

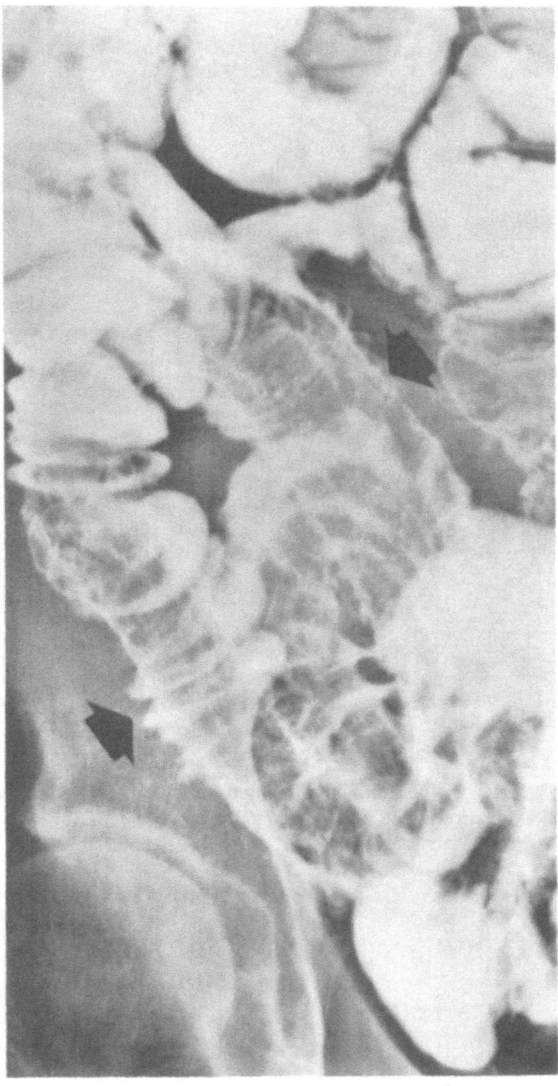

Fig. IV.84. Deceptive pattern of an invagination caused by a surgical gauze 70 cm in length that was left behind in the abdominal cavity and perforated into the intestinal lumen.

folds and dilated loops that are present in a quarter of patients with celiac syndrome.

Modern enteroclysis technique has now completely eliminated the hindrance of flocculation. The transit in celiac disease may be so rapid that, even with this technique it is hardly possible to obtain adequate filling of the intestinal loops (fig. IV.94). Therefore, when celiac disease is suspected, it is essential that the flowrate of the contrast fluid be in excess of the normal 75ml/min. A rapid flow is also necessary for detecting a slight decrease in the number and any flattening of the mucosal folds in the proximal jejunum (fig. II.1). In some cases a well filled jejunum may show the haustral-like pattern caused by spasm, resembling normal colon (fig. IV.62).

5.3.3. Lambliasis. Patients with a disturbed gammaglobulin synthesis are highly susceptible to infectious diseases such as lambliasis. In this condition hypermotility, dilatation and tendency to flocculation can all be just as pronounced as in celiac syndrome. Diagnosis on grounds of the X-ray photos alone is often not possible (fig. IV.95).

5.3.4. Pancreatic insufficiency. In pancreatic insufficiency disturbance of digestion results in an increase of 'bulk' in the intstinal lumen. This large amount of content stretches the intestine and thus enhances peristalsis (fig. IV.96). The intestine is but mildly dilated and a similarly slight tendency to increased flocculation is manifest. There is a marked tendency to dilution of the contrast medium in the large volume of digestive juices present (figs. IV.97 and IV.177).

5.3.5. Naish syndrome. This disease is based on degenerative changes in the mesenteric plexus resulting in severe dilatation with little peristalsis in the proximal portion which gives inadequate mixing with the intestinal juices and thus impaired digestion. Further, a marked tendency to flocculation of barium suspension is observed on the X-ray films (fig. IV.98). Very active non-propulsive and retro-peristaltic movements can occur occasioning severe colicky pain. Histological examination reveals considerable hypertrophy of the innermost muscle layer in the bowel wall. The

complaints, is sometimes unaware of his illness. The cause of the disease is a genetically determined pathological reaction to the gluten fraction in wheat.

Some decades ago the radiological findings were characterised and also limited to the single observation of marked flocculation of the contrast fluid. This situation changed when Marshak, by rapid administration of large volumes of contrast medium, was able to demonstrate the mucosal

114

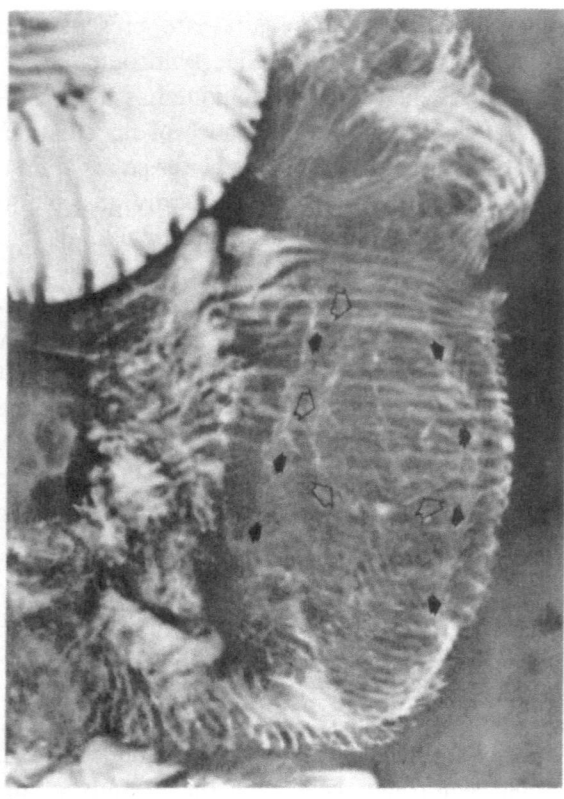

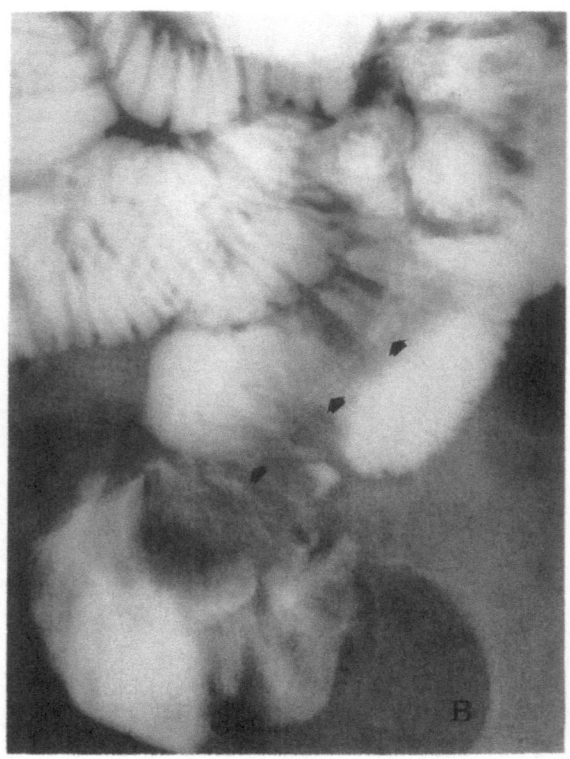

Fig. IV.85B. Stretched-out longitudinal course of folds in the centre of the intussuscipiens of an invagination.
(courtesy Dr. M. Riha – Stadskanaal)

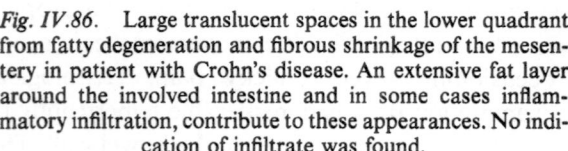

Fig. IV.85A. Intussusception of jejunum into jejunum, caused by a lipoma ± 2 cm in diameter (lower); the latter can be seen in the intussuscipiens (open arrow). The mucosal surface of the intussuscipiens is also just visible (solid arrows) about 0.5 cm inside the wall of the enclosing intestinal loop (upper)

Fig. IV.86. Large translucent spaces in the lower quadrant from fatty degeneration and fibrous shrinkage of the mesentery in patient with Crohn's disease. An extensive fat layer around the involved intestine and in some cases inflammatory infiltration, contribute to these appearances. No indication of infiltrate was found.

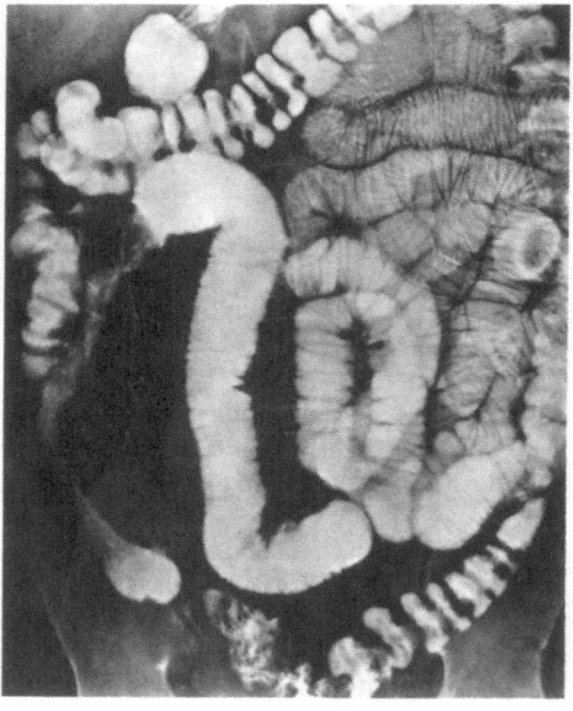

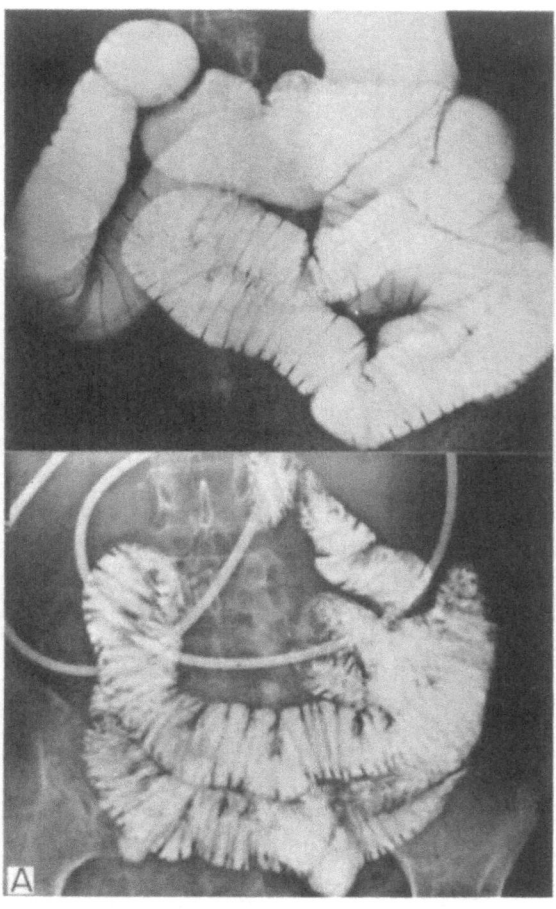

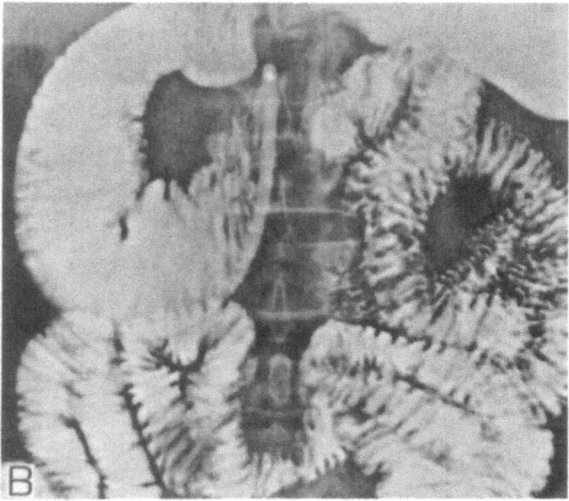

Fig. IV.87B. In this very thin patient, even the moderate use of antispasmodics caused passage to be retarded in the duodenum at the point where it crosses the aorta so that frequent vomiting developed. In the rest of the small intestine fairly active motility was still present.

Fig. IV.87A. Hypomotility and pronounced dilatation of the entire small intestine from prolonged use of antispasmodics and analgesics. The abnormality is noted during the first few minutes of the examination. The impression of the aorta on the duodenum is often clearly visible in these patients. Retroperistaltic movements in the duodenum are common and there is usually marked reflux of the contrast fluid into the stomach. One year after the above-mentioned drugs had been discontionued almost completely, the motility in the jejunum had returned to normal. Some slight dilatation was still visible.

condition shows a gradual increase in severity with age. Without observation of the very pathological contractions under screening, differentiation from scleroderma or amyloidosis is not always possible (fig. IV.6).

5.4. Intestinal dilatation with anatomical abnormalities
Few or very variable peristaltic changes.

5.4.1. Congenital lymphedema.
In lymphedema, the lymphatic channels in the mucosa and submucosa are dilated, usually from impeded drainage somewhere in the mesentery or paralumbar region. The condition can result from imflammatory processes, tumor growth or irradiation fibrosis. In the congenital form the lymph vessels in the mesentery and periphery are hypoplastic. The lumen is usually dilated and the mucosal folds become shorter and thicker. On X-ray the mucosal surface in the jejunum may appear spiculated and can be likened to a coarsely toothed saw. When the lymphedema is acquired, the swollen intestine appears somewhat stiff and tube-like; both on X-rays and under fluoroscopy it is obvious that the contractions are impeded and less frequent (fig. IV.99AD).

5.4.2. Zollinger-Ellison disease.
In Zollinger-Ellison's disease, solitary or multiple adenomas or slowly growing carcinomas involving the gastrin-secreting cells in the pancreatic islands of Langerhans, cause markedly increased secretion of gastric acid.

The mucous membrane in the various parts of the digestive tract cannot tolerate this large quan-

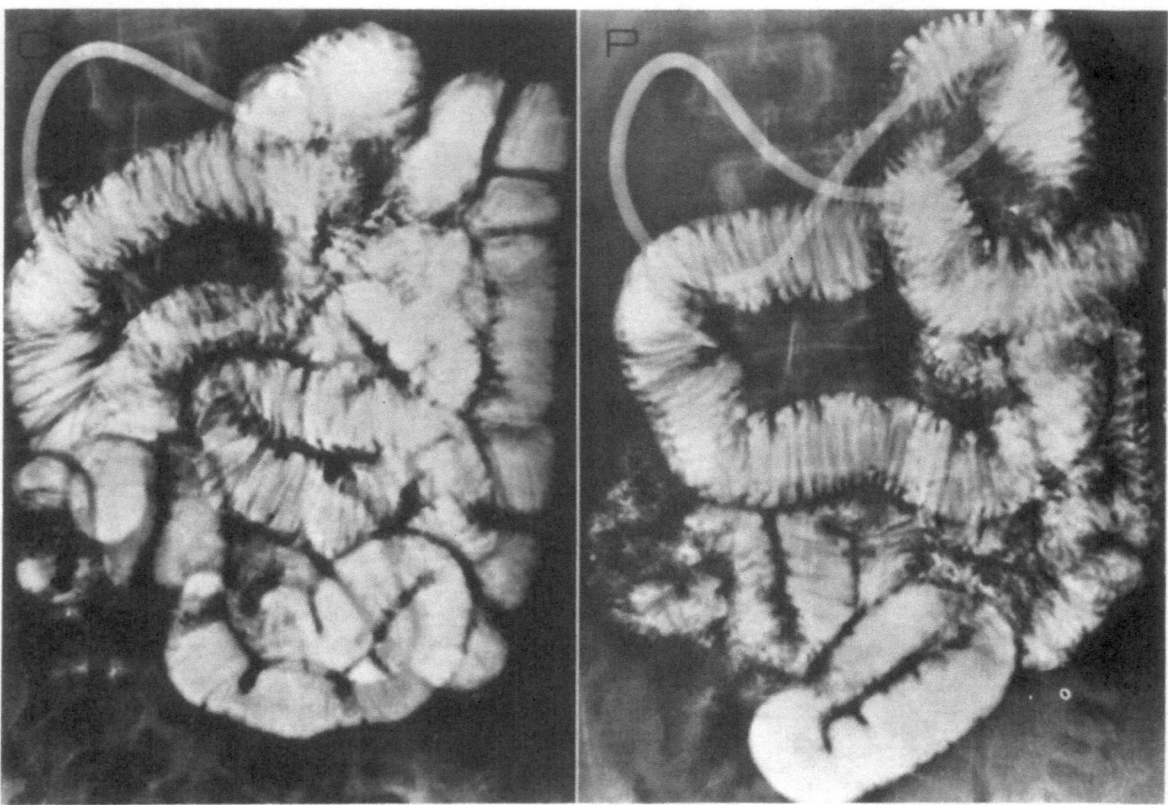

Fig. IV.88. (o) Mild case of drug-induced atony. There are fewer loops in state of contraction than in normal cases, but no dilatation of the lumen can be seen. (P) Several weeks after the use of tranquillizers was discontinued, the number of intestinal loops in a state of contraction is again normal.

tity of gastric acid. This leads to broadening of the mucosal folds in the jejunum as well as in the stomach and duodenum. This disease should be considered as a chemical enteritis. Ulcers with secondary stenosis can be found in the jejunum and the distal half of the duodenum, similar to those developping as result of the action of gastric acid on esophageal mucosa. Because of the high acidity in the duodenum the enzymes for digestion of fats and proteins are inactivated and steatorrhea develops. In less severe cases there is only 'intestinal hurry' and a watery diarrhea. During the radiological examination, the unusually strong tendency towards flocculation of the contrast fluid is striking (fig. IV.100). In some cases the loops of the small intestine are markedly dilated (fig. IV.101). The cause of this dilatation is not clear.

5.4.3. Amyloid disease. Amyloid is a protein substance that can be deposited in tissue by an unknown mechanism without demonstrable cause. It is assumed that an immunologically determined disturbance of plasma cell function is involved. In addition to this so-called primary amyloidosis, there is also secondary amyloidosis. These amyloid deposits occur in conjunction with various diseases such as chronic infections, multiple myeloma and lymphoreticular malignancies. Amyloid deposits are commonly local but may also be spread diffusely in all layers of the wall throughout the digestive tract. The deposits may be small or quite large. In the latter case they can form nodular masses and bulge into the contrast column so that differentiation from lymphoreticular malignancy may be difficult (fig. IV.102). Depending upon localization of the deposits, resorption and motility can be disturbed, leading to a malabsorption syndrome and fairly severe meteorism.

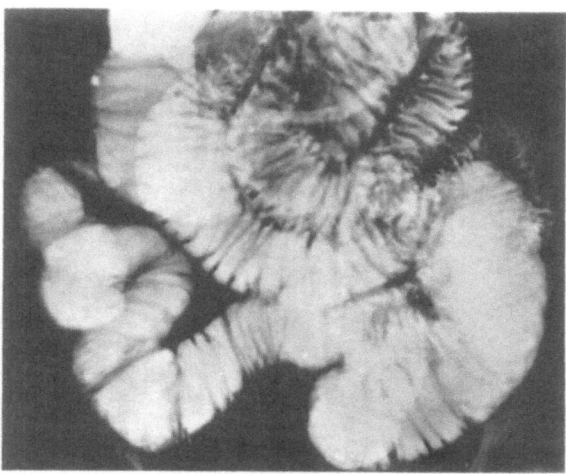
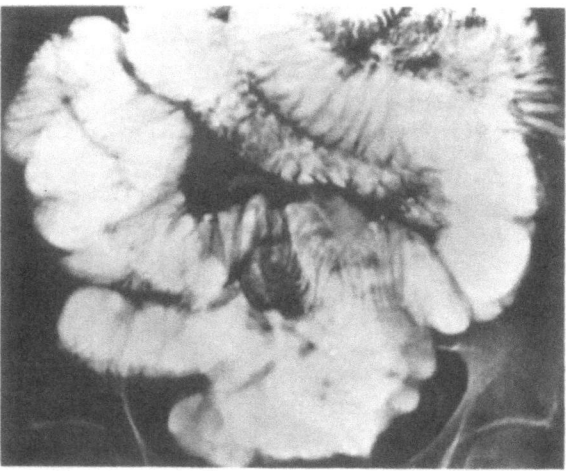

Fig. IV.89. Pseudo-obstruction of the small intestine from disturbed motility in a patient with amyloidosis. There are diverse contractions, especially in the jejunum. Although differentiation from scleroderma or drug-induced atony is most difficult, the presence of sacculations would suggest scleroderma. This degree of dilatation of the ileum and a more pronounced decrease in peristalsis in the jejunum would indicate a drug-induced atony.

The complaints from localization in the small intestine consist mainly of painful cramps. This is accompanied either by diarrhea as a result of gas accumulation, or by a pseudo-obstruction (fig. IV.89). The lumen of the small intestine may be obviously dilated, the intestinal wall thickened and the mucosa atrophied. Severe atrophy of the mucosa in the ileum produces a completely smooth mucosal surface without folds, similar to that seen in reflux ileitis, in ulcerative colitis or after remission of Crohn's disease. Smooth walls in the jejunum are usually from celiac disease.

5.4.4. Scleroderma. As a result of fibrosis, the skin becomes smooth and tightly stretched so that the face resembles a mask. Fibrin deposits in the intima of the walls of the small arteries cause stenoses with consequent ischemic necrosis in the fingertips (Raynaud's phenomenon) and diverse internal organs, including the small bowel. In the digestive tract the layers of smooth muscle become atrophied and are replaced by fibrous tissue. This leads to a decrease is pertistalsis, hypotonic dilatations and sometimes finally to stenosis.

The most frequently recognized characteristic, occurring in 80% of cases, is reduced peristalsis and a slight dilatation of the esophagus. Less well known but none the less encountered in one-half of the patients is a decreased peristalsis and dilatation of the small intestine. The degree of

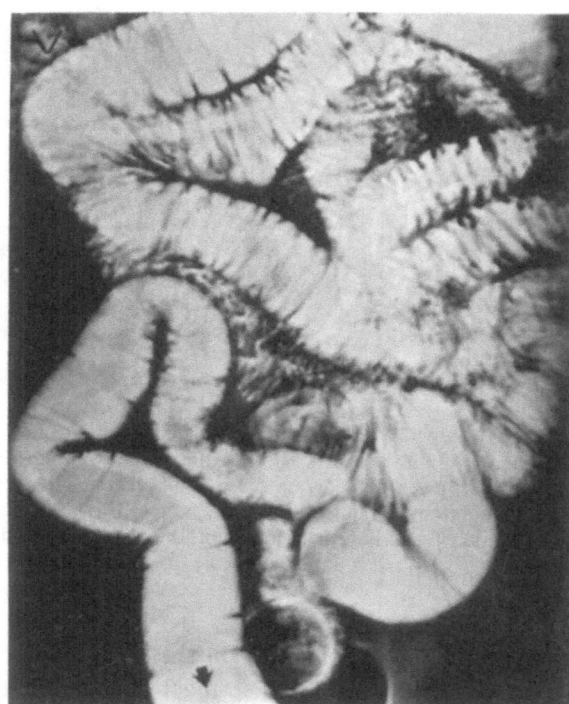

Fig. IV.90. Strikingly pronounced increase in dilatation of the distal ileum, apparently from stagnation of the flow of contrast fluid occasioned by a tumor in the cecum. Motility in the jejunum was completely normal.

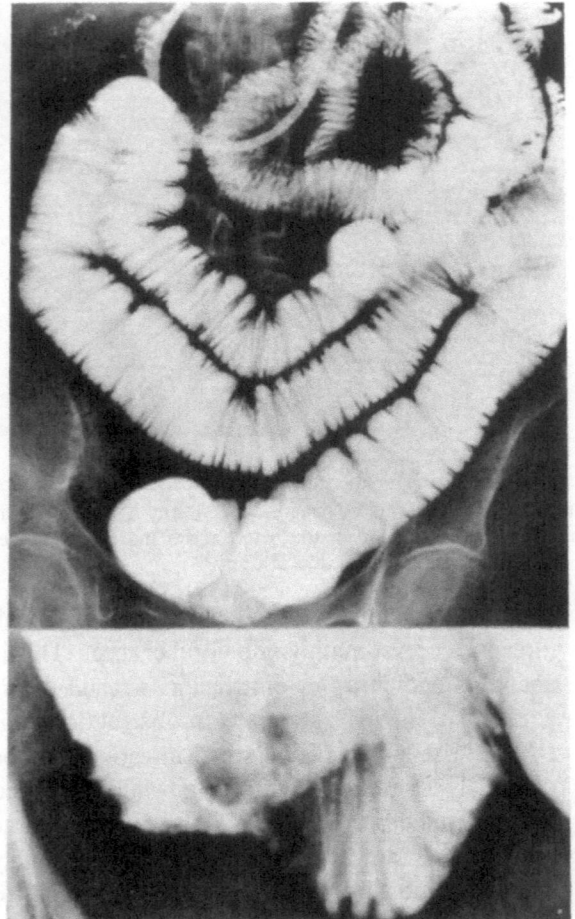

Fig. IV.91. Mechanical obstruction from Hodgkin's disease in the ileum in the lower abdomen. Note the dilatation that increases distally and the normal motility in the proximal jejunum. On this basis, the possibility of a non-obstructing ileus, caused by certain drugs could be eliminated within the first 60 sec of the examination.

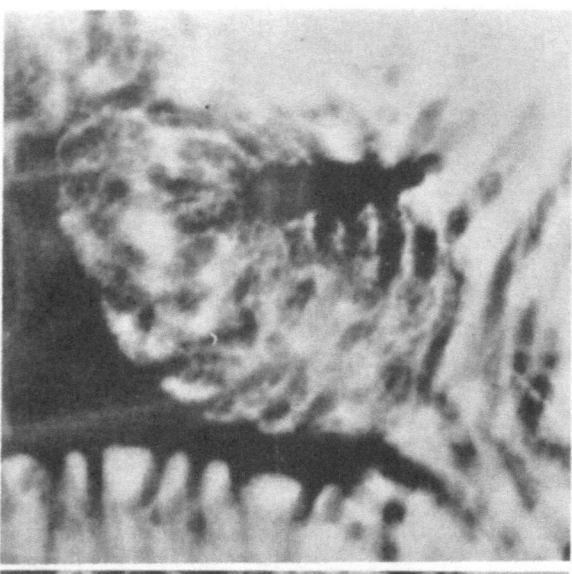

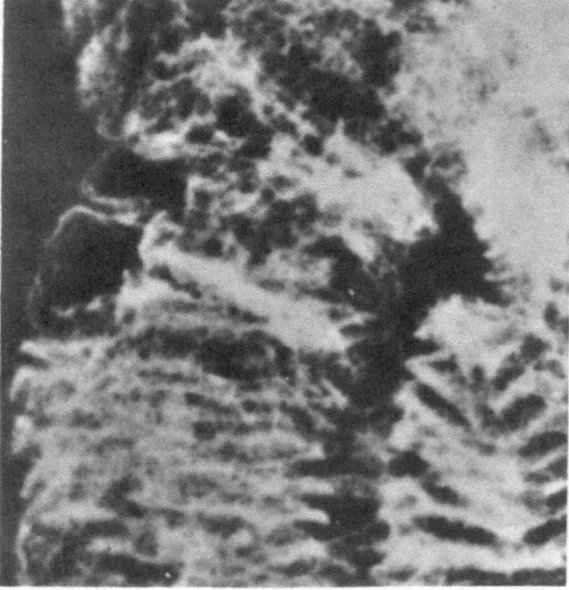

Fig. IV.92. In Whipple's disease the villi can be swollen to some ± 0.5 mm and are visible to the naked eye on endoscopy. On the röntgenogram these villi are difficult to differentiate from foaming of the contrast fluid (fig.III.29). The bubble-like villi, however, interrupt the contours of the intestinal wall.

dilatation can vary and is sometimes so local that sacculations are observed (fig. IV.71). In this stage the patients complain of a 'full stomach' and troublesome flatulence. Obstipation can be so marked that obstruction sometimes develops. The duodenum and jejunum are the most affected so that in a later stage malabsorption may also occur. Obstipation may then be replaced by steatorrhea. Less common, and often not recognized if the other classical symptoms of the disease are missing, are the abnormalities of the stomach. In most cases, a definite atony is seen with gastric dilatation and a decrease in peristaltic movement,

just as in the esophagus. On the other hand, a change in the wall of the stomach due to scleroderma can resemble a linitis plastica or even a local stenosis of the antrum or pylorus. An uneven dilatation of the jejunum together with sacculations is not necessarily due to scleroderma. This

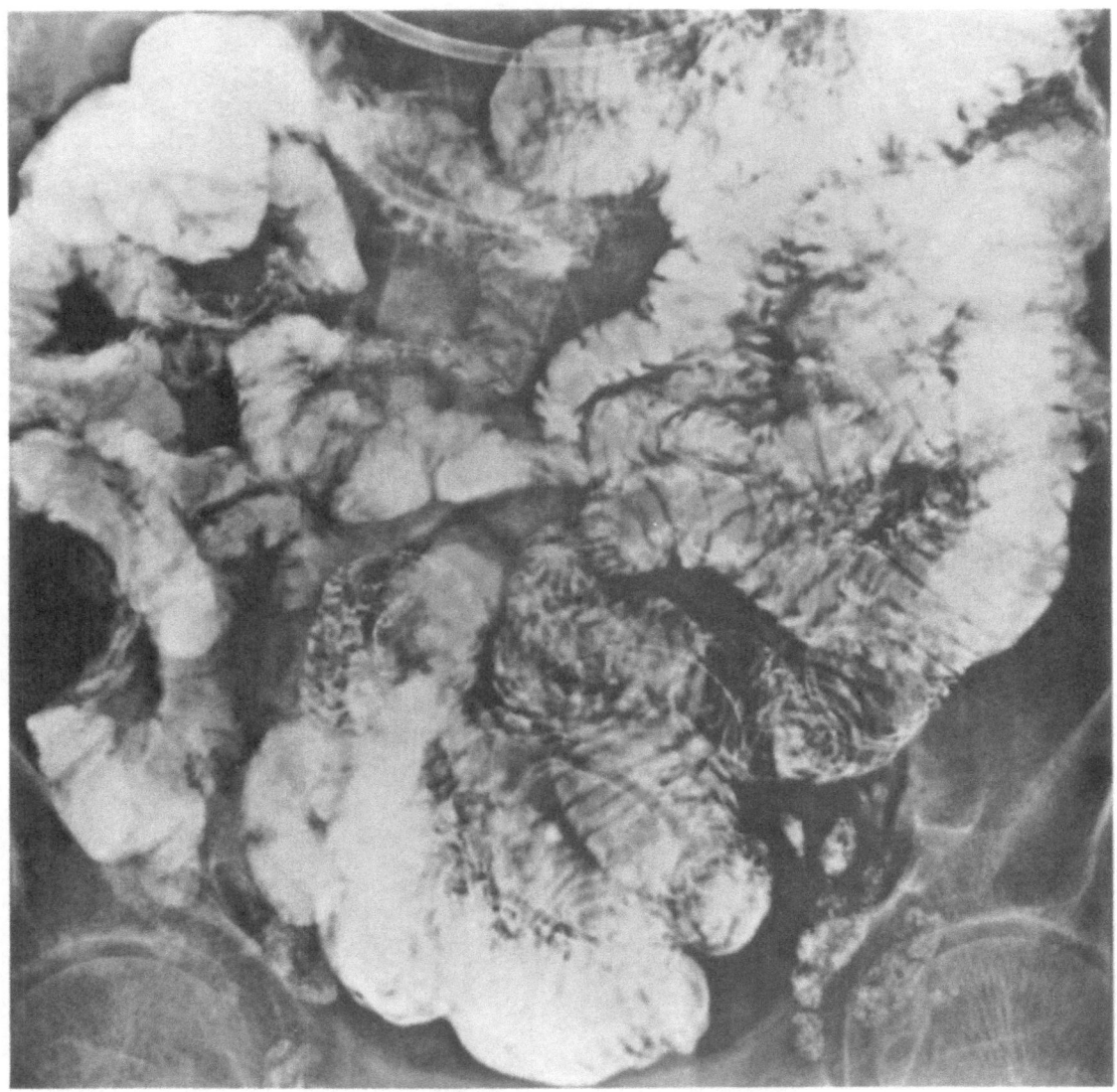

Fig. IV.93. Whipple's disease with increased calibre in the jejunum and ileum as the only sign; normal motility and mucosal relief. The probable diagnosis by biopsy on the basis of the röntgen examination was confirmed. Because motility was normal, and the barium suspension did not flocculate, drug-induced atony and celiac disease were considered unlikely.

combination has been observed in a chronic alcoholic with Wernicke's syndrome (fig. IV.103).

5.4.5. Tropical sprue. Mucosal atrophy in the jejunum is seen in about half the cases of celiac syndrome, but in tropical sprue mucosal atrophy is mainly seen in the ileum. Moreover there is dilatation of the ileum increasing distally and in the jejunum the folds are less pronounced than normal. Clinically serious absorption disturb-

ances are manifest (fig. IV.104).

5.4.6. Post-resection (extensive). Where repeated resection has been performed and the abdominal cavity must be filled with the remaining 1 to 2 metres of small intestine, the bowel compensates this by increasing somewhat in calibre. Motility is normal or slightly increased but medication is often administered to reduce this so that absorption of nutrients is enhanced.

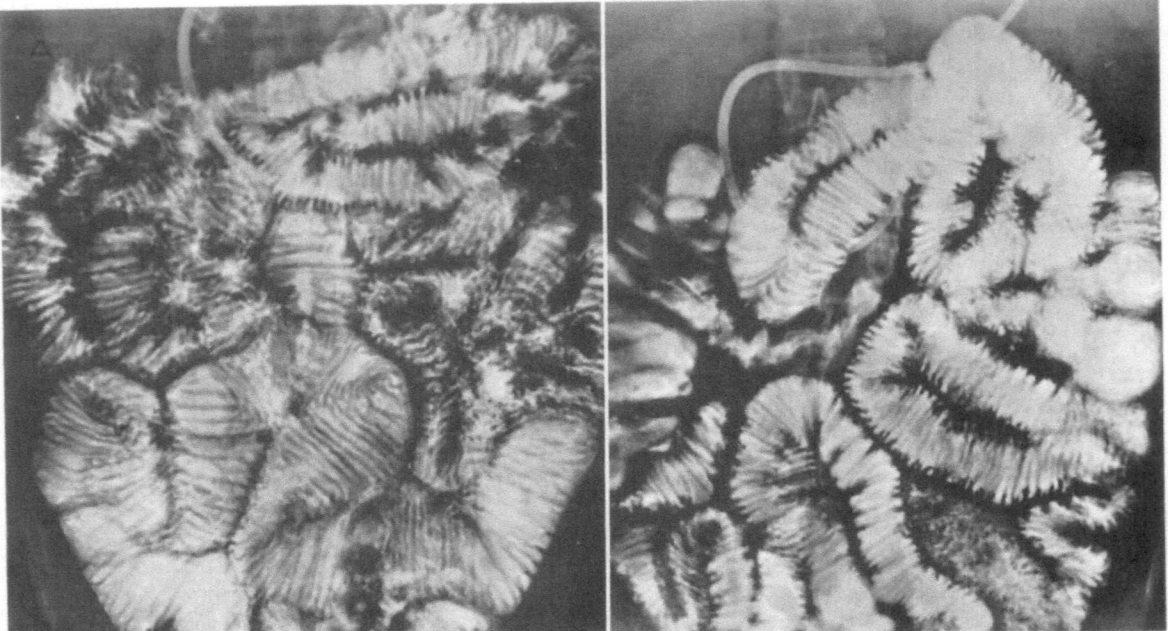

Fig. IV.94. Celiac disease with highly dilated loops in the jejunum and especially the ileum. Transit was so rapid that it was not possible to fill the intestine adequately (left). Radiological improvement after treatment (right).

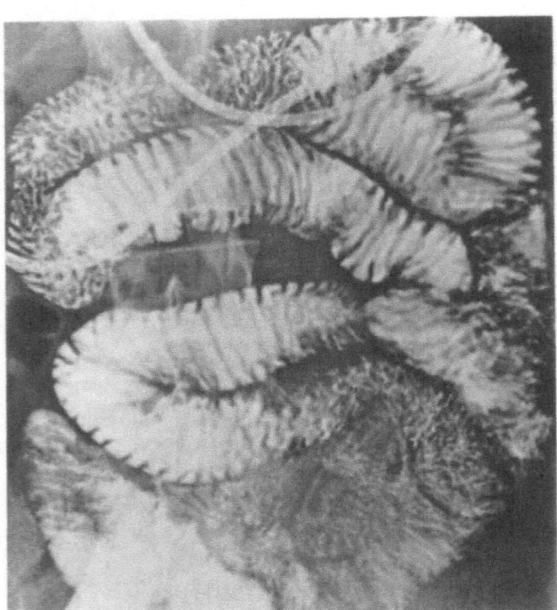

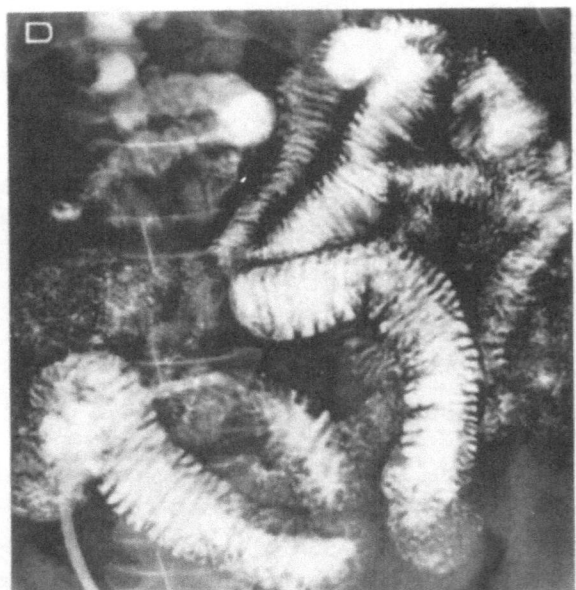

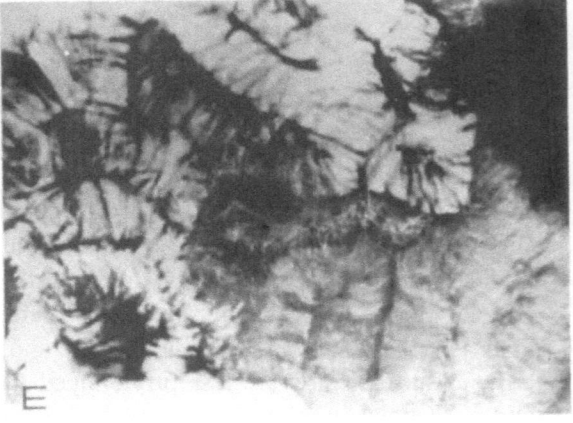

Fig. IV.95. Dilatation of the jejunum and hypermotility, caused by lambliasis. Differential diagnosis should include celiac disease and Whipple's disease. Dilatation is rather usual in lambliasis.

Fig. IV.96. Hypermotility of the intestine accompanied by a dilated lumen in pancreatogenic steathorrea (D). The conventional examination of the same patient showed only dilution and marked flocculation of the contrast fluid (E).

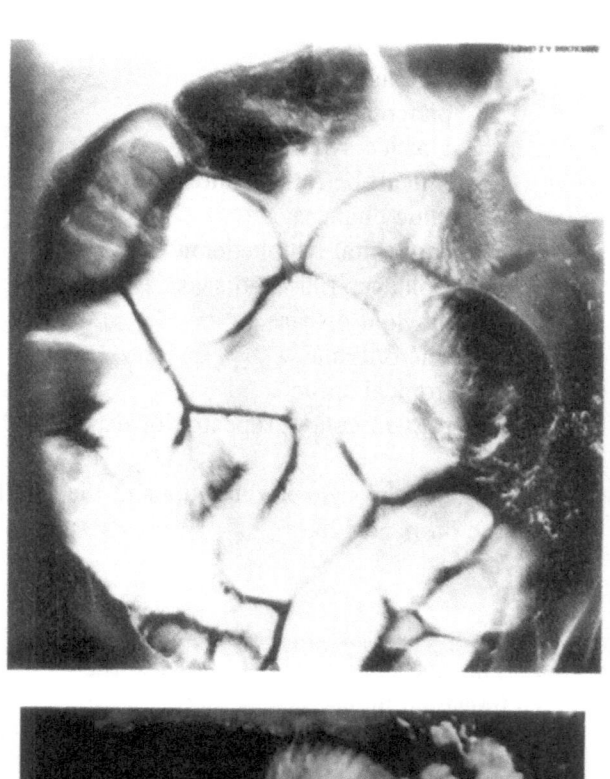

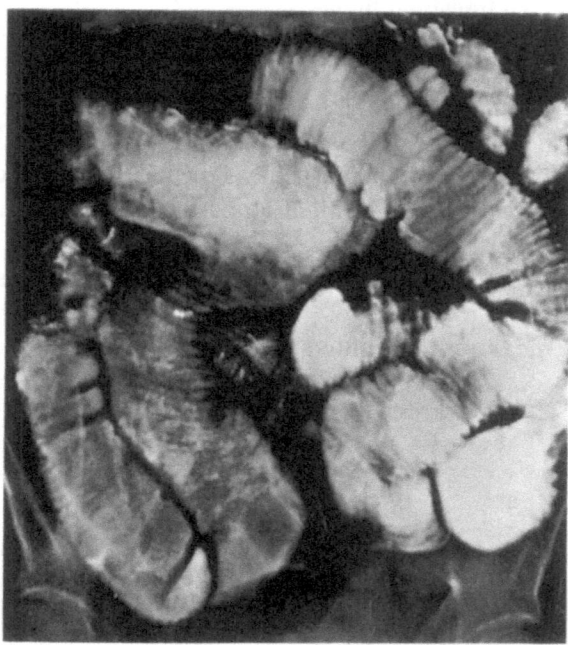

Fig. IV.98. Pronounced flocculation of the contrast fluid in Naish's syndrome. The intestinal loops are markedly dilated, as in the patient in fig. IV.6.

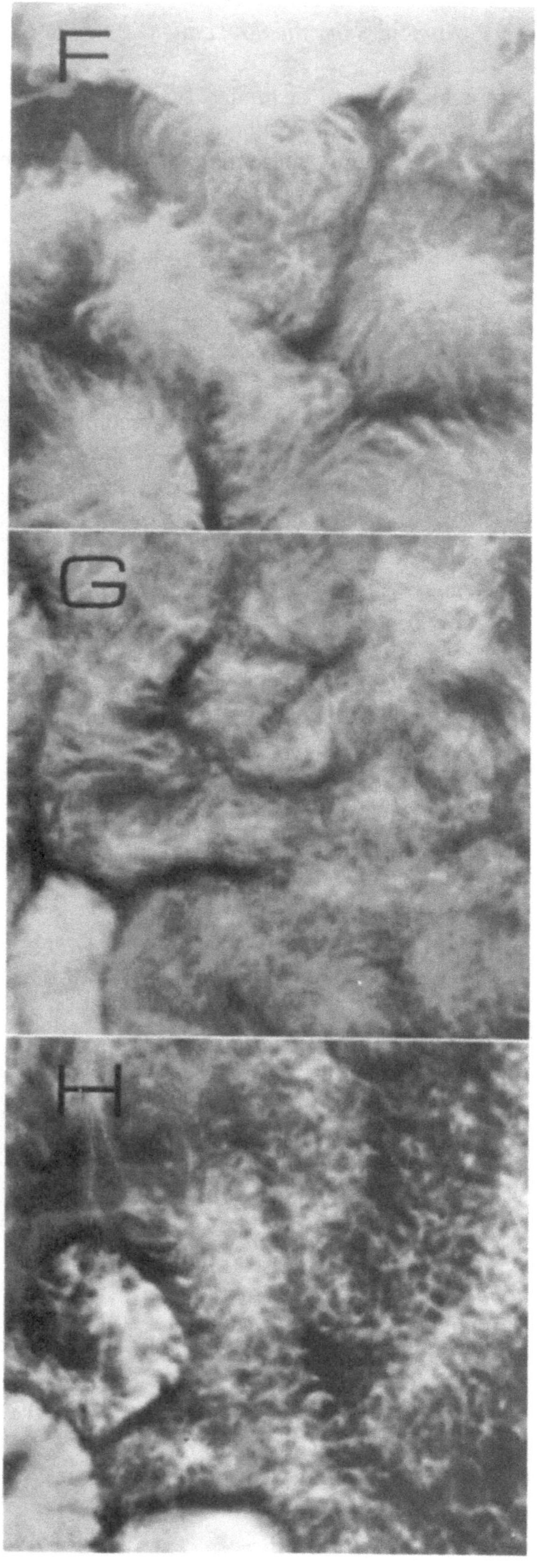

Fig. IV.97. Contrast column with vague margins due to a combination of movement of the intestinal wall, caused by hypermotility, and dilution of the contrast fluid, caused by hypersecretion or disturbed resorption of fluids (F and G). With the infusion technique this vagueness or haziness was less pronounced (H) than during the preceding follow-through examination (F and G).

6. *Summary intestinal dilatation*

Involving a short or limited segment.
    no alteration in mucosa
        superior mesenteric artery syndrome
        crossing bands
        extraluminal carcinoid lesions
        mesenteric fibrosis
        adhesions
        scleroderma
        internal hernia
    thickened mucosal folds
        Crohn's disease or tuberculosis
        post-resection
        vascular insufficiency
        crossing bands
        radiation enteritis
    loss of mucosal pattern
        Crohn's disease or tuberculosis
        tumor growth
        vascular insufficiency
    irregular mucosal pattern
        Crohn's disease or tuberculosis
        radiation enteritis
        tumor growth
        carcinoid disease
    mucosal destruction
        malignant tumor
        non-specific ulceration
        skip lesions in Crohn's disease
    extra-luminal mechanical obstruction
        extramural foci
        adjacent organs
        intramural intestinal foci
    intra-luminal mechanical obstruction
        food residue in distal ileum
        perforating gallstone
        post-operative foreign body in the bowel
        invagination from polyp or tumor
    spasm
Involving a longer segment
    reduced motility
        infusion rate too high
        atony from medication
        amyloid disease
        paralytic or obstructive ileus
    increased motility
        Whipple's disease
        celiac disease

        lambliasis
        pancreatic insufficiency
        Naish's syndrome
    anatomical aberrations and minor or variable
    peristaltic changes
        congenital lymphedema
        Zollinger-Ellison disease
        amyloid disease
        scleroderma
        tropical sprue
        post-resection, repeated or extensive.

Scheme of X-ray signs in dilatations of the small intestine on page 123.

D. The spaces between and outwith the intestinal loops

1. Increased wall thickness

The bowel wall is normally 1-11/2 mm thick, measured on radiographs as the half of the space between two intestinal loops lying in juxtaposition.

    The thickness of the intestinal wall can increase from a variety of causes and thus also the measured loop interspace. These causative factors can be specified as follows:

X-ray signs occurring in:

Dilatations of the small intestine

refers to dilatation · refers to lesion

Diseases	Long segment	Short segment	Solitary	Multiple	Esp. duod. + jejunum	Especially ileum	In entire length	Normal motility	Hypomotility	Hypermotility	Normal mucosa	Fluid levels	Causative lesion	Spasms	Narrowing, stenosis	Edema, thickened wall	Nodular lesions, cobblestones	Abnormal course of folds	Fold destruction	Fold pattern lost
Crohn's or T.B.	●	●	●	●		●	●	●				●	●	●	●	●	●	●	●	●
Non-spec. ulcer.		●	●	●			●	●			●		●	●		●				
Whipple's dis.	●						●	●			●	●								
Giardiasis	●						●				●	●								
Malignant tumor	●	●	●				●	●	●				●		●	●	●	●	●	
Carcinoid		●	●	●	●					●			●					●		
Short bowel	●						●	●			●									
Internal hernia		●	●				●	●	●		●	●	●		●	●		●		
Intussusception		●	●				●	●		●		●			●	●		●		
Bands-ligaments	●	●	●	●		●		●	●		●	●	●	●	●	●		●		
Massive adhesions	●					●	●	●	●				●	●				●		
Ischemia		●	●				●		●				●	●			●			
Mesenteric fibrosis		●	●	●			●						●		●			●		
Radiation enteritis		●	●	●		●	●	●	●				●	●	●	●		●	●	
S.M.A. thrombosis	●					●			●				●	●				●	●	
Too rapid infusion	●				●			●				●								
Drug induced atony	●				●		●	●				●								
S.M.A. syndrome		●	●		●			●	●			●			●		●			
Cong. lymphedema	●						●	●	●								●			
For. body-galstone	●					●					●	●	●		●					
Obstructive ileus	●						●		●		●	●	●		●	●		●	●	
Paralytic ileus	●						●		●		●	●	●			●				
Adult celiac dis.	●						●			●	●									●
Tropical sprue	●					●		●	●											●
Scleroderma	●	●		●			●	●	●	●	●									
Pancreatic insuff.	●						●				●	●								
Naish's syndrome	●						●		●		●	●	●		●					
Zollinger Ellison	●						●	●	●	●							●			
Amyloid disease	●						●	●	●								●	●		●

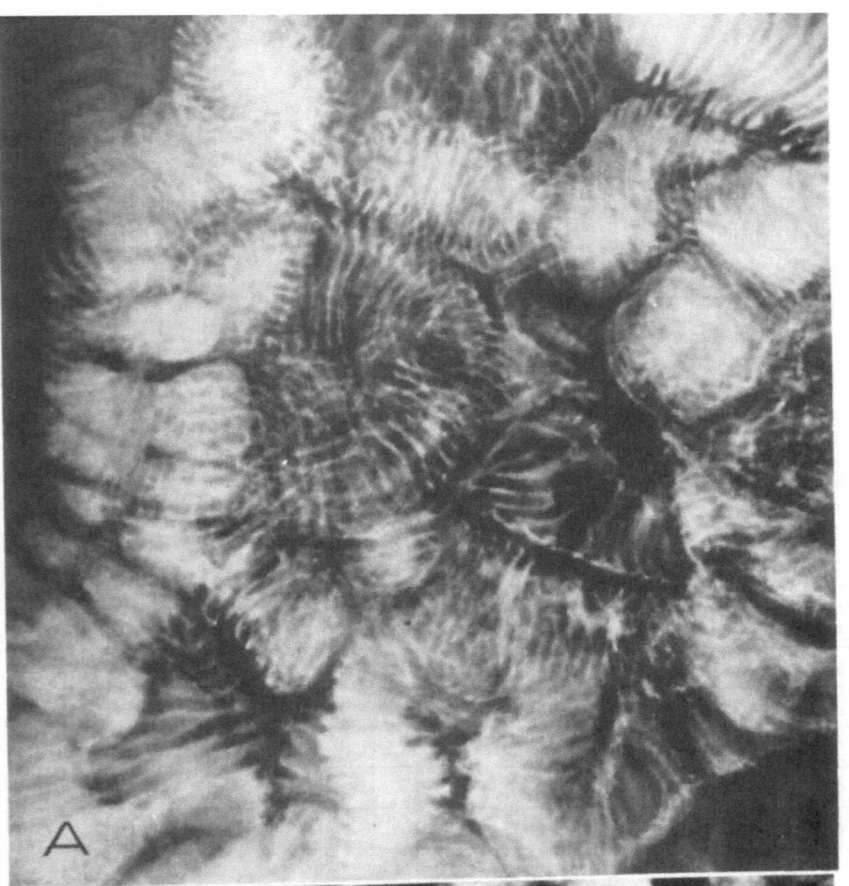

Fig. IV.99A: Lymphedema of congenital origin. It may be difficult to differentiate this pattern from certain forms of celiac disease (fig. IV.94). In celiac disease, however, there is increased motility and in the absence of hypoalbuminemia or secondary infection, the mucosal folds are not thickened.

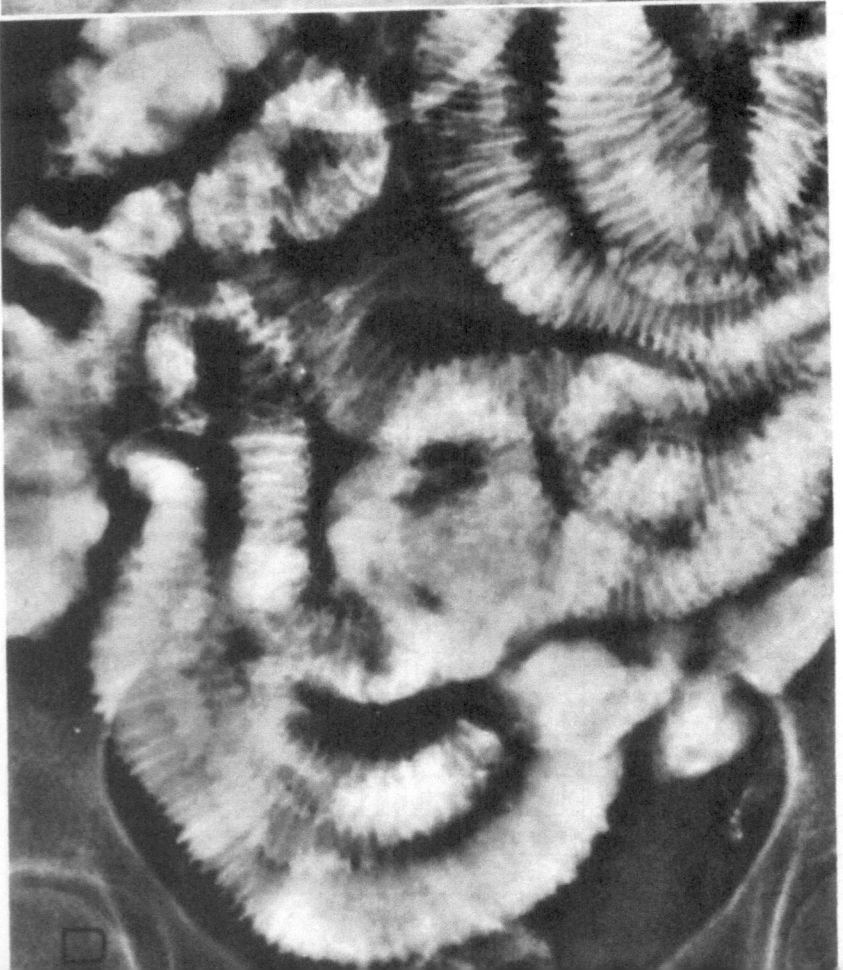

Fig. IV.99D: Post-irradiation lymphedema. Because this edema has developed more acutely than a congenital lymphedema, the mucosal folds are thicker, the wall of the intestine is more rigid and therefore there is less peristaltic activity.

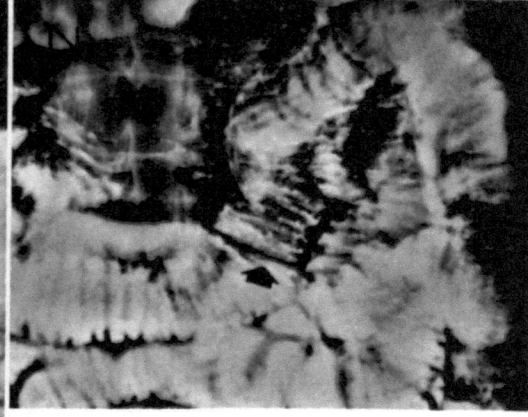

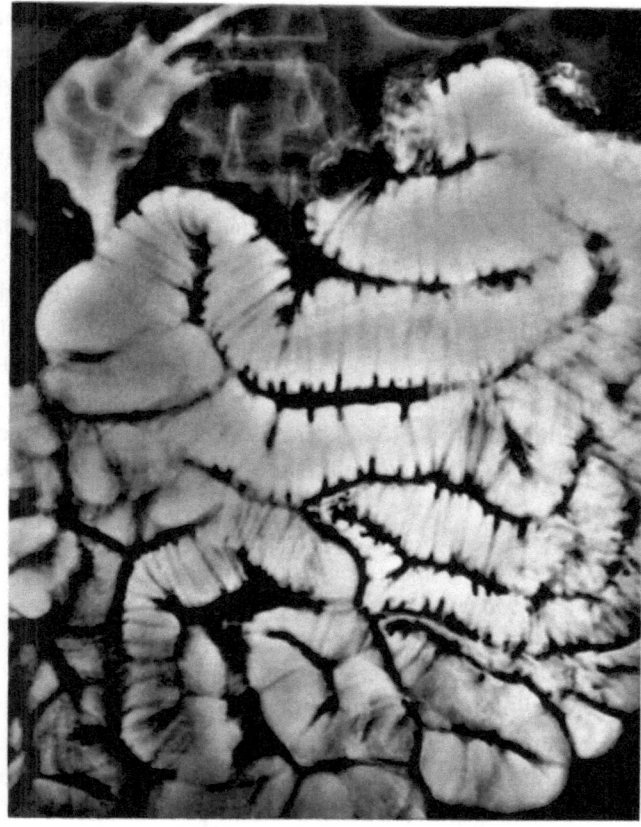

Fig. IV.100. Zollinger-Ellison disease. Moderately dilated intestinal loops in both, ileum and jejunum. Normal motility. Mucosal folds normal; only in the proximal duodenum are they obviously too coarse (M). In spite of the administration of large quantities of contrast fluid to counteract the effect of the responsible intestinal secretions, flocculation developed immediately after termination of the infusion (N).

1.1. Hypoalbuminemia

Loss of protein, whether from disturbance of protein metabolism, inflammatory processes or tumor, results in edematous swelling of the mucosal folds and often, but not inevitably, to thickening of the intestinal wall (fig. IV.105). The space measured between two adjacent loops may increase to some 4 or 5 mm.

1.2. Inflammatory processes

In a number of conditions the thickness of the wall can increase not only from the associated hypoalbuminemia but even more so from interstitial inflammation of the intestinal wall itself. Frequently encountered examples of this are Crohn's disease, paratyphoid (fig. IV.43) or yersinia enterocolitica infections. In Crohn's disease moreover, marked thickening can arise from fatty degeneration of the bowel wall and hypertrophy of the circular muscle (fig. IV.106). A very marked increase in space between the columns of contrast medium in the distal ileum and directly adherent cecum can be seen in the presence of appendicular or other infiltration in this area (fig. IV.107).

1.3. Vascular abnormalities

A similar markedly thickened and also very rigid intestinal wall develops in the presence of impaired arterial or venous blood supply, initially from congestion and edema but in its further course also from necrotising enteritis (fig. IV.34).

Thrombosis with its more severe congestion and inflammatory component gives rise to the most marked thickening of the bowel wall and in addition more pronounced dilatation, but in this case complete recovery can occur (fig. IV.108). Radiation 'enteritis' also shows markedly thickened folds and intestinal wall which, in this considerably more gradually developing process, are for a great deal the result of fibrosis. The mucosa shows as a rule superficial ulcerative changes. Recovery is excluded, increasingly severe stenoses develop in the final stages.

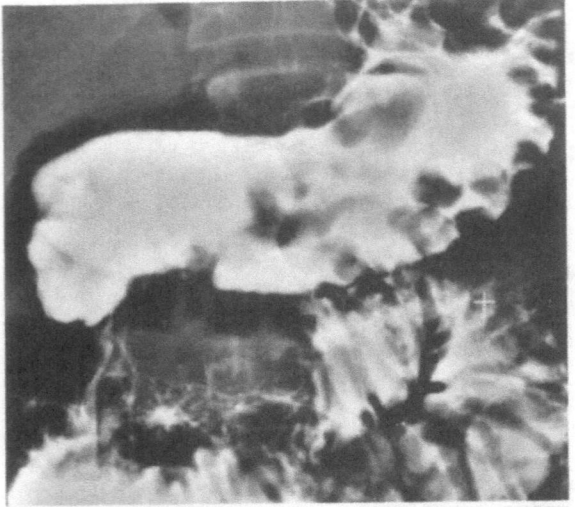

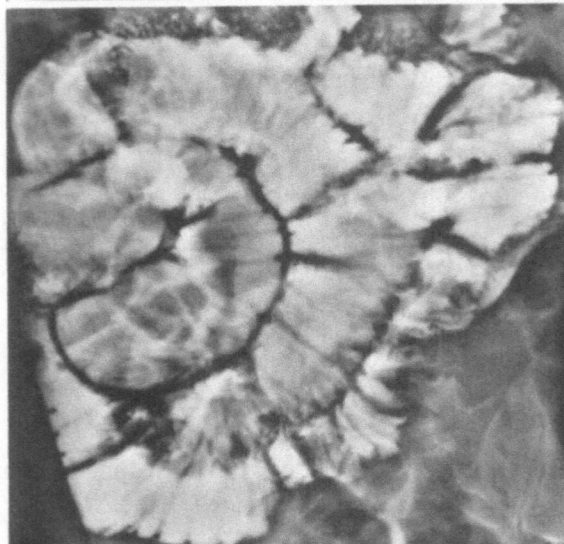

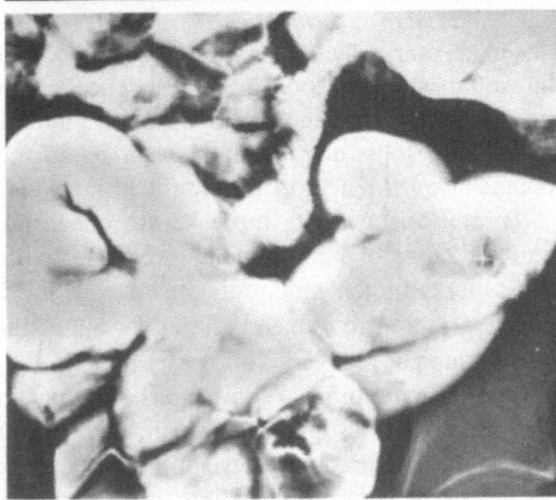

1.4. Tumor growth

Tumors extending in the bowel wall without direct narrowing of the lumen and marked destruction in their vicinity can present as obviously thickened intestinal wall and in the case of malignant lympfomas this can involve quite a long segment (fig. IV.109). Metastases from linitis plastica give a similar picture but it is here more focal with intervening normal areas (fig. IV.41). Such superficial involvement is rare in carcinoid disease and is then in any case confined to a short segment (fig. IV.78). When a superficially growing tumor suddenly assumes a more aggressive character, this gives rise to very irregular and unpredictable increase in width of the intestinal wall (fig. IV.III).

2. Empty spaces between or outwith the bowel loops

2.1. Peritoneal and mesenteric fat

A voluminous omentum can result in lacunae central in the abdomen or scattered among the intestinal loops (fig. III.12). A convolution of the intestinal loops in the minor pelvis is but very rarely seen in the pyknic somatype (fig. IV.112).

2.2. Mesenteric fibrosis

Kinking or angulation of intestinal loops as well as extensive mutual fusion or adhesions can be seen in retractile or sclerosing mesenteritis. This rare disorder is also accompanied by pronounced fatty degeneration and post-infectious shrivelling of the mesentery (fig. IV.5). As a result of the pronounced shortening and increased contracture of the mesentery, there are only a few intestinal loops in the centre of the abdomen. The lumen of the intestine can vary in size, the mucosal relief remains rather unchanged.

2.3. Inflammatory disease

A degeneration or contracture of the mesentery can also lead to empty spaces in the central abdomen. Together with an increase in mesenteric

Fig. IV.101. Zollinger-Ellison disease. Very coarse mucosal folds in the stomach, duodenum and jejunum with pronounced dilatation of the loops in the jejunum and the ileum.

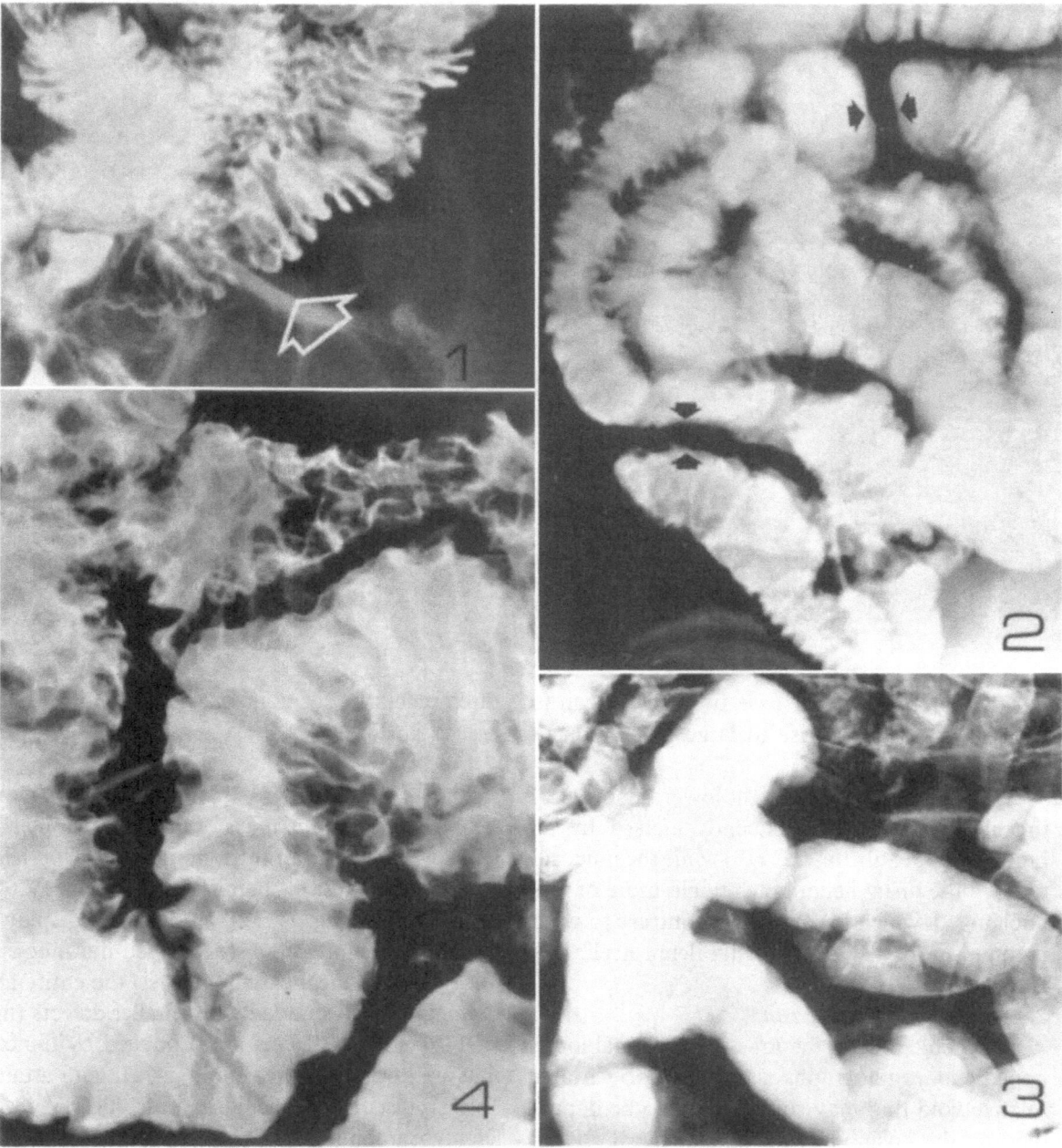

Fig. IV.102. Abnormalities, increasing in severity, in four patients with primary amyloidosis of the small intestine. (1) Decreased motility in the small bowel and mucosal folds with a slightly undulant course in some regions (arrow). (2) No clear-cut abnormalities in the jejunum (not shown). In the ileum the mucosal relief is flattened and the intestinal wall is thickened. Differentiation from a lymphoma is not really possible. After remission of Crohn's disease the intestinal wall is neither as thick nor as rigid (stiff). (3) Flat mucosal relief throughout almost the entire small bowel. (4) Greatly thickened intestinal wall and broad irregular mucosal folds that in places can no longer be recognized. There are multiple nodular amyloid deposits and unequal dilatation of the intestinal lumen.

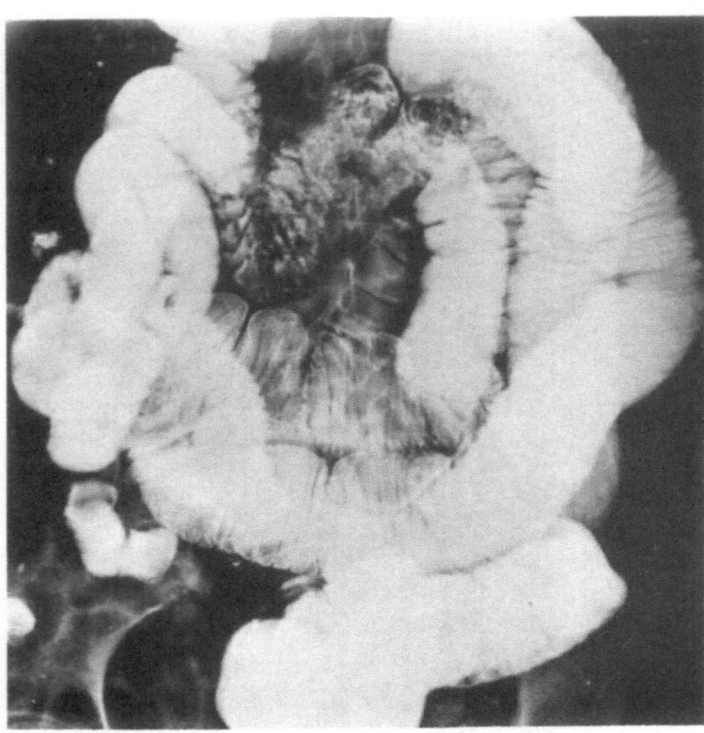

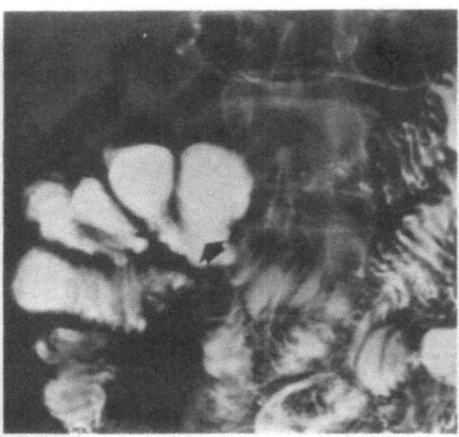

Fig. IV.103. Unequal dilatation of the jejunum and the ileum with sacculations (arrow) in a chronic alcoholic with Wernicke's syndrome. Normal stomach. Mucosal folds in the proximal jejunum are broadened (not visible here); This is a normal finding in alcoholics but has not been encountered in patients with scleroderma.

fat, the combination of these two factors can in Crohn's disease give rise to large empty spaces (fig. IV.86).

An empty space in the right lower quadrant of the abdomen is very frequently caused by an inflamed appendix (fig. IV.113) while the mucosal folds in the distal ileum may remain more or less unchanged, which is completely contrary to what is found in disease of the distal ileum itself.

2.4. *Adhesions and spasm*

A contractile area in the mass of intestinal loops appears on radiographs as a sort of variable relative void that may sometimes also be dependant on the position of the patient (fig. IV.114).

Adhesions are characterized by extended feather-like fold patterns arising from passive extension due to contraction of neighbouring adherent loops (fig. IV.115). Since adhesions have a pronounced preference for the lower abdomen, contractile areas can here and particularly after repeated surgical intervention, sometimes be very extensive (fig. IV.58). Somewhat vacuous areas caused by local contractility from carcinoid foci are infrequently seen (fig. IV.64). A similar pic-

ture, regularly seen, is provided by irradiated areas (fig. IV.117).

2.5 *Tumors*

Lesser defects in the mass of intestinal loops can be caused by ,e.g. an intra-murally growing leiomyoma (fig. IV.28), a carcinoid focus (fig. IV.65) or metastases (fig. IV.39), all of which display a picture of compression or stretched-out mucosal folds. In peritoneal carcinomatosis the entire abdominal area is studded with smaller defects (fig. IV.116). Larger defects are produced by tumors that are known for their rapid growth and attainable size such as reticulosarcoma (fig. IV.48z), leiomyosarcoma (fig. IV.48Y) or Hodgkin's disease (fig. IV.42).

2.6. *Cysts and organs*

A mesenteric cyst (fig. IV.118) shows a sharply defined ovoid defect that is better visualized with the auto-compression of the prone position than in the supine. A similar sharply defined defect, but positioned marginally, can be caused by an enlarged prostate (fig. IV.33), liver or spleen, or a transplanted kidney (fig. III.10).

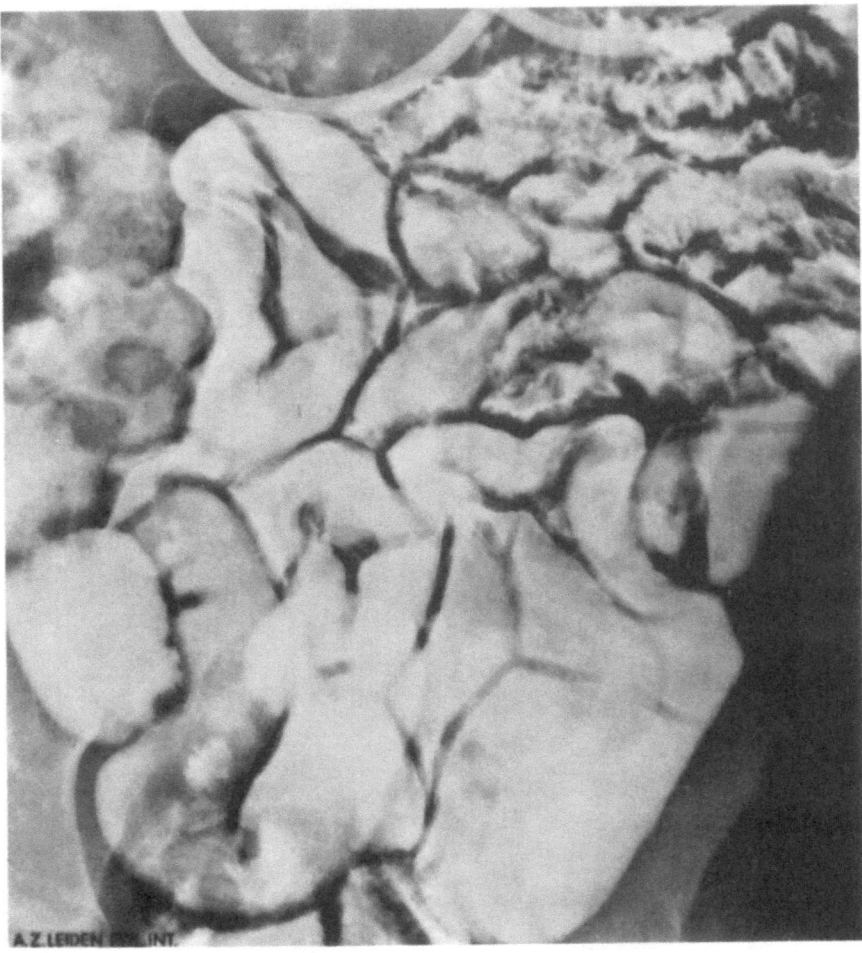

Fig. IV.104. An eight-year-old boy with a growth deficiency of several years'duration. The röntgenogram showed pronounced mucosal atrophy. In the ileum absolutely no folds were visible. In the jejunum they were noticeably shortened. Moreover, there was an increased tendency towards flocculation of the barium suspension and a marked dilatation of the ileum. The nature of these abnormalities that caused a disturbance resorption remained unknown. While definitely not celiac disease, it may well have been some similar condition such as tropical sprue (see also page 61 and 119).

2.7. Perforation of the bowel

Perforation should be considered where all available spaces between the loops in the lower abdominal region are filled with a vague milky shadowing (fig. IV.120). It should further be borne in mind that the patient may be completely unaware of the condition as clinical symptoms appear only after several hours.

2.8. Diverse causes

In case of doubt in the assessement of filling defects or impressions on the bowel lumen Chapter III.C2 should be consulted.

3. Barium configurations projecting from or lying without the normal bowel

3.1. Adhesions

Although an adhesion can be somewhat flattened (fig. IV.57) the majority are pointed and sometimes even very long (figs. IV.57 and IV.59). They occur very frequently and are far and away most common in the lower half of the abdomen.

3.2. Ulcers, fistulous tracts and abcesses

Large ulcers, malignant or not, are rarely seen and present mainly in the duodenum (fig. IV.121), the

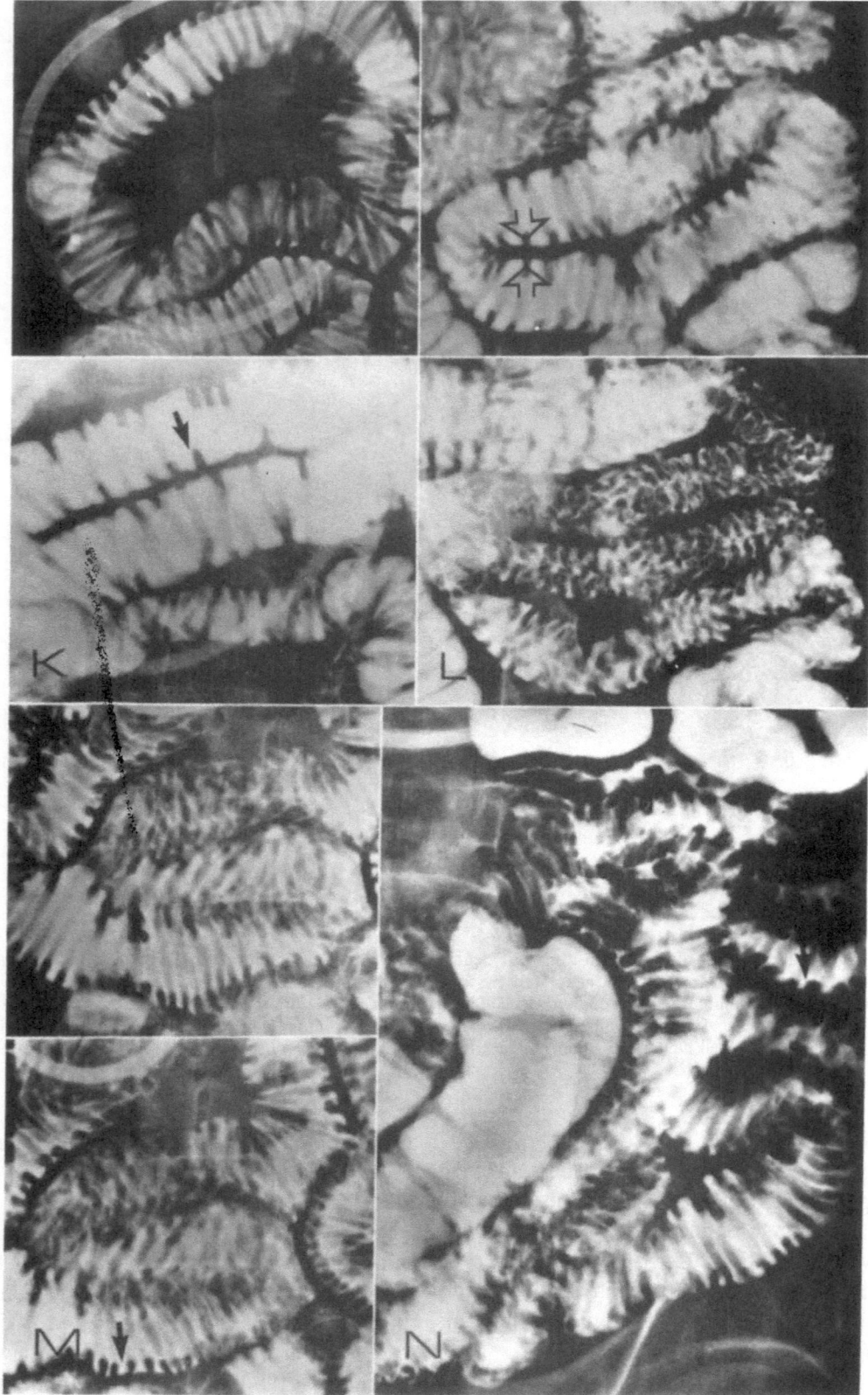

Fig. IV.105. Four patients with edematous swollen folds due to hypo-albuminemia. (K) Swollen folds only, no thickening of the intestinal wall. (L) Swollen folds and thickening of the intestinal wall. (M) Biconvex or omega-shaped folds but no thickening of the intestinal wall. The patient has Crohn's disease of the colon. (N) Omega-shaped folds and thickened wall in the bowel of a patient with celiac disease.

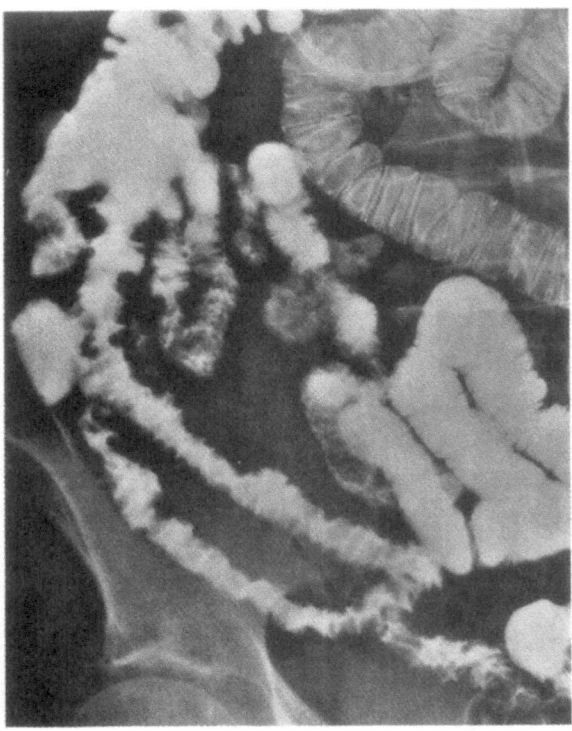

Fig. IV.106. Larger translucent spaces between intestinal loops as a result of an inflammatory infiltrate or a layer of fat encircling the intestine in Crohn's disease.

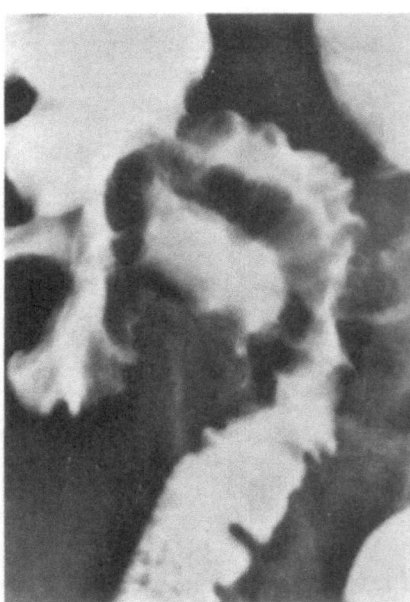

Fig. IV.107. Infiltrate of unknown origin in ileocecal region. Surgery revealed that the large oval accumulation of contrast medium was an ulcer crater. No indications of appendicitis or Crohn's disease.

ileocecal region and at the site of a Meckel's diverticulum. A remarkable picture is formed by very pointed projections, at least a centimetre long, at the site of a non-specific ulcer that has become stenotic by contracture. The appearance is probably due to prolapse of normal bowel mucosa between two fibrous rings (fig. IV.31κ). Small ulcers are very frequently seen and in practice mostly in Crohn's disease. Generally these are quite small projections, some 1 to 2 mm deep, outside the contrast column (fig. IV.122). If the projections are deeper (5-10 mm), then the bowel wall is already perforated and a fistula canal or its beginning is present (fig. IV.123). Fistulas may be very extensive and sometimes require special techniques for their effective visualization (figs. II.16 and II.17).

Abcesses occur regularly in the abdominal cavity but usually lack open communication with the gut so that they are not visualized in an examination with contrast medium. Two examples of an abcess with open communication into the gut are shown in fig. IV.124; an amoebic abcess in the right lower quadrant and another in the pouch of Douglas.

3.3. Diverticula and sacculations
3.3.1. Meckel's diverticulum.
Enteroclysis technique has certainly improved the disappointing results in X-ray diagnosis of a Meckel's diverticulum. However, it is still overlooked in the majority of cases, in particular if other conspicuous abnormalities are found during the examination. This diverticulum is located on the anti-mesenteric side of the intestine, usually about 80 cm (20-100) from the ileocecal valve. Its length can vary from negligable to several centimetres and it is freely mobile in the abdominal cavity.

To discover a Meckel's diverticulum, it is essential that several spot films be made of the diverse ileal loops in different projections with assistance of a good compression technique. During the examination these films must be studied carefully so that further detailed studies can be carried out in case of doubt. If this is neglected, most Meckel's diverticula, even the large ones, will assuredly be missed (fig. IV.125). In particular the presence of a diverticulum should also be suspected if suggestive configura-

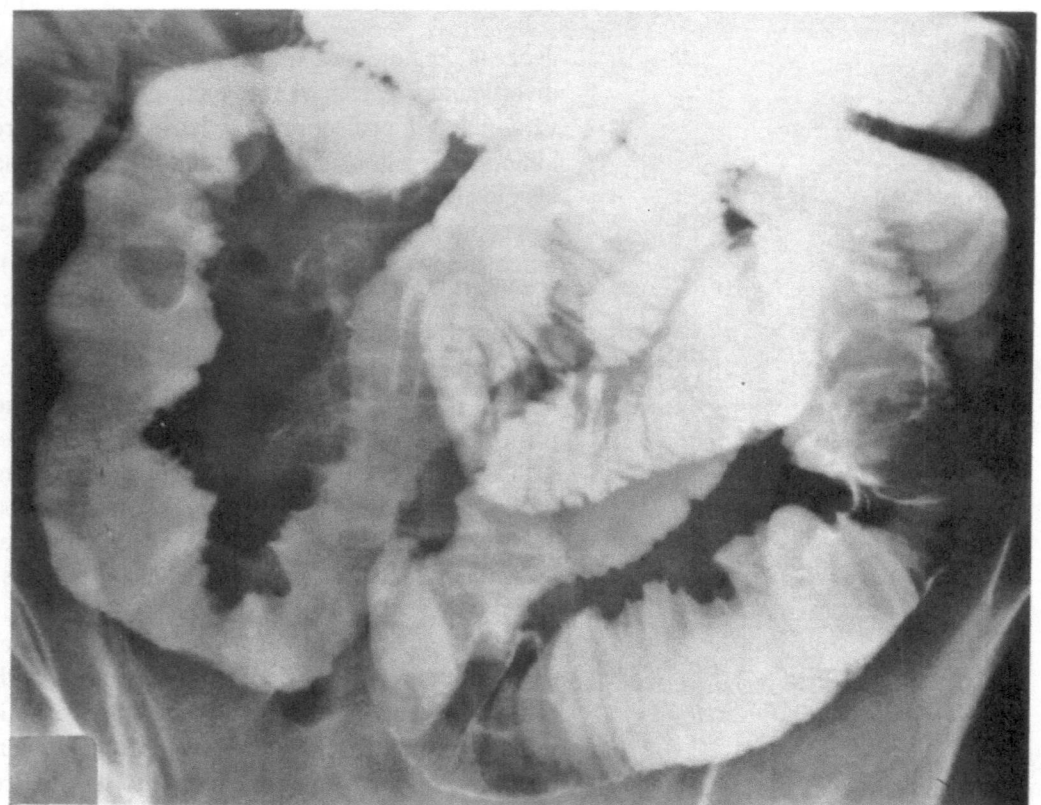

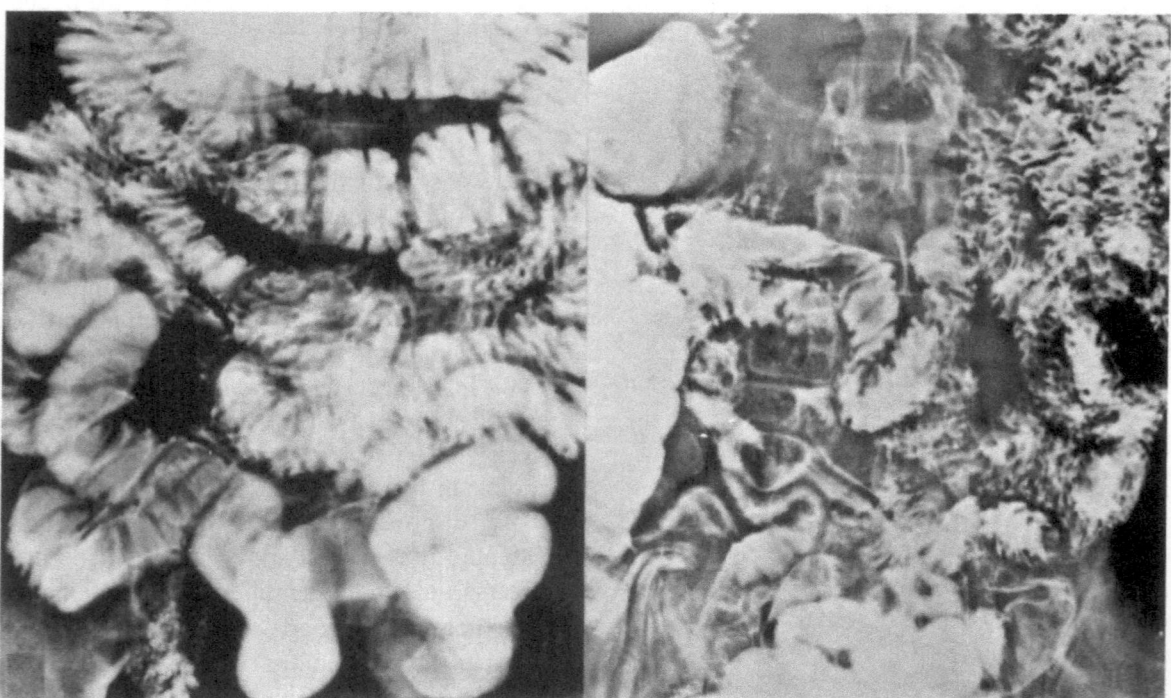

with an elevated erythrocyte sedimentation rate and a leucocytosis of 12,000/mm³. The X-rays show dilated loops with thickened walls, markedly broadened mucosal folds and 'thumbprinting'. Several weeks later a laparotomy revealed a white, markedly hyperemic ileal loop, which was 1 m long, and numerous mesenteric lymphomas. Resection was not carried out and the patient gradually recovered spontaneously. A follow-up X-ray taken several weeks later showed excellent recovery with few residual phenomena, at the most, fewer folds in the ileum (below).

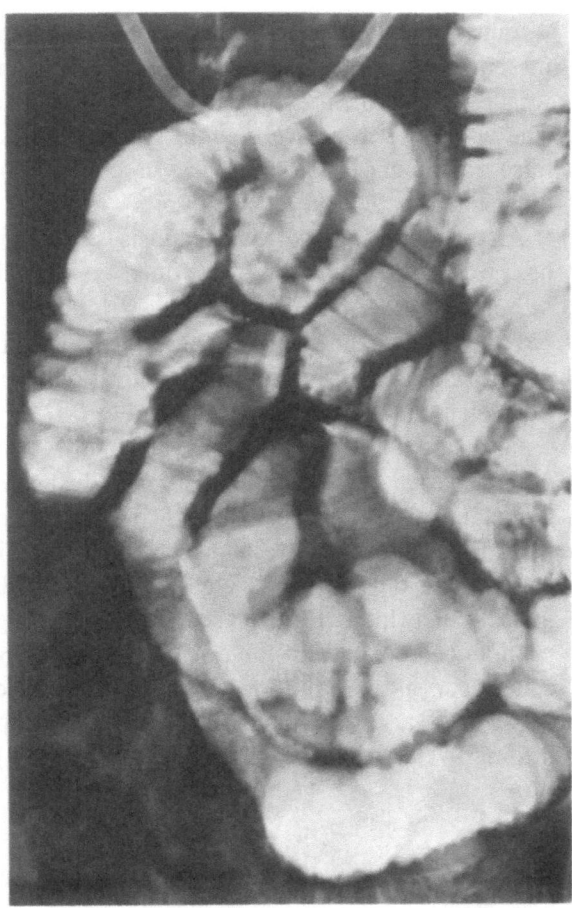

Fig. IV.109. Malignant lymphoma involving almost the entire ileum with thickened rigid intestinal wall and obliterated mucosal folds. The lumen of the intestine is slightly dilated.

tions, showing no signs of mucosal ridges, are visualized (fig. IV.126).

If a triangular shadow, as seen in fig. IV.127 is encountered anywhere in the mucosal patterns of the intestinal loops, then this is certainly the junction with the omphalo-enteric duct. A Meckel's diverticulum is therefore present, even if it cannot be visualized further on the X-rays. Two other examples are shown in figs. IV.128 and IV.129. A frequently encountered misleading pattern is the round diverticulum shadow that is in fact an axial projection of an intestinal loop (fig. IV.130). Another fake pattern is the configuration that resembles a blind sac but actually is the front of the advancing column of barium suspension (fig. IV.131).

3.3.2. Congenital diverticula and acquired diverticula. Congenital diverticula are situated on the anti-mesenteric side of the intestine. They involve the tunica muscularis and are therefore contractile.

The mucosal folds in the intestinal wall can be followed through the neck of the diverticulum (fig. IV.132). In practice however, this cannot always be determined with certainty so that differentiation between a congenital anomaly and an acquired diverticulum is usually not possible.

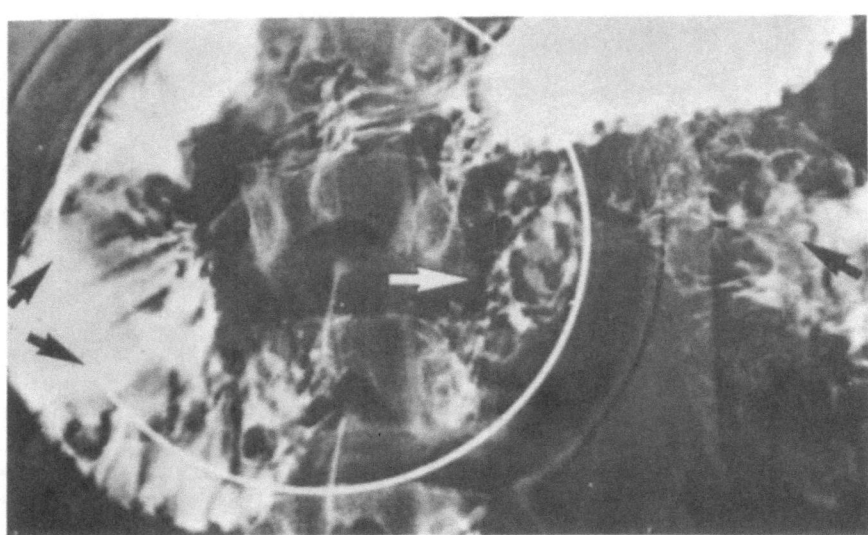

Fig. IV.110. Polyps of differing size in the duodenum in a patient with Peutz-Jeghers syndrome. (Courtesy Dr. J.R. Achterberg – Leiden).

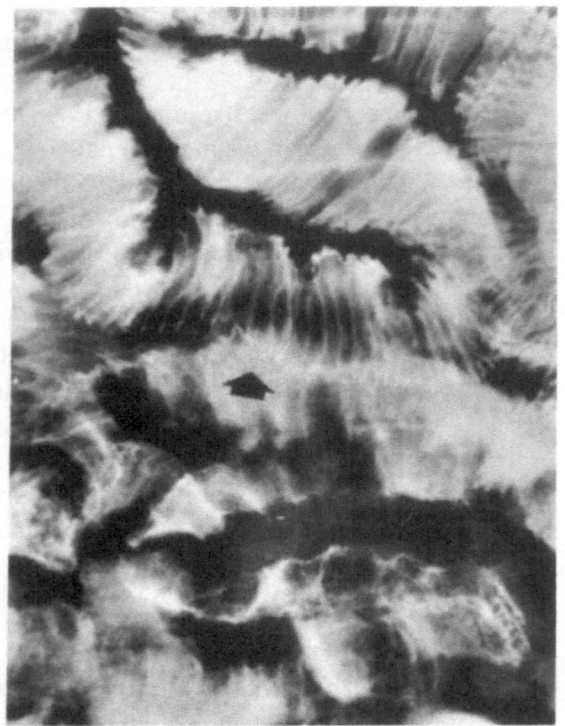

Fig. IV.111. Pronounced edema and obviously thickened wall of the intestine in a case of lymphoreticular malignancy.

Acquired diverticula are usually located on the mesenteric side of the intestine where the wall is weakest due to the presence of vascular openings. The wall of such a diverticulum is thin and like false diverticula in Crohn's disease, contains no muscular layer.

An example of jejunal diverticulosis is shown in fig. IV.133. Normally there is a decrease in their size and number distally.

Diverticula in the distal ileum are small and rare and are chiefly the result of hypertonia and hyperperistalsis (figs. IV.77 and IV.112).

Occasionally a volvulus may develop or in other cases a diverticulitis or dyspeptic complaints, arising from disturbance in the bacterial flora as a result of stasis. Mechanical complications can develop especially if the diverticula are extremely large. If the mesentery is extra long, pronounced changes in the position of the loops can occur as a result of changes in posture. Torsion of a diverticulum may easily develop, leading to necrosis and perforation (fig. IV.134).

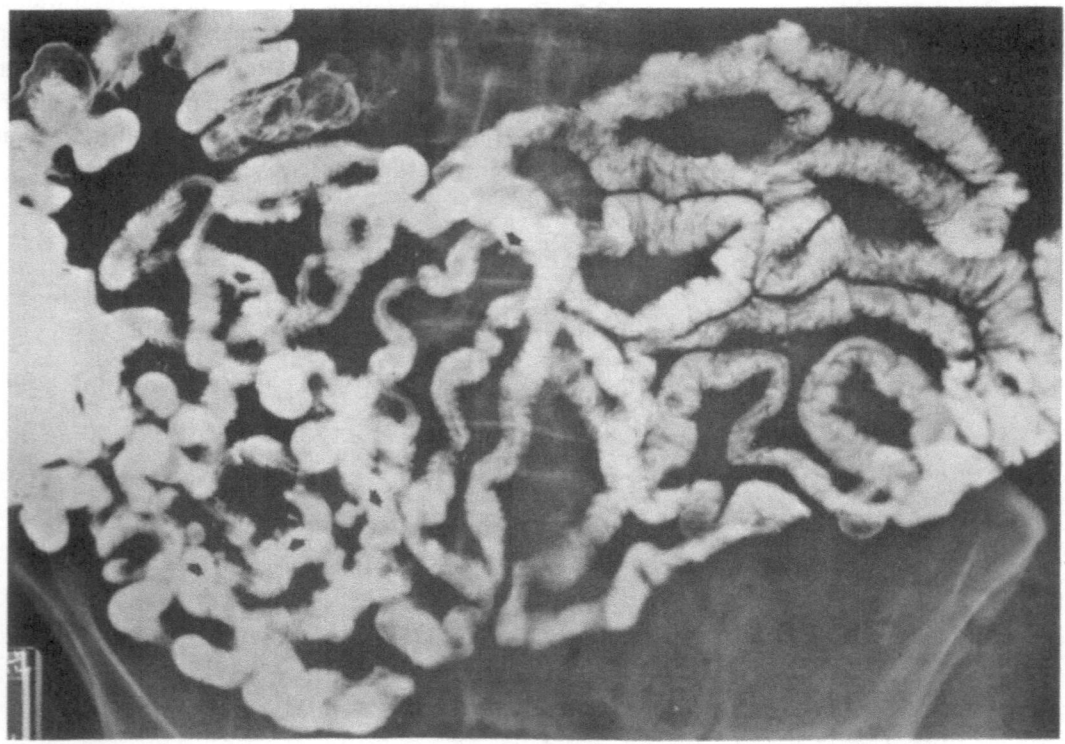

Fig. IV.112. Hypertonicity of the small intestine with decreased diameter of the lumen in a very obese patient. This hypertonicity, which is usually caused by a diminished arterial blood flow, is also the cause of the numerous diverticula of different size that can be seen in the ileum.

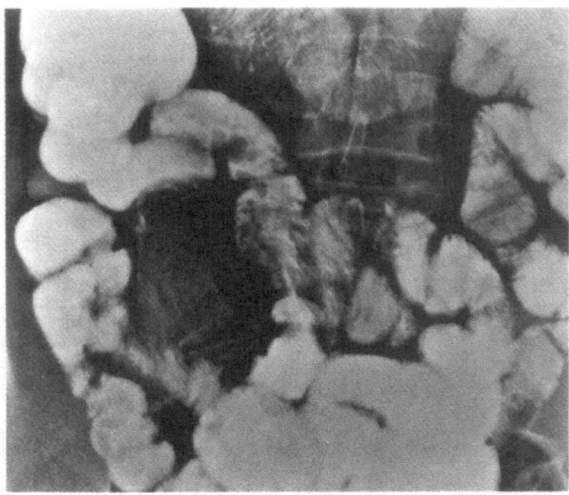

Fig. IV.113. Translucent space between the intestinal loops in the right lower abdomen as a result of an appendicular infiltrate.

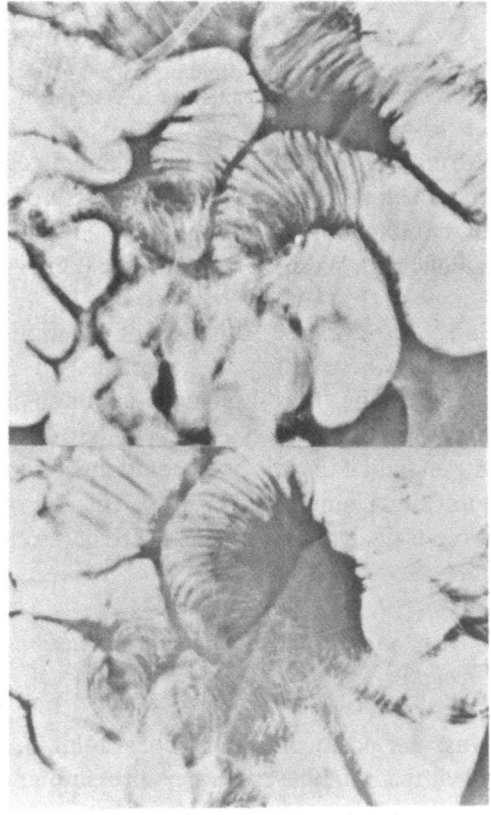

Fig. IV.114. Fusion of intestinal loops to an abcess on the abdominal wall, not or barely visible on the plain film (upper). The compression spot film shows that the mucosal folds in the intestinal loops are definitely stretched and that fusion prevents contraction of these loops (lower).

Perforation can occur during duodenal intubation if the location of the diverticulum is unfavorable (fig. IV.135).

3.3.3. False diverticula. False diverticula in Crohn's disease are easily differentiated from other diverticula because they form in an obviously diseased intestinal wall. There is pronounced hypertrophy of the muscular layers in the wall of the intestine. This hypertrophy causes prolonged spasms in the involved intestinal segment. An intraluminal increase in pressure in these loops may lead to herniation of the intact mucosa through the intestinal wall. Fluoroscopic examination shows that these so-called 'false diverticula' alternate in size (fig. IV.136). False diverticula are lined with mucosal tissue only and consequently are extremely thin walled. They are situated on the mesenteric side of the intestine and have to be differentiated from yet another type of diverticula, the so-called pseudo-diverticula (fig. IV.137 and IV.119).

3.3.4. Pseudo diverticula – Fibrotic sacculations. Pseudo diverticula are usually situated on the anti-mesenteric side of the intestine and contain all layers of the intestinal wall. They are formed by contractions or fibrotic rings originating in the intact intestinal wall opposite the site of an ulceration at the mesentery attachment that has healed with fibrous degeneration and contracture. In contrast to false diverticula which are spherical with a narrow and sometimes long neck, they usually appear to be much larger, vary in shape and are attached to the wall of the intestine by a more or less broad base (fig. IV.137 and IV.119).

Ulcers due to ischemia or from skip lesions in Crohn's disease can heal with pronounced asymmetric contracture. Especially in the distal ileum this can result in a bizarre sacculation between two sites of severe stenosis, resembling a scallop and called therefore the 'shell sign' (fig. IV.32).

3.3.5. Auto amputations. Care must be taken not to consider all multiple sac-like bulges in the intestine as diverticula. One such case for example, is illustrated in fig IV.138. Four or five diverticula – like formations are seen originating from one point and appearing to vary in size from

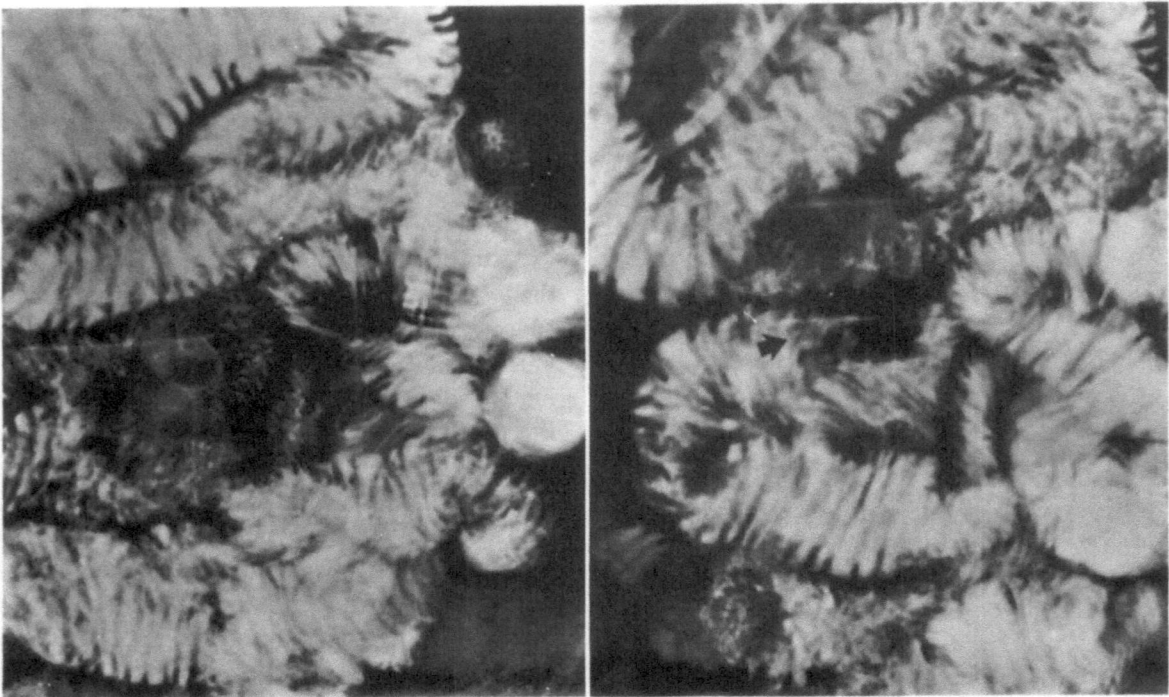

Fig. IV.115. Adhesions after abdominal surgery; displacement of these loops by means of compression and palpation was not possible. In one of the two segments in the contraction phase, the feathered mucosal pattern (arrow) is clearly visible.

2 to 20 cm. It was found that they had developed from multiple auto-amputations after surgical treatment of a hernia during adolescence. It was no longer possible to determine the role played by erroneously placed sutures in the development of this peculiar anatomical phenomenon

3.3.6. *Sacculation in scleroderma and Wernicke's syndrome.*

In scleroderma the layers of smooth muscle in the digestive tract become atrophied and are replaced by fibrous tissue. This leads to decreased peritalsis, hypotonic dilatations and finally sometimes to stenosis. Not well known but still encountered in one-half of patients is a descreased peristalsis in and dilatation of the small intestine. The degree of dilatation can vary and is sometimes so local that sacculations are observed (figs. IV.139 and IV.71). In this stage the patients complain of a 'full stomach' and troublesome flatulence. Obstipation can be so marked that obstruction may develop. The duodenum and jejunum are the most affected so that in a later stage malabsorption may also occur. Obstipation may then be replaced by steatorrhea.

An uneven dilatation of the jejunum together with sacculations need not be due to scleroderma. This combination has been noted in a chronic alcoholic with Wernicke's syndrome (fig. IV.103).

3.3.7. *Duplications.*

Although duplications can occur anywhere along the entire length of the small intestine, they are most common in the ileum. The duplication may become filled with contrast fluid if there is open communication with the intestinal lumen. (fig. IV.140). This is however not often the case and the space remains closed.

4. *Gas shadows outside the contrast fluid column*

In vascular accidents the mucosal folds become swollen from increased venous pressure and the subsequent development of edema. The impressions of these broadened mucosal folds on the contrast column are called 'thumbprinting'. In the ileum the folds are so scanty and short that the pattern resembles a stiff tube with smooth walls.

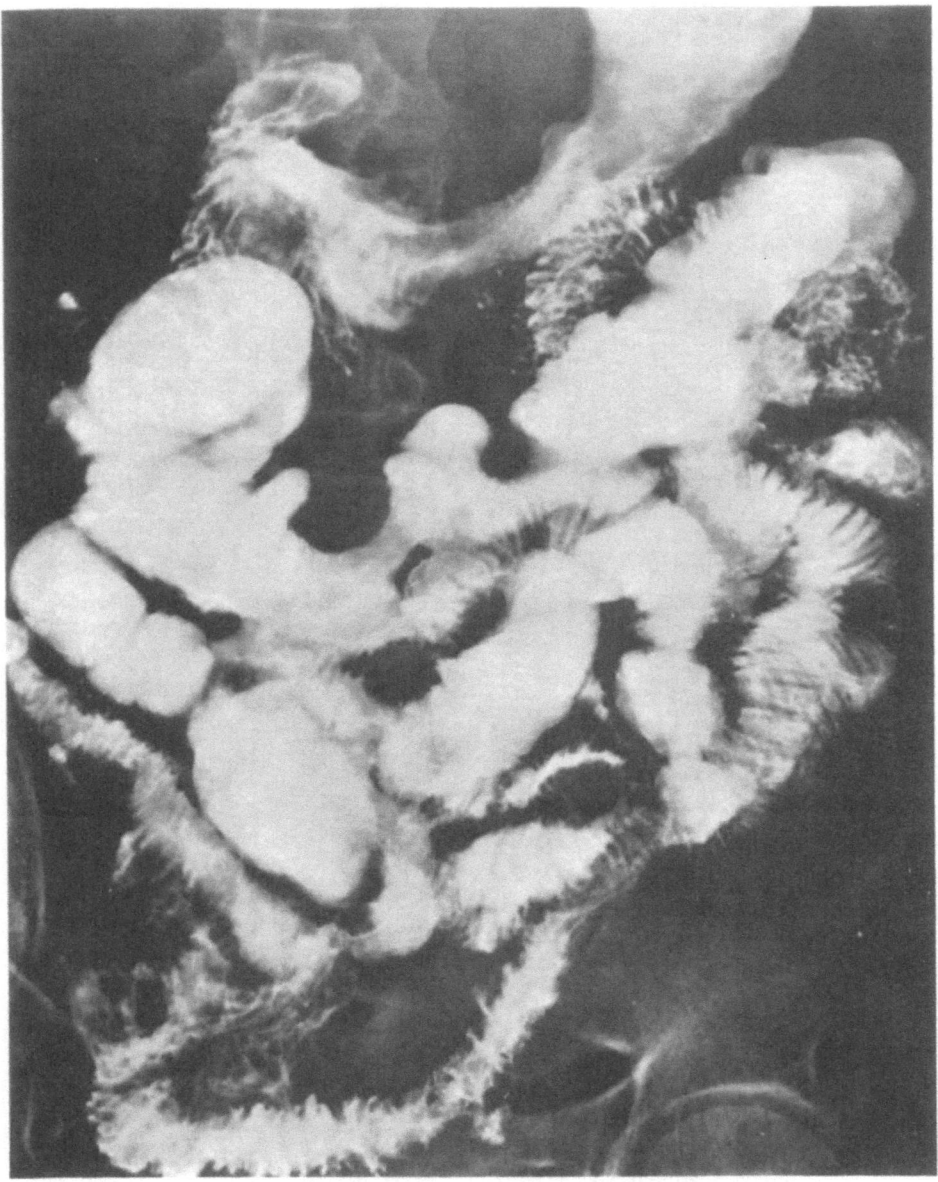

Fig. IV.116. Tumor of the stomach with an extensive peritoneal carcinomatosis.

The first films routinely made are plain abdominal survey films without contrast fluid. These films show a solitary air filled loop which remains unchanged on repeat films. The increased vulnerability of the intestine resulting from vascular insufficiency can lead to secondary infection and mucosal ulceration. In a later stage a necrotizing enteritis develops and bacterially produced gas accumulates within the intestina wall (fig. IV.56AB). This gas pattern can be differentiated from the gas seen in pneumatosis intestinalis as the latter develops in an intestinal wall of normal thickness and with a normal mucosal pattern. Small quantities of gas appear on the X-rays as thin lines (fig. IV.141), large accumulations of gas can assume bizarre shapes (fig. IV.56AB). The ragged contours of these latter gas patterns are easily differentiated from fake patterns of gas outside normal mucosal folds (fig. IV.142).

138

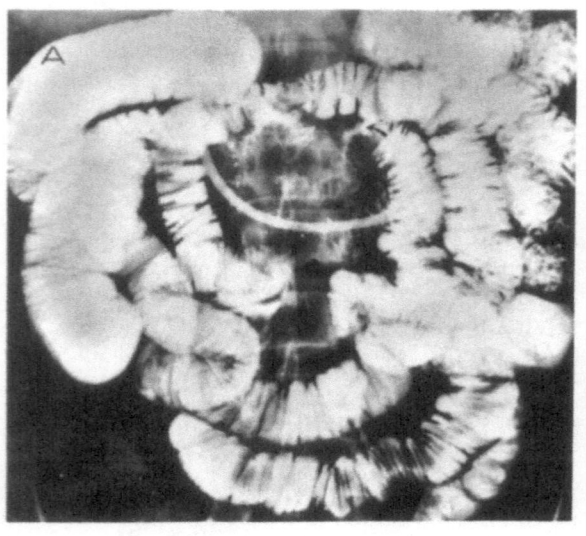

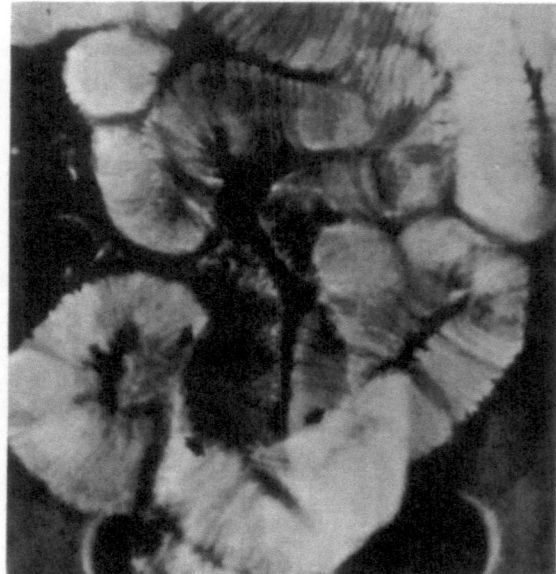

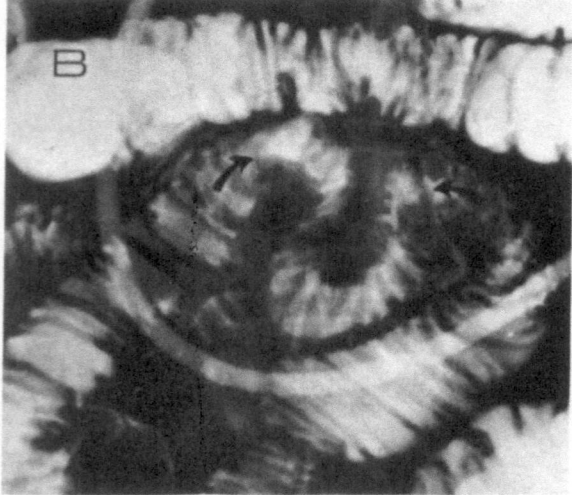

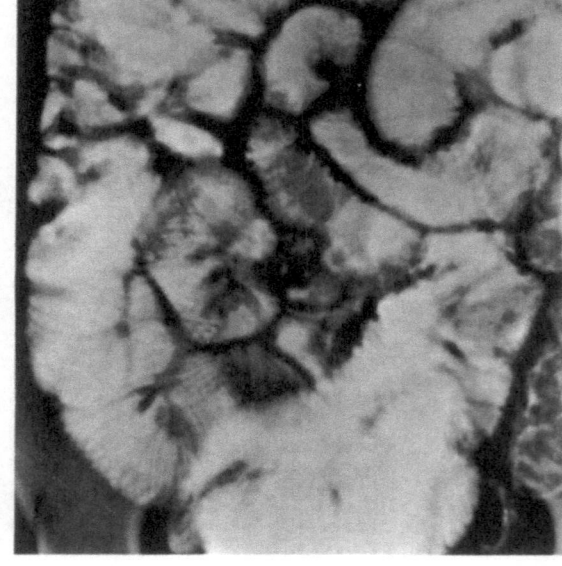

Fig. IV.117. X-rays of a patient with very local enhanced motility of the small bowel without visible abnormalities of the mucosal folds. (A) Radiation enteritis, shortly after irradiation for Hodgkin's disease. After a laparotomy staging procedure, the involved intestinal loops fused with the surroundings and as a result were more susceptible to X-ray damage. (B) A follow-up examination two years later showed that the position of the involved intestinal loop had not changed. Now, however, mucosal changes can be seen. The fold relief has become irregular, the intestinal wall is thickened and rigid, and total dilatation is no longer possible.

Fig. IV.118. Mesenteric cyst, visible when the patient is in the supine position (upper) and hardly visible in the prone position (lower).

5. *Schematic summary of abnormalities between and outwith the bowel loops*

intestinal mucosa thickened as result of hypoalbuminemia
    disturbance of protein metabolism
    inflammatory processes
    tumors
interstitial inflammation of the intestinal wall
    appendicular infiltrate – including possible abscess
    yersinia E.C.
    paratyphoid
    Crohn's disease – wall further thickened from:
        fatty degeneration
        hypertrophy of circular muscle
vascular disease
    superior mesenteric vein thrombosis- predominantly → congestion
        in all cases → edema
    radiation enteritis predominantly → inflammation and fibrosis
    ischemia
tumor growth
    lymphomata – long continuous segment
    linitis plastica – extensive but focal distribution
    diverse tumors – local- sometimes stretched-out folds
empty spaces among the bowel loops
    excess mesenteric fat
    voluminous omentum
    mesenteric fibrosis – with associated severe fatty degeneration
    mesenteric cysts – difference in prone and supine positions
spaces outwith the mass of intestinal loops
    enlarged prostate
    transplanted kidney
    enlarged liver or spleen
relatively spaces in the mass of loops
    adhesions and spasm (variable) – mainly lower abdomen
    feather-like mucosal pattern
unusual auto-compression phenomenon – (see chapter III.(1 and 2)
pointed projections from the column of contrast medium
    adhesions – sometimes very elongated- commonly found
    contracture of non-specific ulcer – ca 1 cm in length – considerable stenosis
    small ulcers (Crohn's) – ca 1-3 mm deep
    fistulous tracts – from a few millimetres to many centimetres in length
round deposits of contrast medium extending from the bowel
    abscess – mainly in lower abdomen
    Meckel's diverticulum – moreover omphalo-enteric duct.
        beware false appearances.
    larger diverticula – chiefly in jejunum
    smaller diverticula – chiefly in ileum – fairly rare
    false diverticula – in severely spastic loop in Crohn's disease
    pseudo diverticula – opposite ulcers from fibrosing – Shell sign
    auto-amputations – rare
sac-like bulging from the intestine
    large ulcer – mainly duodenum
    scleroderma or Wernicke's syndrome
bifurcation or side-branch of intestinal canal
    omphalo -enteric duct – plus Meckel's diverticulum
    reduplicated bowel
    surgically created bypass
gas configurations outside the column of contrast fluid
    intramural from necrotising enteritis after vascular accident
        thin lines or bizarre forms
    beware false or misleading patterns!
intestinal pneumatosis

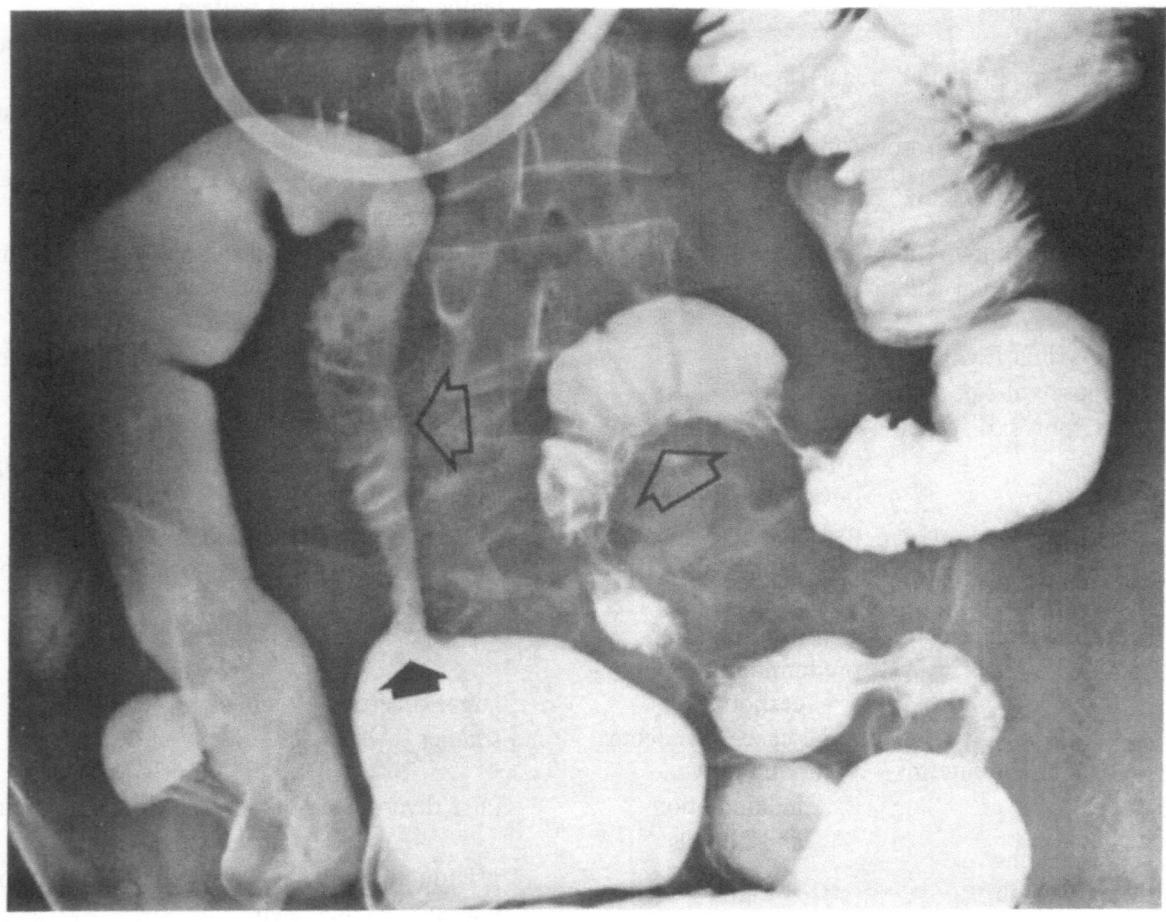

Fig. IV.119. Longitudinal ulcers with contracture (open arrows) and an obvious prestenotic dilatation (solid arrow) are present. The history included several resections (Crohn's disease).

E. Mucosal relief

1. General remarks and misleading patterns

Maximum adhesion to the mucosa and therefore the sharpest patterns are obtained when the contrast fluid flows past a 'dry' intestinal wall. When the intestinal wall is coated with mucus that is not immediately flushed off by a contrast fluid with a lower viscosity, the outer margins of the contrast column are less sharp. Sometimes it is seen that the difference in viscosity between the barium suspension and mucus is so great that mixing does not occur and the mucus remains visible as poorly defined threads.

Flocculation of the contrast fluid is a phenomenon still seen regularly in a conventional follow-through examination in cases of severe malabsorption. As soon as flocculation occurs, anatomical representation of the intestinal mucosa is impossible and the radiological examination should be terminated. In an adequately executed enteroclysis examination, flocculation of the contrast fluid does not occur within the period required for the actual examination – even in cases of severe malabsorption. Flocculation may occur at the beginning or the end of the contrast column where the barium suspension has the most intense contact with the contents of the intestine (fig. IV.143).

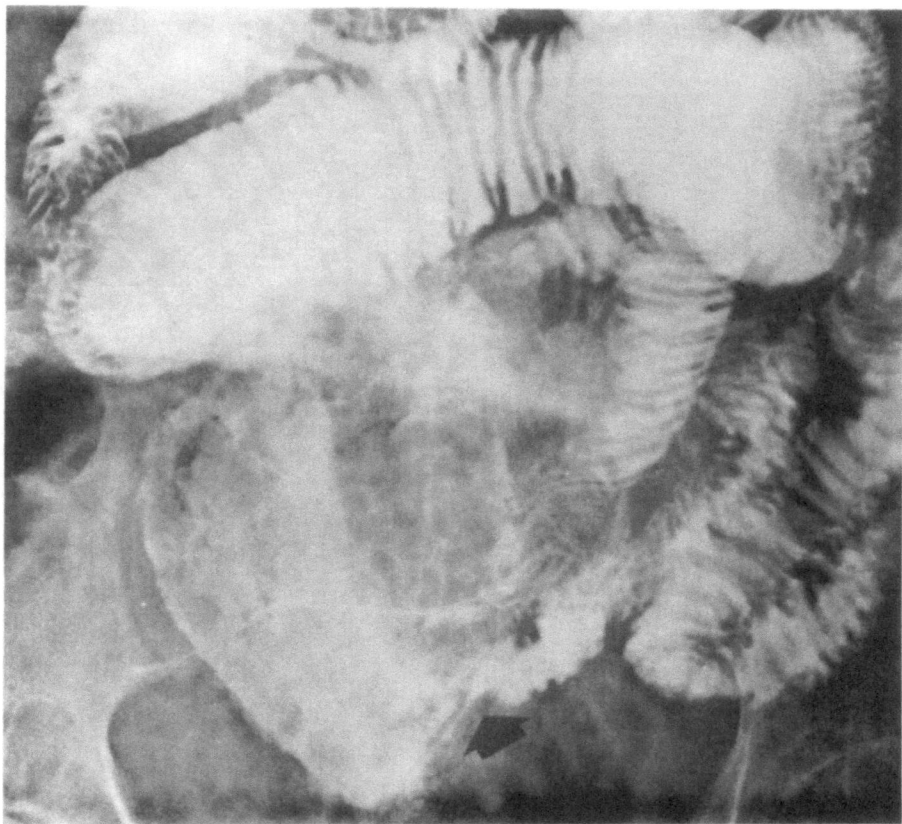

Fig. IV.120. Perforation of the jejunum due to postoperative ischemia. Both mesenteric arteries were occluded. There is contrast fluid in the abdominal cavity and effacement of mucosal folding proximal to the site of necrosis.

This disintegration is observed only when there is sufficient penetration of the contrast fluid by the röntgen rays, it can be masked entirely by underexposure.

Contrast medium that has flocculated is much more viscous than intact barium suspension and is no longer able to retain the impression of the folds of the soft intestinal mucosa. Disintegration of the barium suspension leads to apparent coarsening of the fold relief (fig. IV.144), failure to recognize this will lead to totally incorrect conclusions.

In the proximal part of the jejunum the tendency to reproduce the mucosal folds more coarsely than they actually are is enhanced when, because of hypermotility, there is only moderate filling of the intestinal loops. The drawing and the in vitro experiment illustrated in fig. IV.145AB show that the mucosal folds appear coarser in a moderately filled than in a well-filled intestine. This same

phenomenon can be encountered in vivo. Figure IV.146 shows mucosal folds in the jejunum that seem very coarse, but assumed a quite different appearance in a second examination made after hypotonia had been induced. Endoscopic examination and biopsy studies revealed no abnormalities. The coarse mucosal patterns in Whipple's disease, so often mentioned in the literature, are also largely due to artifact (fig. IV.147AB).

Evaluation of the shape of the mucosal folds should therefore not be based on the patterns obtained at the beginning or at the end of the contrast column, and certainly not if it is obvious that the contrast fluid has lost its original structure. Mucosal patterns should be evaluated on those films taken during or preferably towards the end of the infusion. When the examination lasts too long, dehydration of the contrast fluid in the distal ileum leads to thickening of the barium sus-

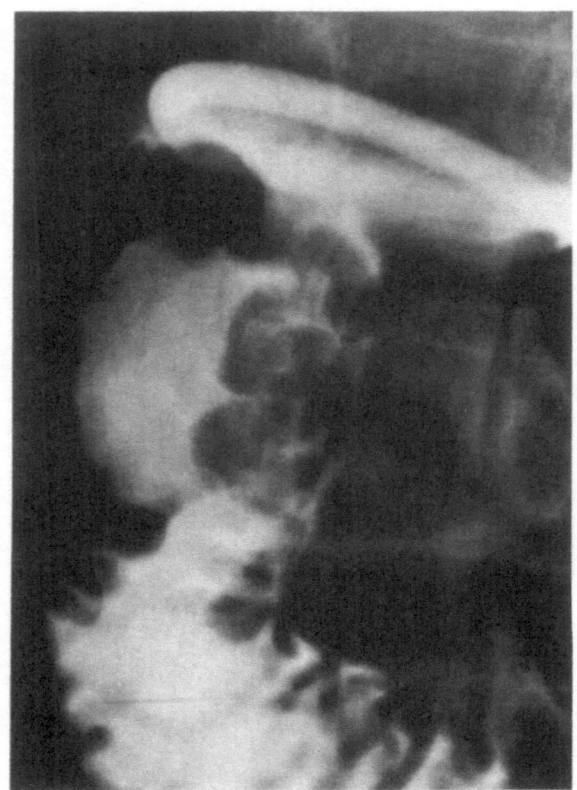

Fig. IV.121. Large ulcerating adenocarcinoma in the descending limb of the duodenum.

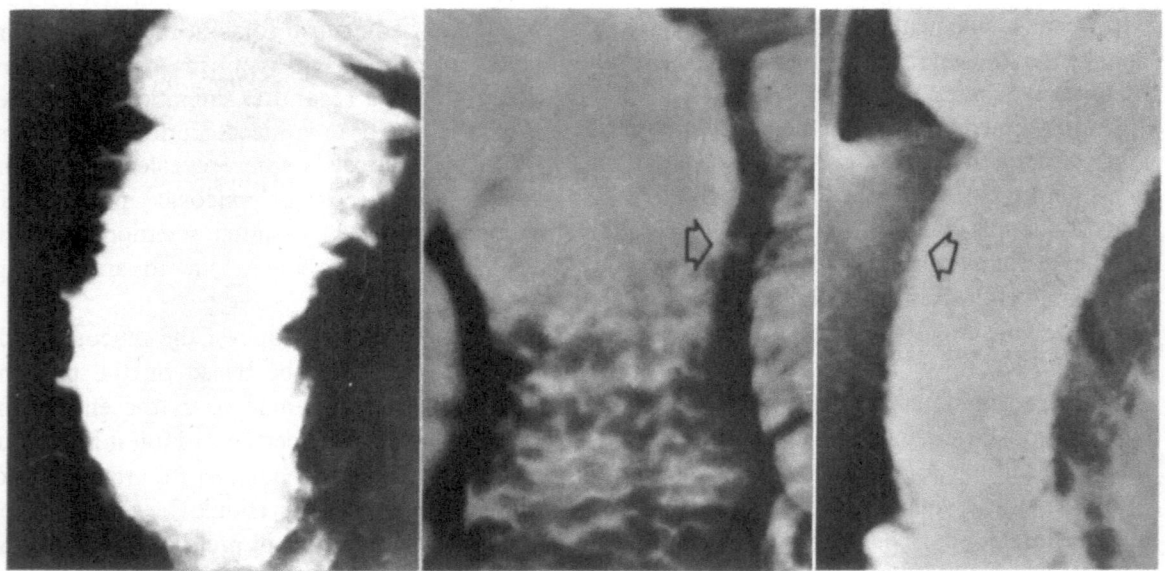

Fig. IV.122. Ulcers in Crohn's disease, some mushroom-shaped (arrows).

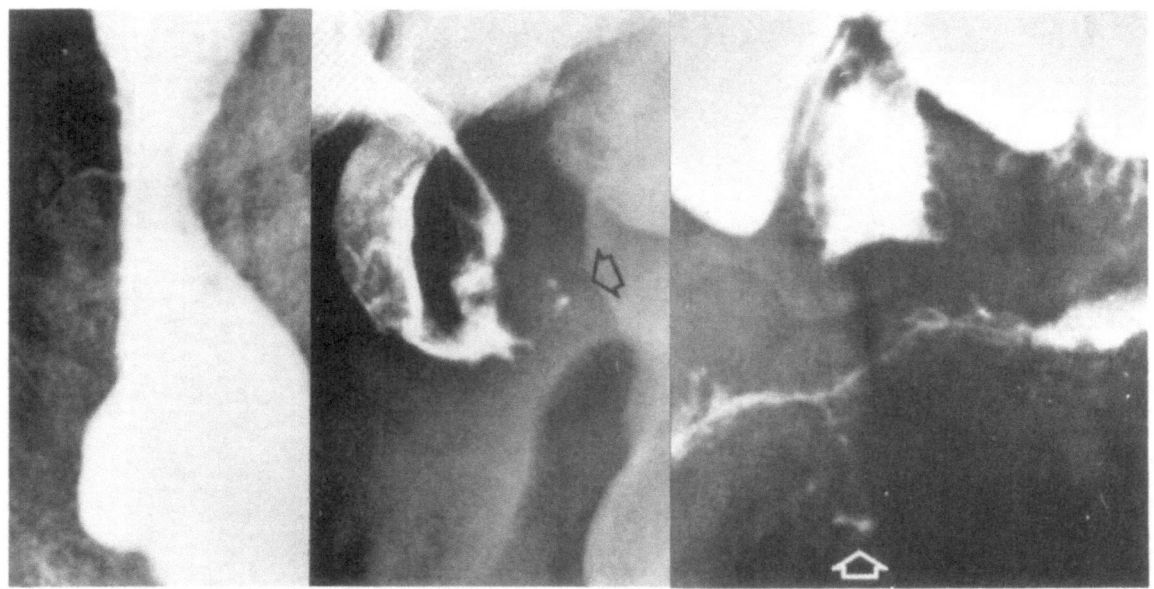

Fig. IV.123. Probably the beginning of a fistulous tract (left). Fistulization towards the bladder (right).

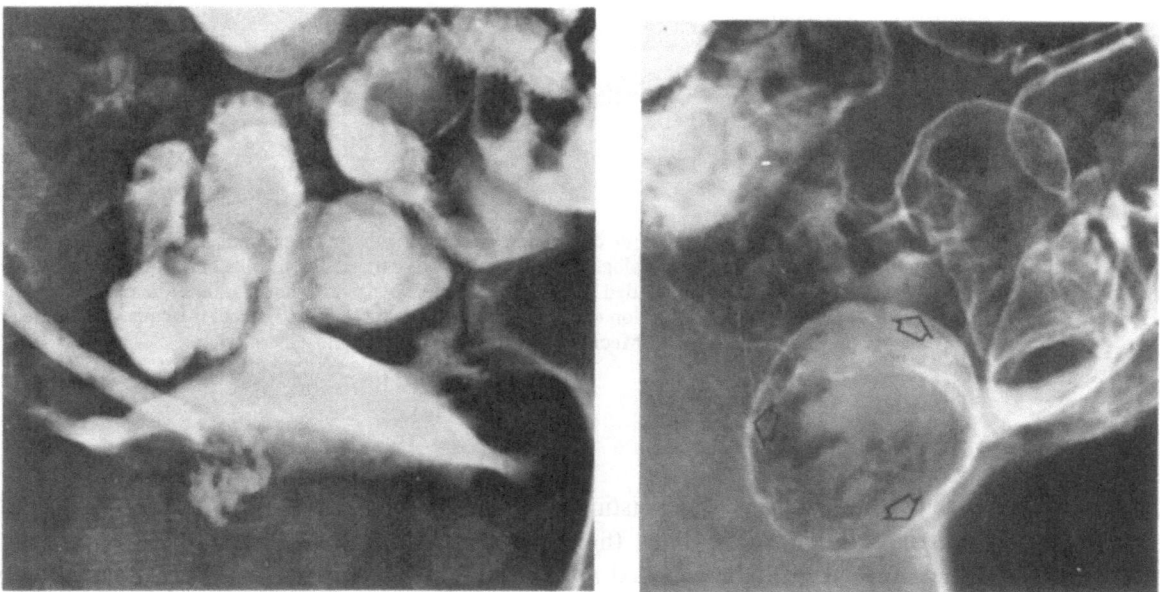

Fig. IV.124. Amebic abscess in most distal part of cecum (left). Appendicular infiltrate with a post-operative perforation into the pouch of Douglas (right).

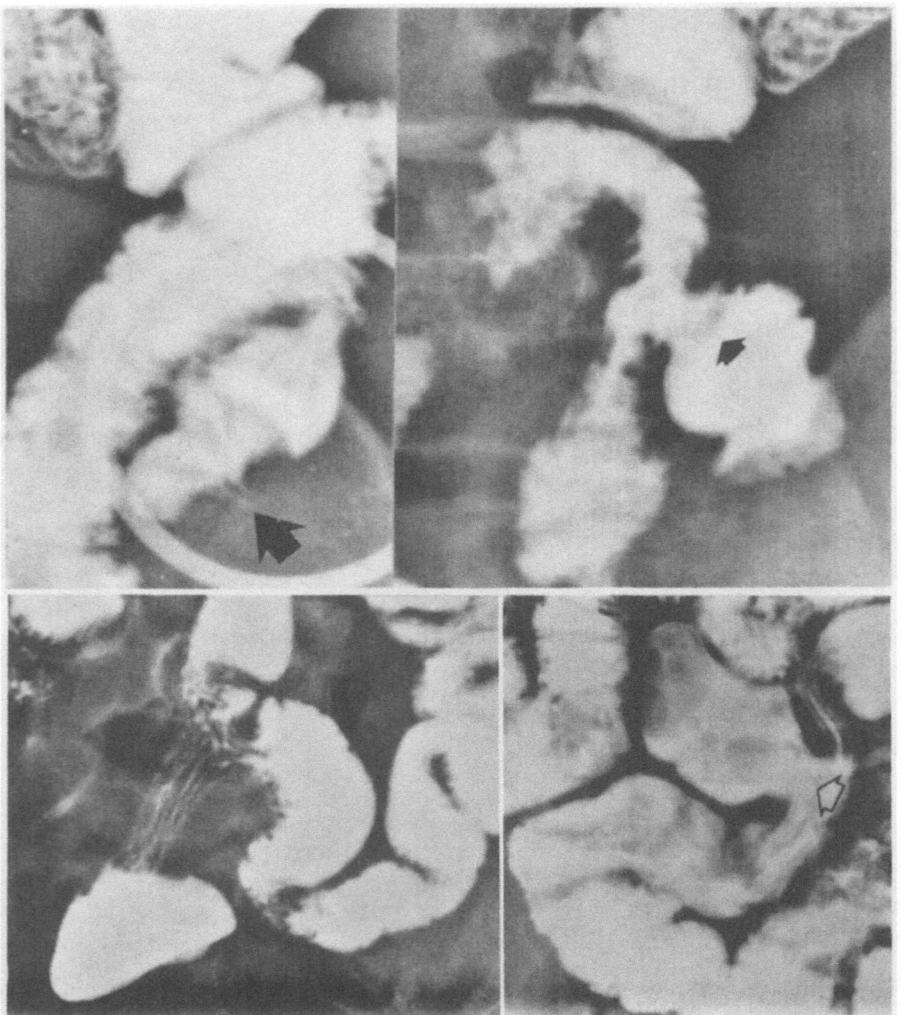

Fig. IV.125. (upper): Bleeding Meckel's diverticulum containing an ulcer with mucosal folds radiating outward. The diverticulum was not demonstrated until a second radiological examination was carried out, in spite of the fact that the entero-clysis examination performed a few weeks before included numerous spot films. Angiographic examination and a technetium scan, as well as endoscopic and radiological examination of the stomach and colon, failed to reveal the cause of the melena. (lower): Another medium-sized Meckel's diverticulum, not diagnosed elsewhere.

pension. A crackle pattern is then seen, consisting of haphazardly arranged thin bright lines (fig. IV.148). These lines can probably be ascribed to residual fold impressions a few minutes old, they are thin because they no longer contain folds. If the contrast fluid in the distal ileum has a grainy structure, the possibility of food residue or reflux of cecal contents in ulcerative colitis can be considered.

2. Edema

Edematous swollen folds are found in diseases associated with *protein deficiency* and *hypoalbuminemia*, such as inflammatory processes and disturbed protein synthesis, and other conditions. The margins of each fold do not then always lie parallel – instead the folds can assume a somewhat biconvex omega – like (Ω) shape whereby

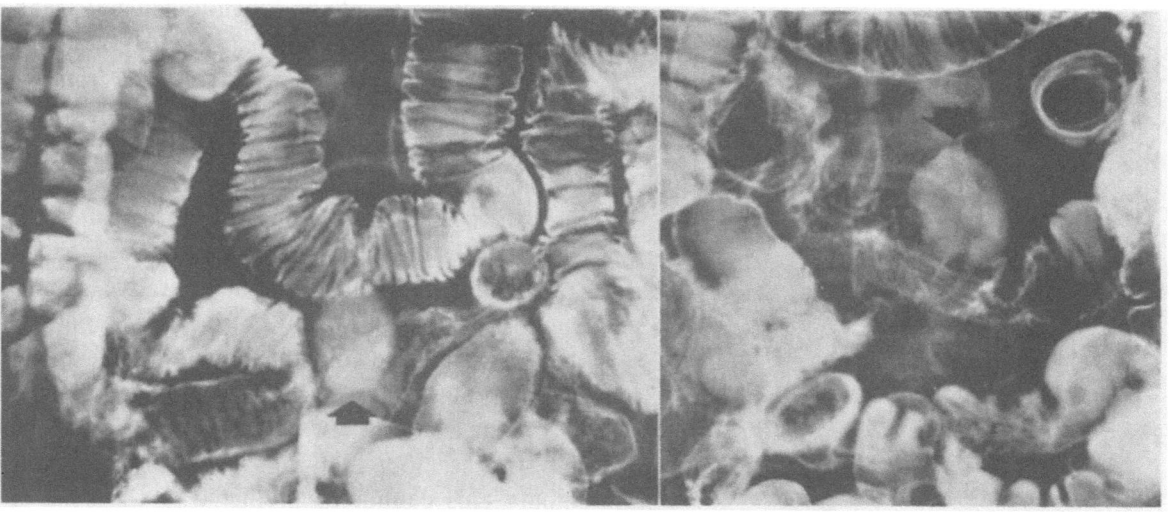

Fig. IV.126 This Meckel's diverticulum (arrow) was not recognized on the survey film of an enteroclysis examination performed elsewhere (left), although the compression spot film taken later also clearly showed a round shadow with no signs of mucosal folds (right).

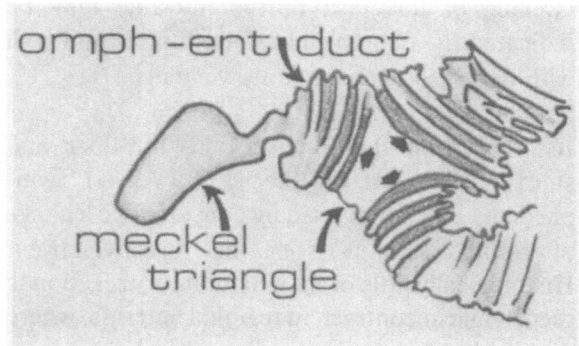

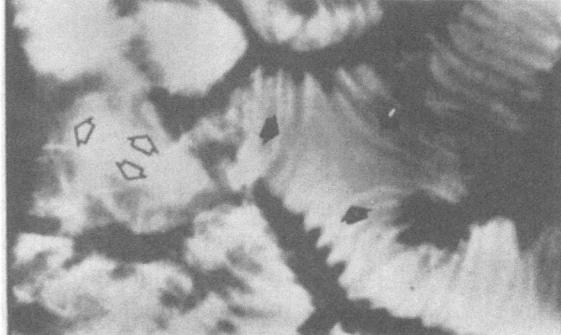

Fig. IV.127. Triangular configuration in the mucosal pattern at the mouth of the omphalo-enteric duct (Meckel's diverticulum).

the base of the fold does not change. The thickness of the intestinal wall is increased only slightly or not at all (fig. IV.105). In the distal ileum, where the mucosal folding can appear longitudinal, the swollen folds begin to follow a twisting course. The mucosal relief appears somewhat disordered, although the continuity of the folds can still be followed, for instance in Yersinia E.C. infections (fig. IV.149). In Crohn's disease, ulceration develops at the bottom of deep longitudinal grooves in the swollen mucous membrane of the ileum and the jejunum. The continuity of these grooves is broken by numerous deep ulcerations that lie perpendicular to the longitudinal folds, causing a cushion-like relief, the so-called '*cobblestone pattern*' (fig. IV.150B). This cobblestone relief, result of a markedly swollen mucosal surface, is however not specific for Crohn's disease but is also encountered in many other disorders such as periarteritis nodosa (fig. IV.46), lympho-reticular infiltration in the mucosa (fig. IV.49) and even after repositioning of an intussusception (fig. IV.45). Cobblestones develop only when pronounced edema and clearly visible circular mucosal folds occur together. Because of the pronounced edema, the mucosa and submucosa –and possibly also the underlying muscular layer – become much thicker and the inner diameter of the intestinal lumen becomes much smaller. The excess mucosal surface must then, of necessity,

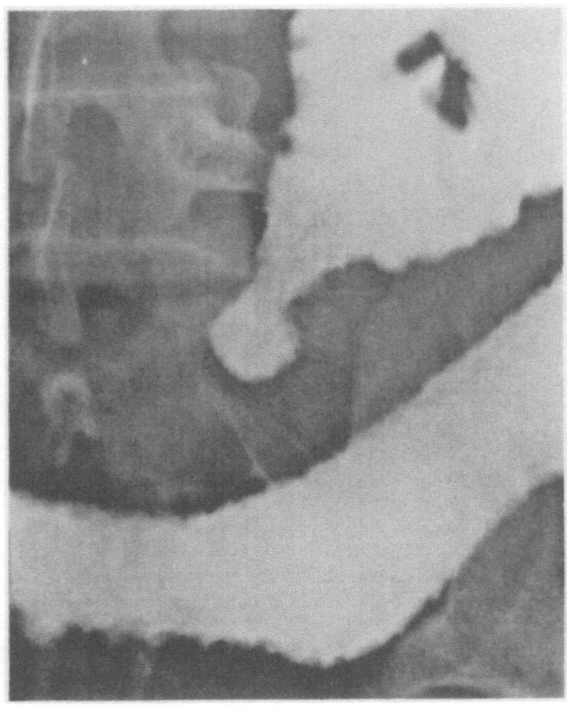

Fig. IV.128. Extensive active Crohn's disease in the distal ileum. The disease has also spread to the fairly small Meckel's diverticulum that was also present.

form longitudinal folds. If the mucosal folds of the involved segment are very small or even absent, the X-ray will show only longitudinal grooves. If there are pronounced mucosal folds, these will swell so markedly that they come to lie very close together and transverse grooves form in between.

The combination of the longitudinal and transverse grooves, which enclose islands of highly swollen mucosa, produces the so-called '*railroad track*' configuration of the cobblestones (fig. IV.150A). It is fairly obvious that the circulation of blood and lymph is disturbed mainly in these grooves so that ulcerations will develop here. If the edema is mainly superficial, as in the so-called reflux-ileitis associated with ulcerative colitis, neither cobblestones nor railroad track pattern will be visualized and the mucosal folds never swell so markedly (figs. IV.150AB and IV.151).

Edema is almost always easier to see when the intestine is moderately filled with contrast medium; This cannot be predicted in the case of ulceration. It is therefore essential that in all cases the intestine should be visualized in various degrees of filling (Fig. IV.152). Because the folds of Kerkring are thinner and farther apart in the ileum than in the jejunum, a slight edematous swelling of this part of the intestine may be indicated by a completely smooth intestinal wall with decreased peristaltic movements.

In *lymphedema* the mucosal folds are thick and short and lie close together (Fig. IV.99D). Lymphedema is accompanied by considerable leakage of serum albumin from the digestive tract. Histologically little or no inflammatory reaction is seen, while in contrast, in regional enteritis, where the lymphatic channels are also dilated, there is an obvious inflammatory reaction.

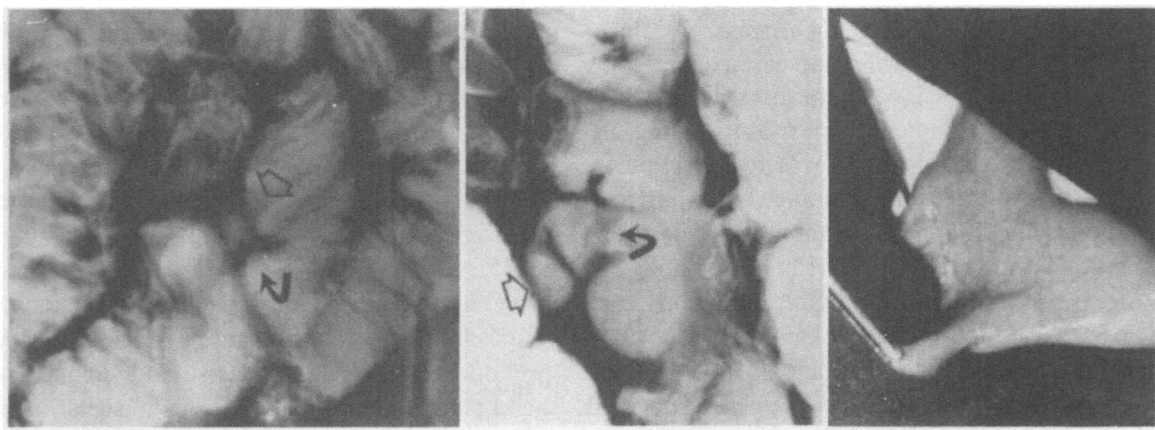

Fig. IV.129. Small Meckel's diverticulum that was scarcely discernible on the detail from the spot film (left) but could be seen on the film taken with compression technique (middle). To the right the surgical preparation.

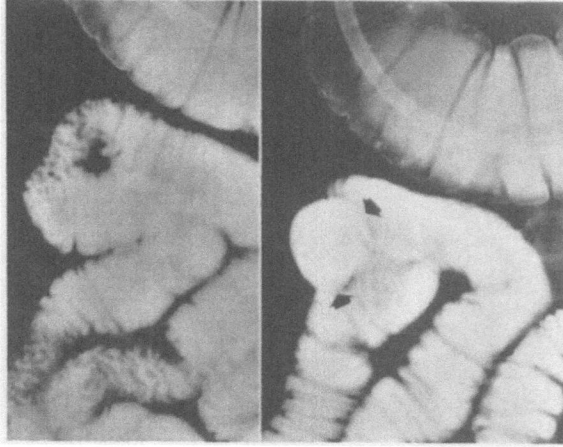

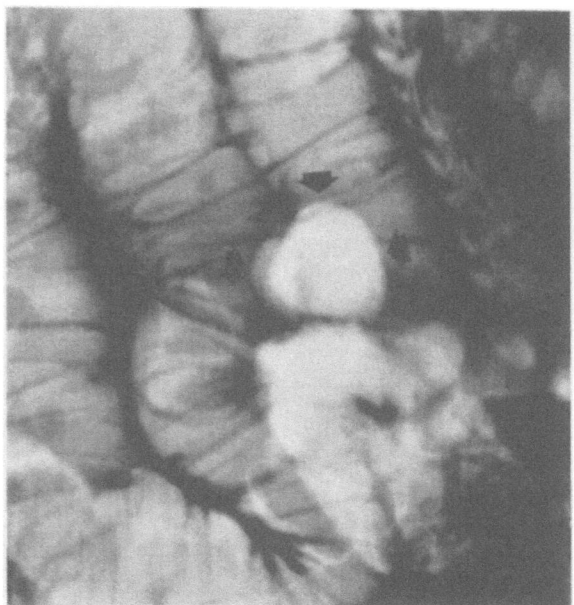

Fig. IV.130. Two patients with a diverticulum-like shadow in the mass of intestinal loops, produced by an intestinal loop visualized in axial projection. For one patient (right radiogram), a repeat examination was necessary for confirmation.

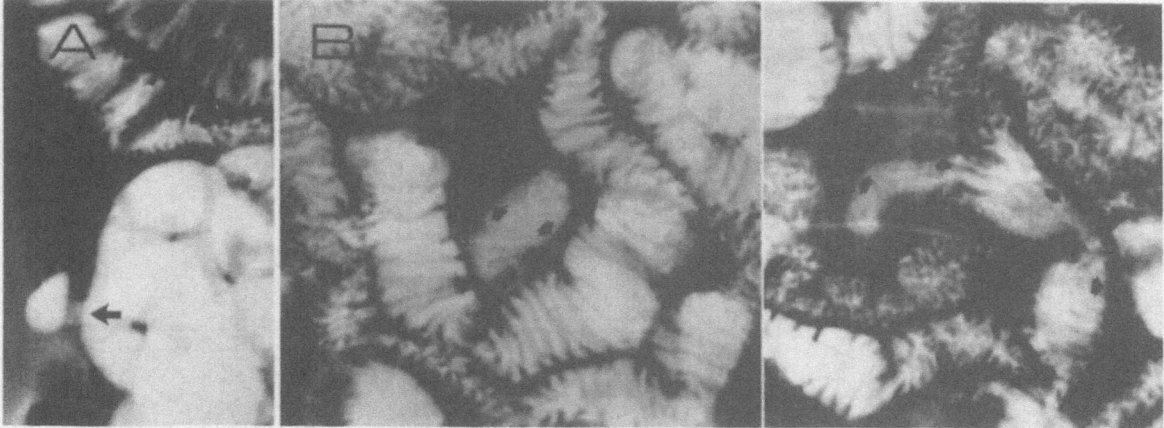

Fig. IV.131. Two patients with a misleading pattern suggesting a (Meckel's) diverticulum. In both cases this is the front of the contrast column. In patient B, disintegration of the contrast fluid is clearly visible. A second exposure taken immediately afterwards revealed that it was a normal segment of the intestine.

Rigidity and reduced peristalsis, thickened mucosal folds and increased space between the intestinal loops are also associated with *vascular disorders* of the intestinal wall. In comparison with lymphedema however, the following radiological differences are found:

1) Thickening of the folds is as a rule much more prominent, while the spaces between are smaller and very pointed. The folds are also wider so that the coarse sawtooth effect is even more pronounced than in lymphedema (Fig. IV.34B), which develops more gradually.

2) Because multiple hematomata are found in the mucosa, the swollen fold relief often appears highly irregular; in addition, multiple swellings bulging out into the lumen may be visible (Fig. IV.56B).

3) The intestinal wall may be markedly thicker than in lymphedema so that the spaces

148

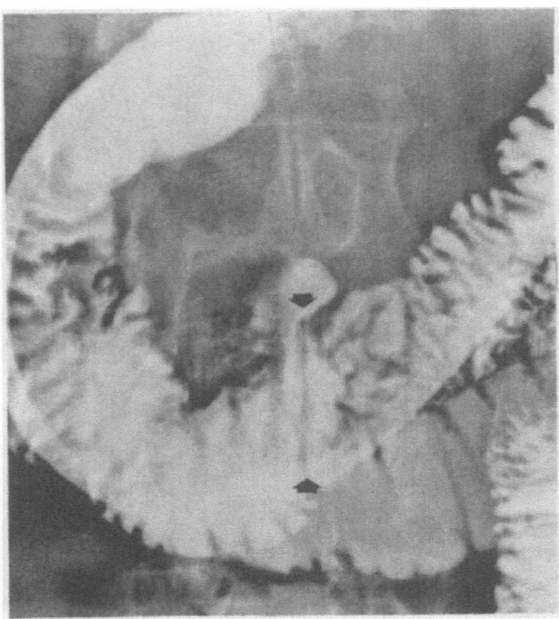

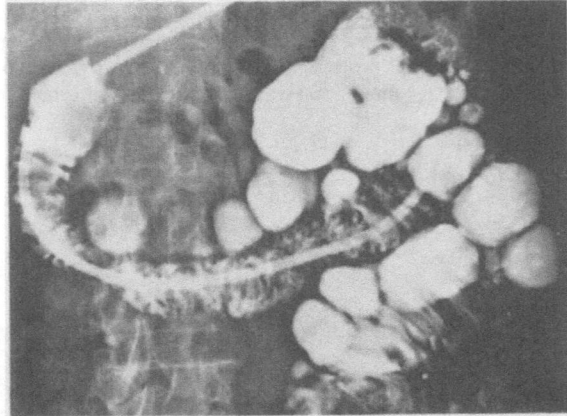

Fig. IV.132. Mucosal pattern at the mouth of a normal diverticulum. The mucosal folds of the intestine extend into the neck of the diverticulum (arrows).

Fig. IV.133. Numerous large diverticula in the duodenum and jejunum. They are visualized most easily when the intestine is in contraction phase and is therefore relatively empty. When the patient is erect, there are numerous fluid levels.

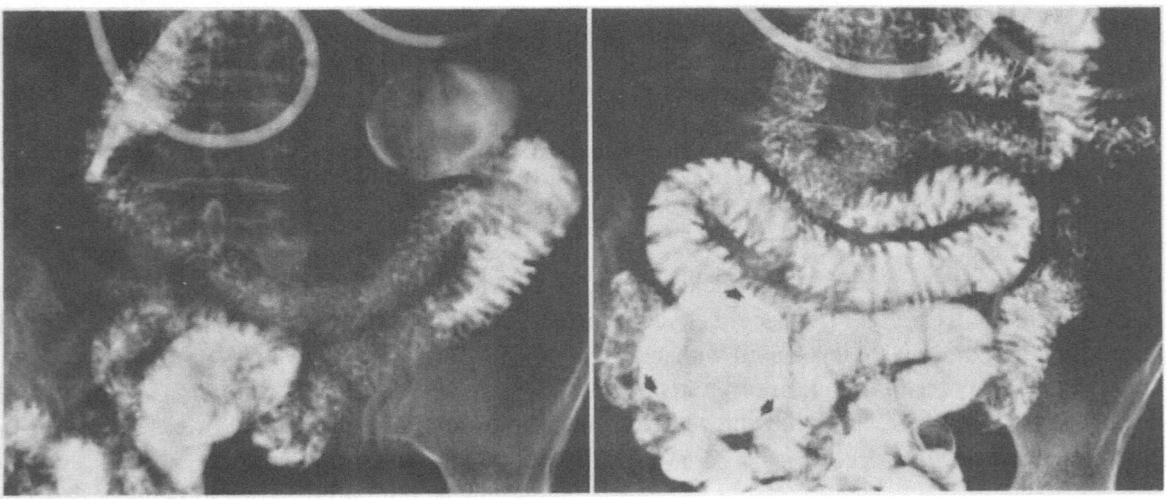

Fig. IV.134. Large highly mobile diverticulum in the proximal jejunum. With changes in the patient's posture, the neck of such a diverticulum can easily twist, producing the symptoms of an acute abdomen. The danger of necrosis and perforation is actual.

between the loops appear on X-ray larger and, as a result of the hematomata, can vary greatly in shape and size.

4) The intestinal lumen is not dilated but often narrowed.

5) In contrast to lymphedema, a vascular accident or celiac disease affects only a restricted segment varying in length from 25 to 50 cm.

6) As a result of inflammatory phenomena in necrotic tissue, the mucosa can show superficial ulcerations and the intestinal wall may contain gas (Fig. IV.56AB).

In cases of vascular accident it is not always simple to differentiate between arterial and venous disturbance and certainly when several days have already elapsed. Both, clinical and radiological differentation are easier in the early stages. The following schematic summary can offer some assistance.

Vascular accident (diff. diagn.)

arterial: acute course
          wall initially thin
          hypermotility
          serositis consistently present

hematoma:
          subacute course
          normal peristalsis
          polypoid morphology
          'mesenteric mass'

venous: gradual course
          wall thickened
          'thumbprinting'
          absent peristalsis

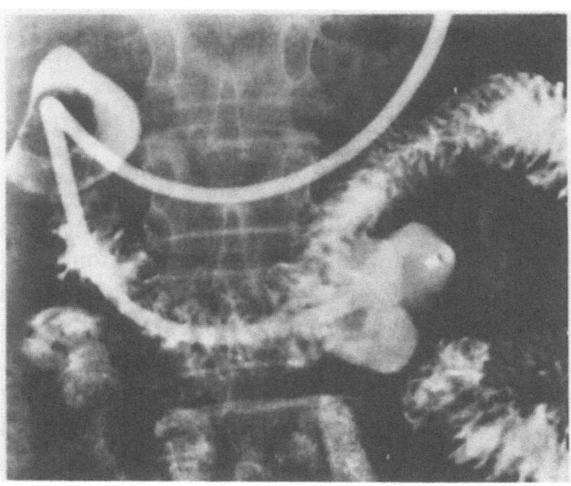

Ischemic infarct (aetiol.)

arteriosclerosis:
        old age or diabetes

thrombosis:
        inflammatory process or irradiation

fibro-muscular hyperplasia

post-operative

mechanical occlusion
        adhesions, bands
        volvulus-internal hernia

micro-emboli
        polycythemia
        valvular defects
        atrial fibrillation
        myocardial infarct

vasculitis
        collagen diseases-Burger's disease
        allergics (Henoch-Schönlein)

medication (ergotamine etc.)

Periodic circulatory insufficiency

falling heart minute volume (e.g. hypotension)

increased demand (e.g. after copious meal)

associated condition: circulation already marginal

X-ray: no abnormality with complaints of only 1 to 2 hours duration.

Hemorrhage in bowel wall (aetiol.)

disturbed coagulation
        anti-coagulants
        phenacetine
        hemophilia
        vitamin K deficiency

'blunt' trauma (from blows etc.)

X-ray: chiefly in duodenum or proximal jejunum where they cross the vertebral column

course: usually rapid and complete recovery occasionally fatal

Disturbance of venous drainage (aetiol.)

thrombosis from inflammatory process

compression (cyst or tumor)

bands or volvulus

cardiac decompensation

portal hypertension

Fig. IV.135. If the tube becomes lodged in the duodenum or falls too far into the descending duodenum, this can be due to diverticula in the outer curve of the duodenum. Beware of perforation!

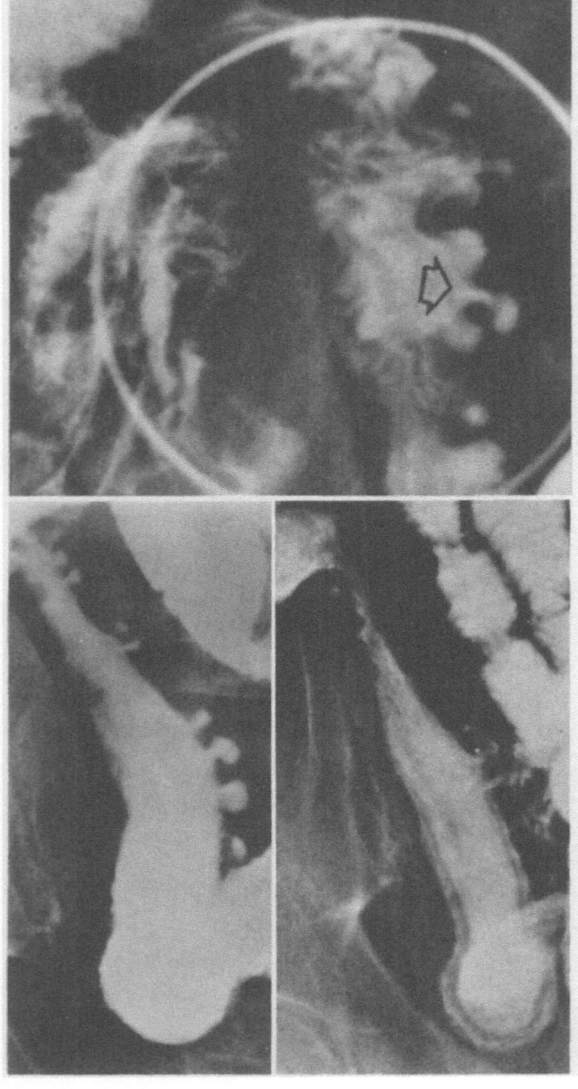

Fig. IV.136. So-called false diverticula in Crohn's disease from herniation of the mucosa through the remaining layers of the wall (right). Compare true diverticula originating in a normal mucosa (arrow).

The *occurrence of edema* can be systematised according to the length of the affected segment:

2.6.1. edema *generalised* or involving very long segments.
- congenital lymphedema – dilated loops (fig. IV.99A)
- acquired lymphedema – calibre normal (fig. IV.99D)
- loss of protein; regardless of cause (fig. IV.105)
- Crohn's disease – colitis variant (c. 5%) (fig. IV.153)
- Whipple's disease – exclude disintegration! (figs. IV.147AB)
- celiac disease – edema result of superimposed infection (fig. IV.43)
- malignant lymphoma – slow superficial growth over long period (fig. IV.154)
- vasculitis – collagen diseases (fig. IV.155)
- cirrhosis of the liver (fig. IV.156)
- thrombosis of superior mesenteric vein – very thick folds + dilatation (fig. IV.108)

2.6.2. edema very *local* or involving limited segments:
- lympho-reticular malignancy (fig. IV.76) irregular folds
- ischemia – sudden onset, frequent spontaneous recovery (fig. IV.141)
- vasculitis – collagen diseases (figs. IV.157 and IV.158).

Collagen diseases are not rare; the most common are scleroderma, periarteritis nodosa (PAN), lupus erythematosus and dermatomyositis. Although these diseases may be encountered in all age groups, the patients are usually between 20 and 40 years of age. With the exception of PAN, which is more common among males, these diseases, and in particular scleroderma, are generally encountered in females. Manifestations in the digestive tract are a frequent finding (50% or more) whereby the incidence in the small bowel varies. It is also possible for the abnormalities to be limited to the digestive tract, with total absence of the characteristic and easily identified skin lesions.

Henoch-Schönlein disease (fig.IV.159).

In Henoch-Schönlein disease, there is an acute arteritis accompanied by pain in the abdomen and joints associated with purpura and nephritis. The intestine shows submucosal edema with moderately swollen mucosal folds. The larger arteries in these intestinal loops, that appear red during surgery, remain unimpaired so that circulation is barely disturbed and generally no necrosis or

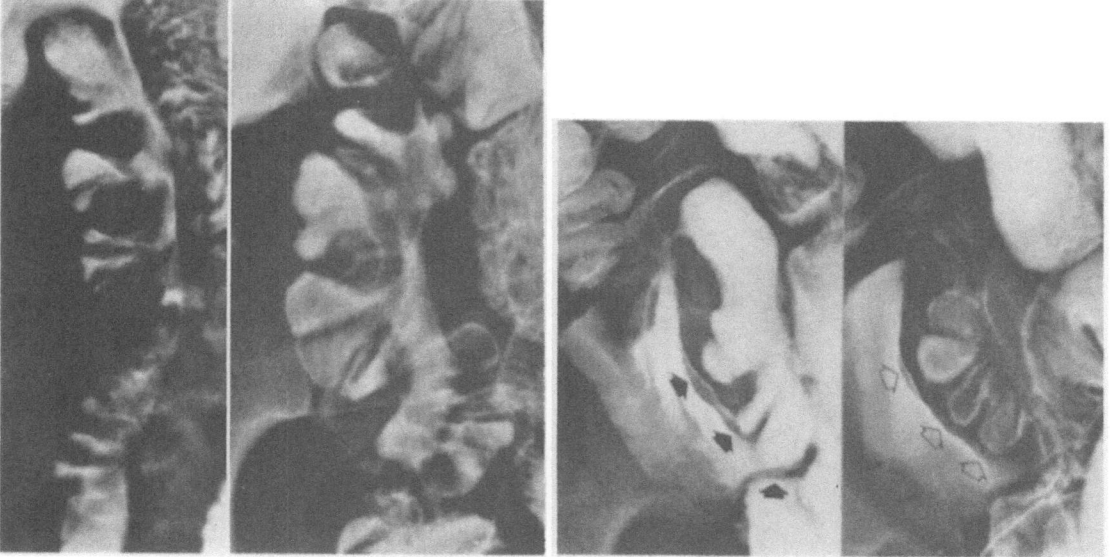

Fig. IV.137. Pseudo diverticula, developed in the intestine opposite shrunken longitudinal ulcerations as a result of spastic or partially fibrotic constrictions. They vary in shape and size. Crohn's disease (left) and vasculitis (right).

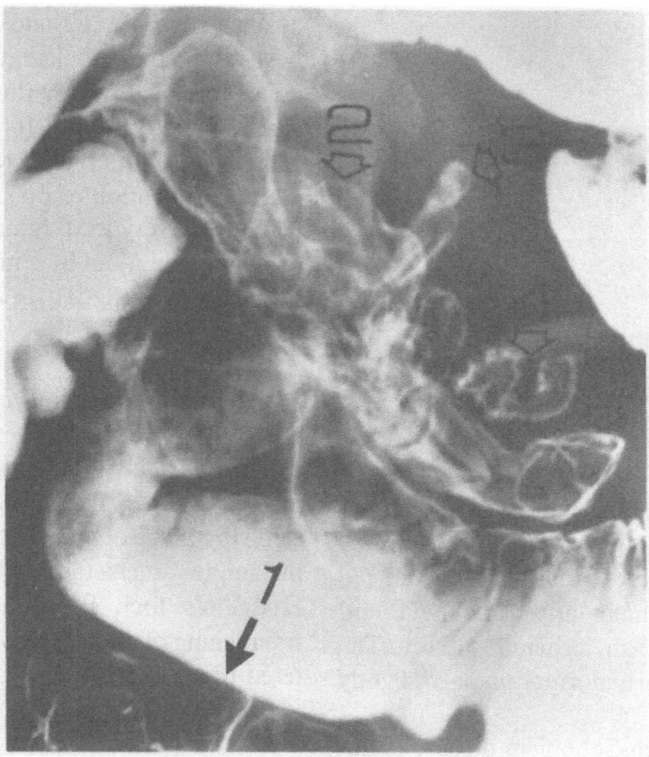

Fig. IV.138. Five sac-like bulges, extending from one point in the ileum. These developed due to constrictions and auto-amputation of the intestinal lumen after an incarcerated inguinal hernia was treated surgically. It is no longer possible to determine whether artificial ligation is involved here.

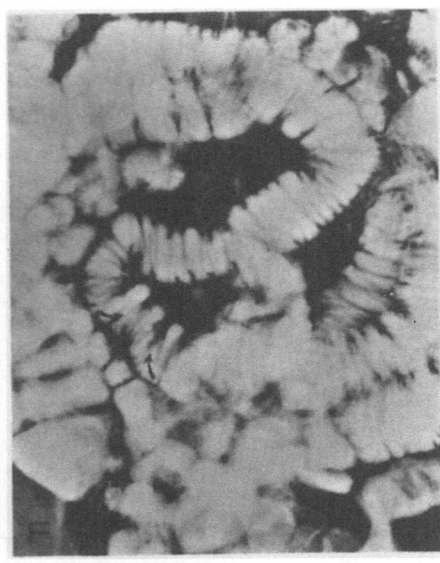

Fig. IV.139. Minimal sacculations (arrows) in the jejunum in a patient with scleroderma. On this radiogram it is not possible to distinguish these appearances which may be incidental and normal from the more subtle abnormalities associated with scleroderma.

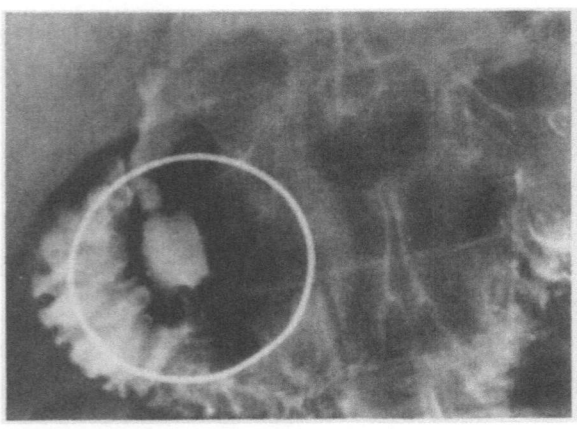

Fig. IV.140. Duplication cyst in the duodenum.

ulceration develops. Here too motility is enhanced but encompasses a segment larger than that found in the early stages of an ischemic infarct. The calibre of the intestine is normal or only slightly decreased.

The etiology of Henoch-Schönlein disease is unknown, but is now considered to be one of the collagen diseases. Unusual for this group of diseases is that Henoch-Schönlein disease is recurrent and self-limiting.

– radiation 'enteritis' – superficial ulcerations (fig. IV.75)
– Crohn's disease – early stage of recurrence (fig. IV.160)
– Yersinia E.C. inflammation – 10-30 cm in distal ileum (fig. IV.149)
– appendicitis – collateral edema or other inflammation in this area (fig. IV.107)
– reflux ileitis – superficial edema in ulcerative colitis (fig. IV.161)
– after reposition of an invagination – extremely thick edema – exclusively in babies, the mucosal tissue here is extremely loose and elastic (fig. IV.45).

3. Interrupted folds

Interrupted folds occur very frequently in Crohn's disease as the result of extremely local destruction of the mucosal pattern. Dependant on the stage of activity of the disease, the remaining intact portions of the folds may become edematously swollen (figs. IV.162 and IV.74). At the site of a healed longitudinal ulcer, the folds, here arranged concentrically towards the formerly active lesion, also terminate abruptly (fig. IV.163). Similar ulcer sites are also found after recovery from ischemia. Abrupt truncation of one or more folds can also result from very local tumor involvement or from local stretching-out by a metastasis growing within the mucosa (fig. IV.164).

4. Local broadening of folds

Folds may show local broadening from aphthoid ulcers (Crohn's, Yersinia), for which they appear to be the place of choice (fig. IV.160), from small melanoma metastases (fig. IV.164) or from Hodgkin's foci. In primary amyloidosis local broadening of already very broad folds is encountered (fig. IV.102).

5. Locally aberrant course of folds

Apart from the type associated with fibrous con-

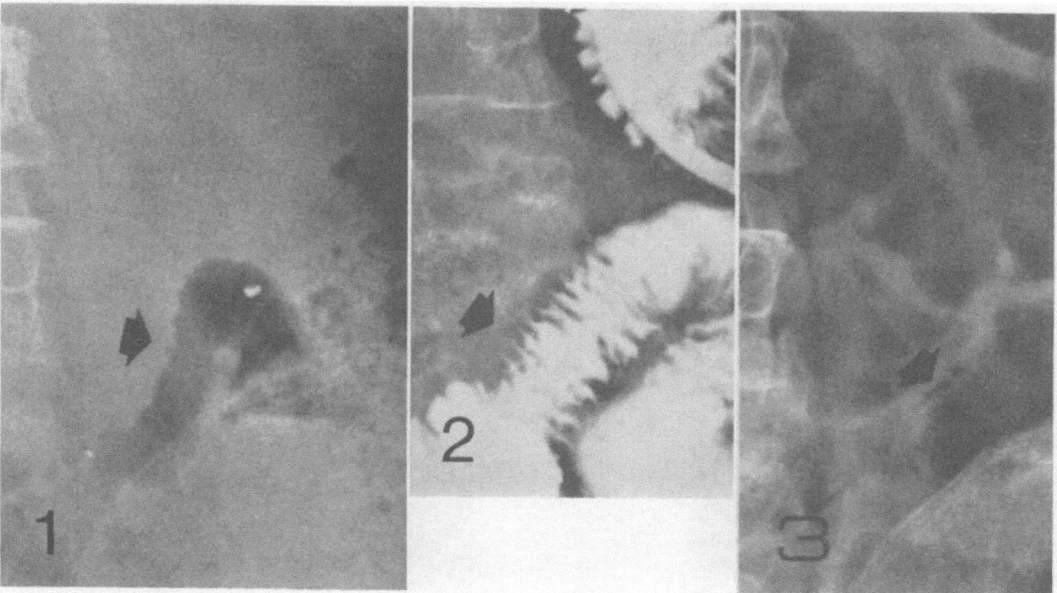

Fig. IV.141. (1): Intestinal loop filled with gas in a patient with acute abdominal pain. The mucosal folds are flattened and obviously broadened. (2): The enteroclysis examination performed the following day shows the same abnormalities in the same loop. The swelling of the mucosal folds has possibly even increased. (3): Several days later an abdominal survey film revealed an intramural film of gas in the intestinal wall at the same site, apparently as a result of local necrosis with limited perforation. Fortunately, because of the contained nature of the lesion, recovery was complete.

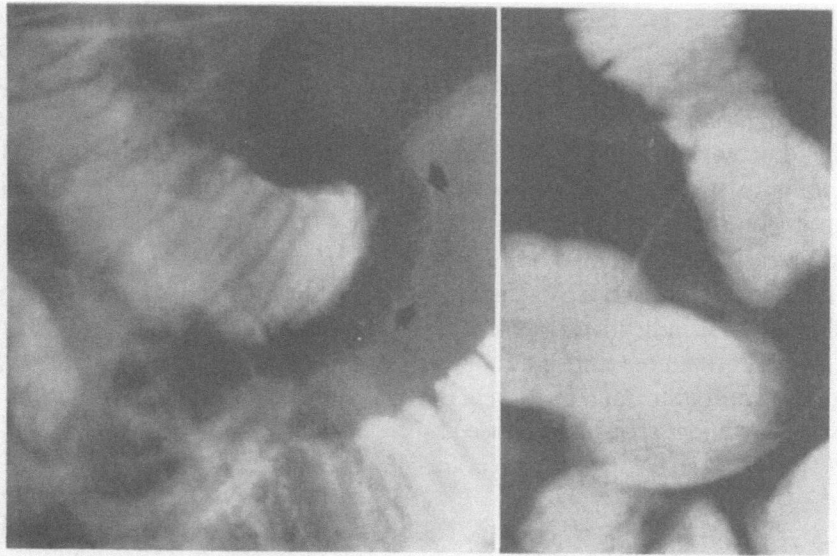

Fig. IV.142. Misleading gas pattern with sharply defined margins in the small intestine.

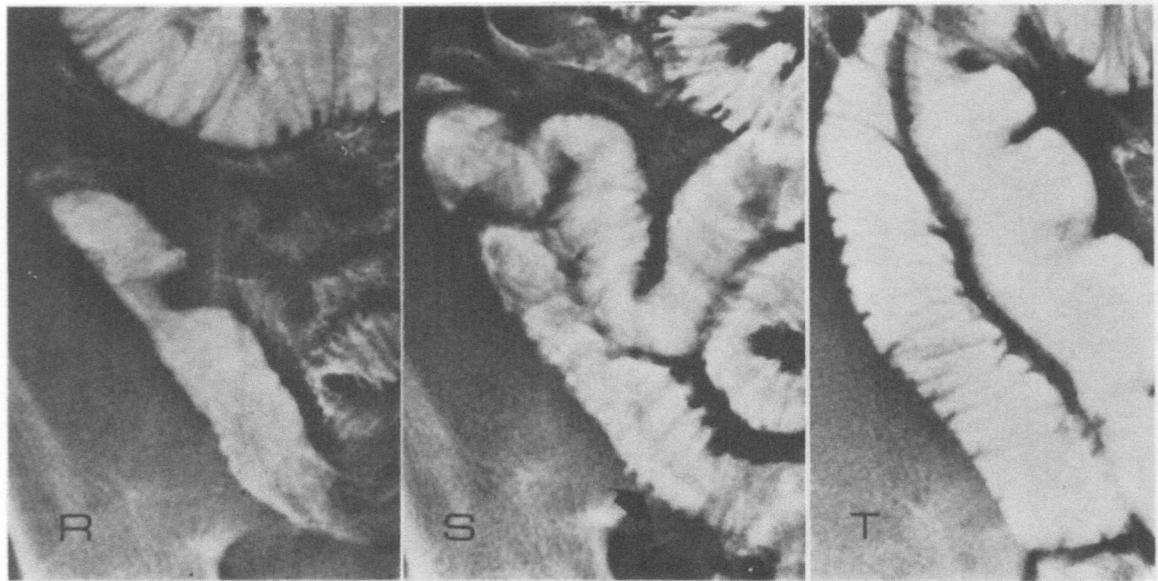

Fig. IV.143. Disintegration of the barium suspension can sometimes occur at the head of the contrast column. Because of the increase in the viscosity of the contrast medium, it is no longer possible to obtain a good reproduction of the mucosal folds (R). At the same location but a few minutes later, disintegration is less and vague impressions of the mucosal folds can already be seen (S)). Still later the disintegrated contrast fluid has moved distally and the completely intact barium suspension gives a normal reproduction of the fold relief (T).

tracture in healed ulcers, described in subsection 3, folds with aberrant course are found very frequently and in numerous variations in association with adhesions (figs. IV.57 and IV.59) and in lesser degree in other conditions coupled with fibrous contracture, such as carcinoid foci (kinking sign), mesenteric fibrosis and sclerosing peritonitis (figs. IV.68, IV.5 and IV.8AB). Further similar findings are a triangular fold complex at the site of an omphalo-enteric duct (fig. IV.127), a concenteric configuration by a hernial orifice, constricting band or volvulus (fig. IV.25) and an extended or roundly stretched-out course from external compression (fig. IV.114) or with intramurally infiltrating leiomyomata or other tumors (fig. IV.48). A very characteristic zig-zag appearance of the fold pattern is indicative of inability of the bowel to dilate in this area and may further indicate a degree of contracture and fixation of the mucosa. These appearances are usually caused by tumor growth (fig. IV.29).

6. Stretched-out course of folds

6.1. Circular course
When this appearance presents as a *long and*

continuous segment in a well filled bowel, the following possibilities should be considered:

a) too *rapid infusion* of contrast fluid.
   Dilatation is here most marked proximally and decreases distally. Motility is normal at commencement of the examination (fig. III.13).

b) *Hypomotility*, usually consequent on the chronic use of tranquillizers, soporifics or some types of analgesic, also shows dilatation most marked proximally and decreasing distally. Even in the initial stage of the examination motility is more or less obviously disturbed (fig. IV.182).

c) *Ileum obstructed* in its distal half.
   Intestinal calibre and motility are proximally only minimally disturbed or normal. Distally there is a gradually increasing dilatation and decreasing motility up to the site of obstruction (fig. IV.90).

A *lengthy segment with intermitting* stretched-out folds generally in a but moderately filled intestine with normal to lively motility is suggestive of:

a) *Celiac* syndrome in patients with poor reaction to therapy, characterised radiologically by lively motility, wide loops and

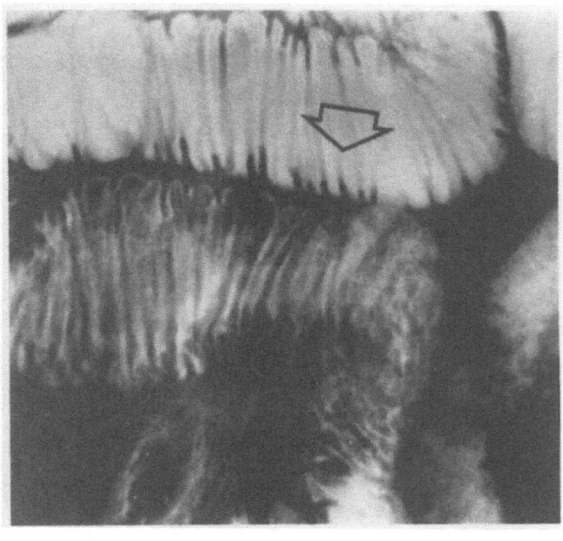 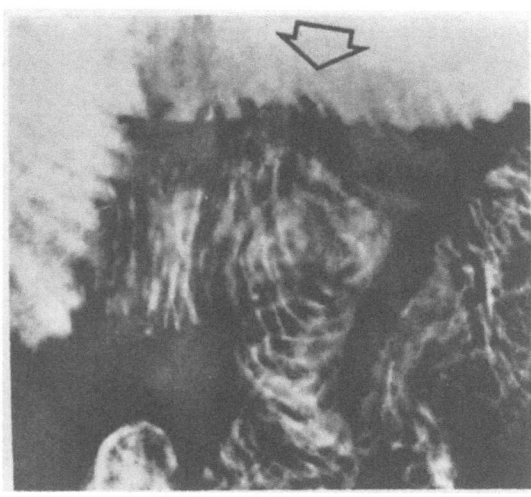

Fig. IV.144. On the initial exposure (left) the mucosal folds appear normal. A subsequent exposure (right) shows that disintegration of the contrast fluid has developed rapidly with flattening and apparent coarsening of the mucosal folds. The structure of the contrast fluid has become granular.

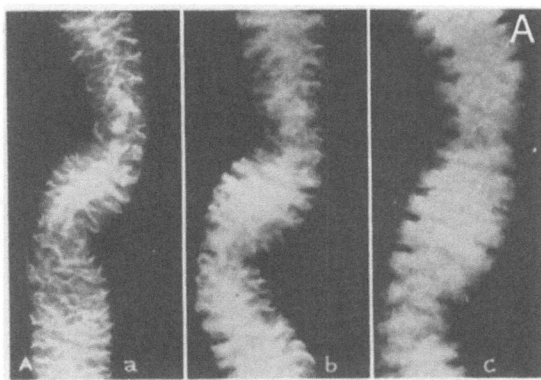

Fig. IV.145A: Sloan's experiments in vitro showing that mucosal folds appear coarser when the intestinal loops are moderately filled with contrast fluid than when the loops are well filled.

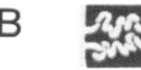 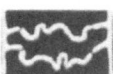 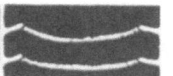

Fig. IV.145B: Schematic representation of a stretched and a contracted intestinal loop. Stretched mucosal folds probably cause thinner clarification lines on the X-ray than those which are more or less folded together.

rapid flocculation of the contrast medium (fig. IV.94).

Giardia lamblia infestations give a pretty well identical picture (fig. IV.95).

b) *Massive adhesions* produce wide but empty intestinal segments resulting from the contraction of adherent neighbouring loops (figs. IV.70A).

c) *Scleroderma* presents with restricted dilatations where intestinal tonus and motility are locally disturbed. Peristalsis is further normal

to sluggish and accompanied by a satisfactory grade of filling (fig. IV.71E).

6.2. Circular, oblique or longitudinal course

More striking is the occurrence of 'stretched-out' mucosal folds involving a *solitary, short segment*. The course of the folds is here mainly circular or oblique (see subsections a and b) while longitudinal folds, so typically associated with severe stretching in adhesions, hernia or invagination (see subsections b and c), are rarely seen but can occur even in the jejunum.

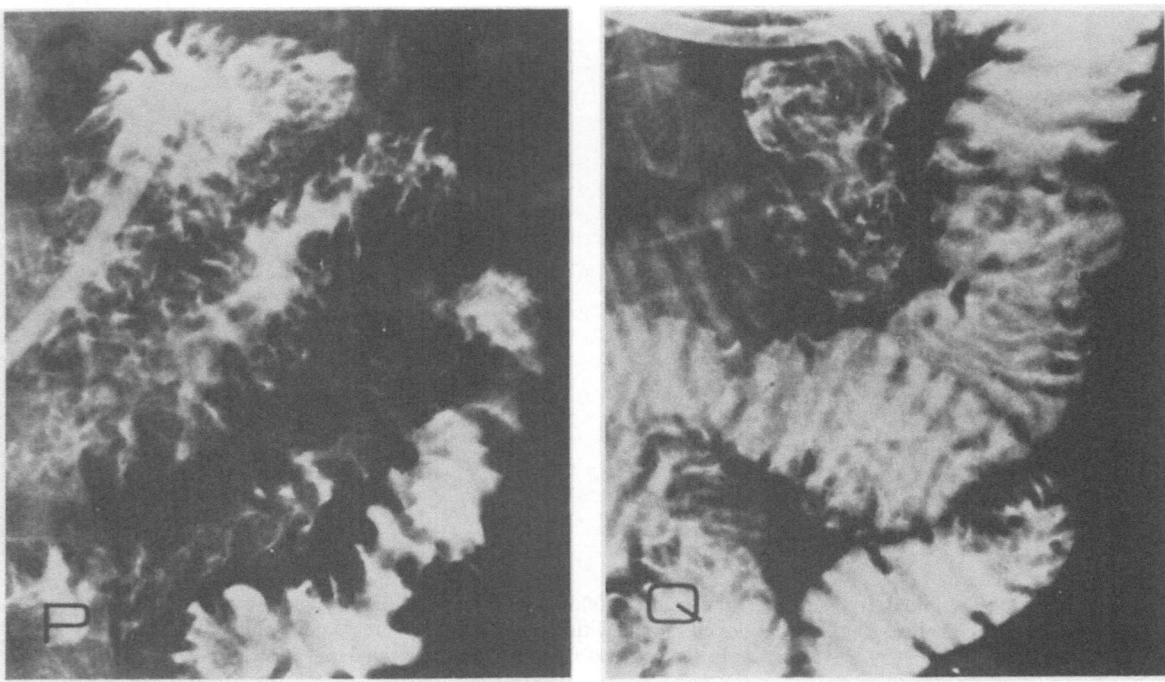

Fig. IV.146. These mucosal folds in the jejunum were judged as definitely too coarse (P). Before the repeat examination, a hypotonic agent was administered. The folds are now seen to be completely normal (Q).

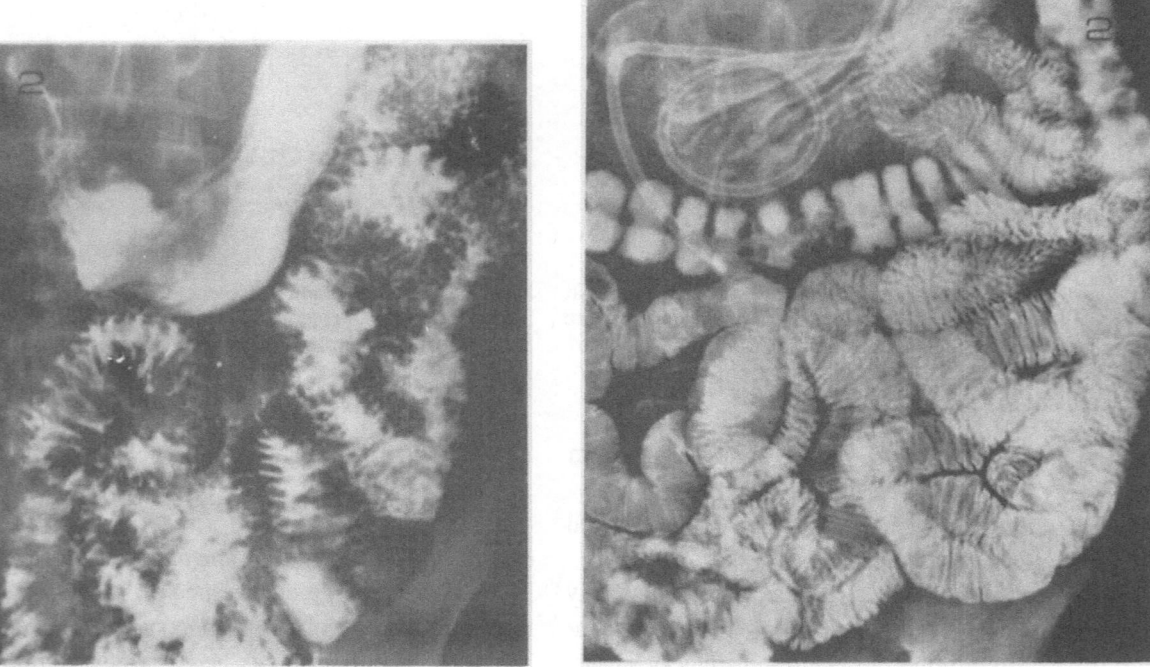

Fig. IV.147. Conventional transit examination of the small intestine in patient with Whipple's disease (left). Coarse mucosal pattern, dilated jejunal loops and rapid flocculation of the barium suspension was observed. The same patient (right) examined by using the enteroclysis method. The mucosal folds now appear normal.

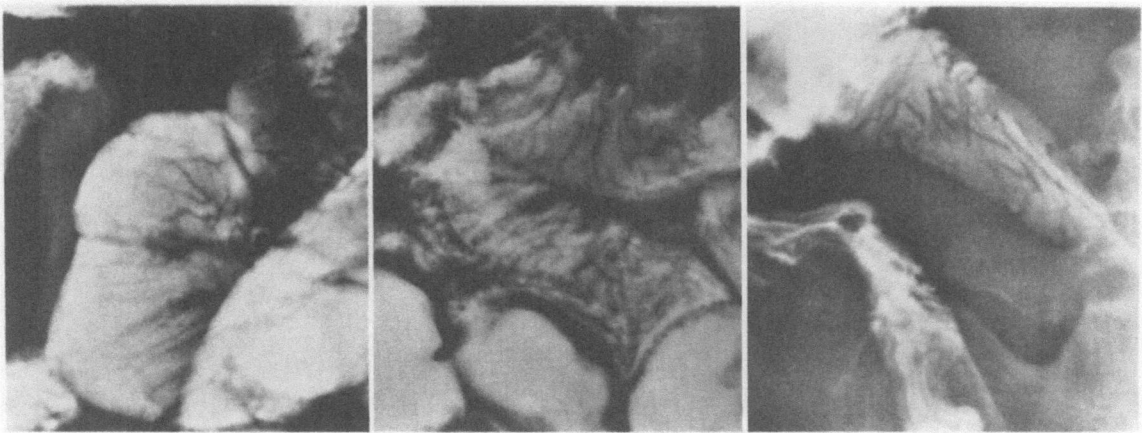

Fig. IV.148. Crackle-like configuration of bright lines in the contrast fluid in the distal ileum. To date these lines have only been observed in the ileum and are presumably caused by residual fold impressions in a thickened barium suspension.

a) Intramural tumors or infiltration on the intestinal wall by a tumor lying outwith the gut (fig. IV.183A), metastases (fig. IV.29) or carcinoid foci (fig. IV.65). Misleading artefacts can be produced by compression. Especially if the compressor is not indicated by a lead marker, the possibility of diagnostic error on the part of a later, independant viewer may arise (fig. IV.183B).

b) Of a completely different nature are the readily recognizable appearances of 'stretched-out' folds in adhesions (figs. IV.115 and IV.6), ligaments (fig. IV.63), hernia (fig. IV.176), fusion with abcess wall (fig. IV.114) and compression by other intestinal loops (fig. III.2B).

c) A further unmistakable form of locally 'stretched-out' folds, longitudinal as well as circular, seen in a more or less empty bowel is that caused by the intraluminally situated intussuscipiens of an invagination (figs. IV.85AB).

d) In the ileum, which is poorly supplied with circular folds, longitudinal mucosal folds frequently appear, resulting even from contractions (figs. IV.125 and III.21A) or severe edema (fig. IV.45).

7. Irregular appearance of the folds (folds still recognizable)

An irregular appearance of the fold borders is nearly always caused by superficial or deeper reaching ulcerative changes, generally from Crohn's disease, radiation enteritis or vascular anomalies. Where the folds have a circular course, whether or not swollen with edema, the irregularities follow this same circular course (fig. IV.161). In the absence of circular folds, as certainly in the presence of edema is the case in the distal ileum, then the irregular appearances, depending on the phase of contraction, consist of complete flattening or of a linear course (fig. IV.151). When the mucosal pattern has totally disappeared, no arrangement of folds can be recognized in such an ulcerative surface. A smooth surface without folds remains after healing (fig. IV.37). In Whipple's disease irregularity of the still recognizable fold borders from swollen villi (fig. IV.92) is seen. Similar changes are found in lymphoid hyperplasia (fig. IV.165) and foaming contrast fluid (fig. III.29). A very local irregular appearance of folds, that can be critically visualised only with the most advantageous filling of the intestine, is found at the site of anastomosis after

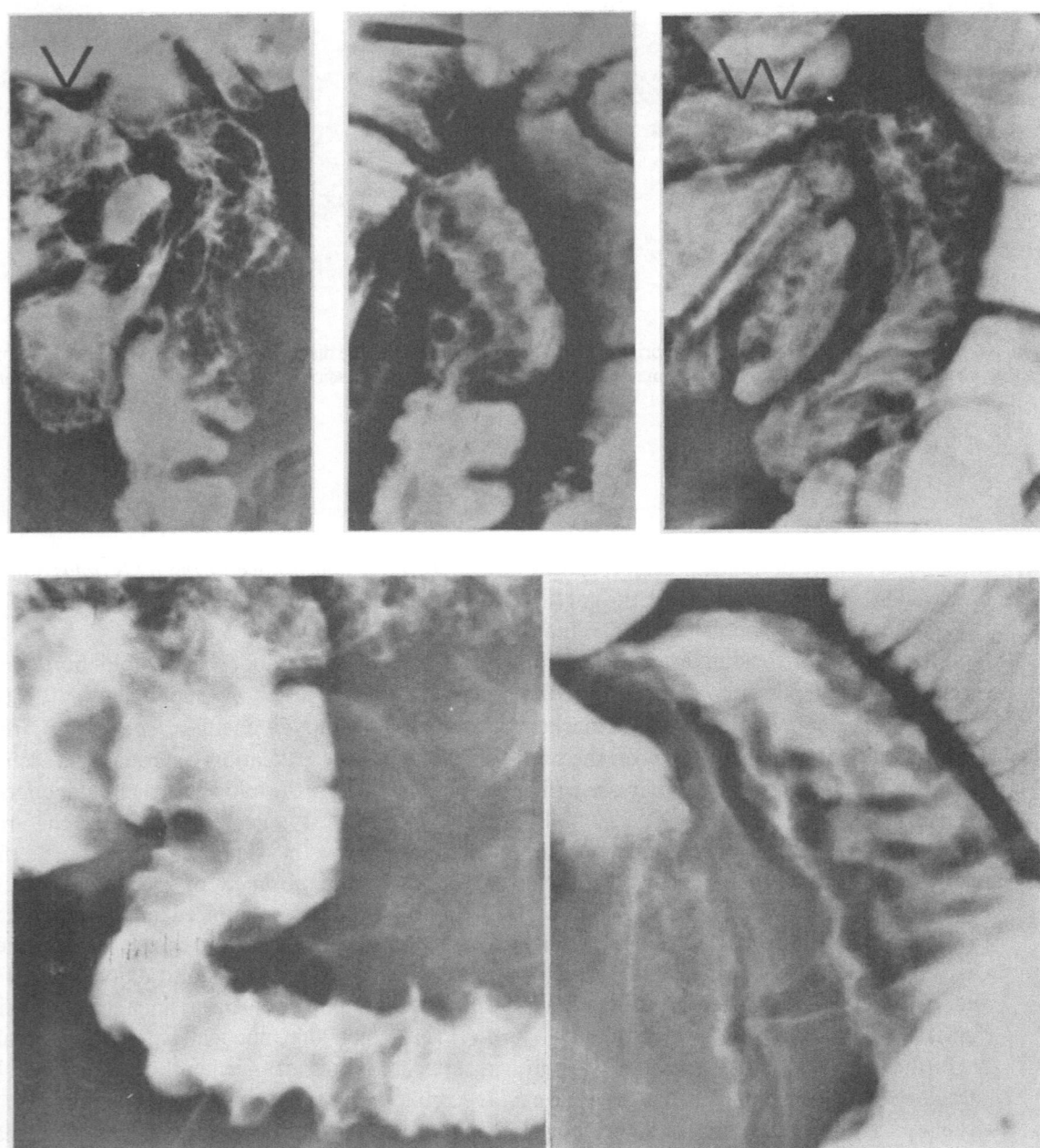

Fig. IV.149. Thick folds with twisting in the distal ileum (upper), voluminous nodular defects (lower left) and thick mucosal folds (lower right) in the distal ileum due to a Yersinia enterocolitica infection.

Formation of Cobblestones
through edema

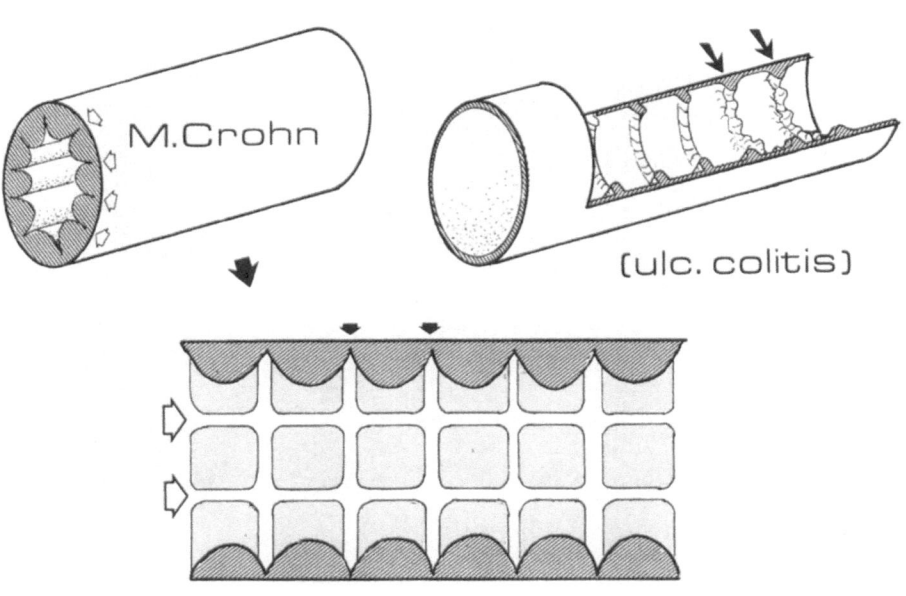

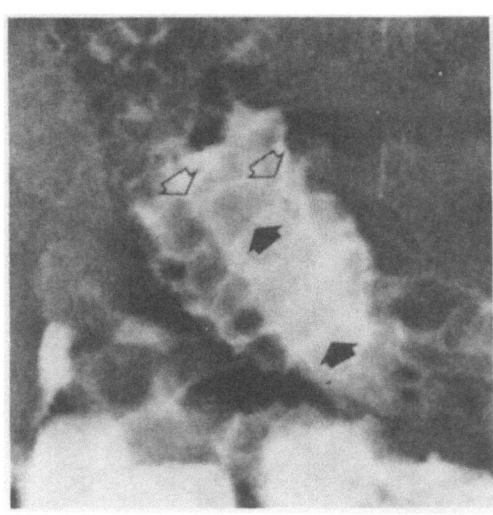

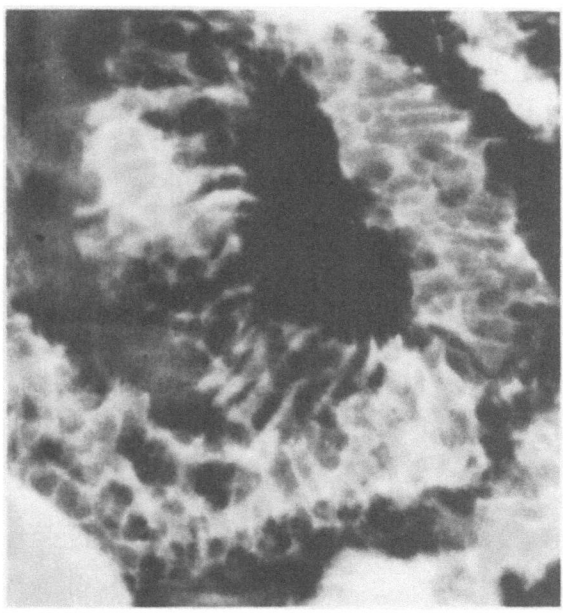

Fig. IV.150A: So-called 'railroad' pattern in Crohn's disease. The longitudinal rails (open arrows) develop because the superficial mucosa is too spacious and must assume smaller dimensions when the mucous membrane swells (see drawing). The ties (solid arrows) are formed by the narrow grooves between the markedly swollen mucosal folds. Between rails and ties is a regular cushion-like pattern (cobblestones).

Fig. IV.150B. So-called cobblestone relief in Crohn's disease caused by longitudinal and transverse grooves in the edematous swollen mucosal surface.

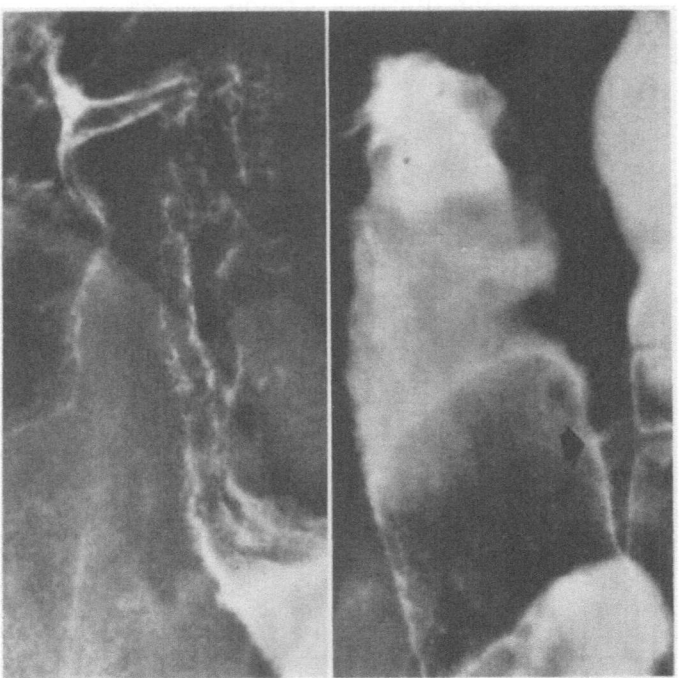

Fig. IV.151. Ulcerative colitis with superficial reflux ileitis in the distal ileum. Rather shrunken cecum and widely opened Bauhin's valve.

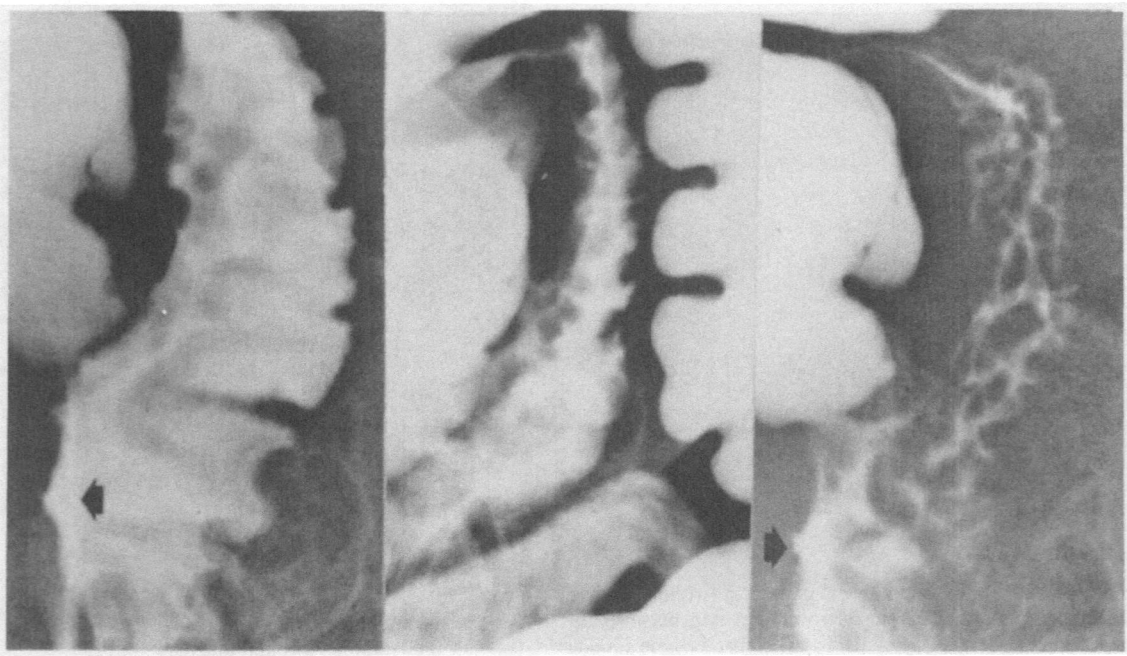

Fig. IV.152. Coarse irregular mucosal relief in the distal ileum with a solitary ulcer (arrow). In this case the abnormalities are as clearly visible in the well-filled as in the empty state and are difficult to evaluate when the intestine is moderately filled. The nature of the abnormality is unknown. X-rays taken two months after removal of a healthy appendix.

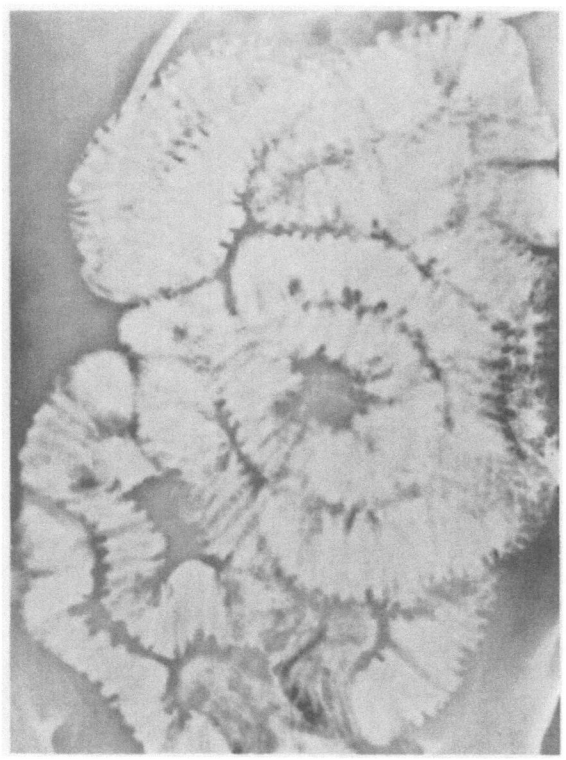

Fig. IV.153. Generalized edema of the mucosa in the jejunum and ileum due, according to the biopsy, to Crohn's disease. As a rule this stage precedes the superficial ulcerative changes seen in fig. IV.37M.

resection (fig. IV.4). Although fairly rarely seen the fold relief in cases of early discovery of mucosal malignancy is still very readily recognizable (fig. IV.76).

8) Destruction of folds (folds no longer recognizable)

Although ulceration can cause such severe destruction that the fold pattern is no longer recognizable (figs. IV.166 and IV.54) this picture is in fact almost universally the result of malignant tumor growth. A few examples are shown in fig. IV.48.

9) Disappearance of fold pattern

Since in the ileum the folds are less pronounced and numerous than in the jejunum and are thus

more readily 'ironed-out', smooth segments devoid of folds appear, if only for this reason, most frequently in the distal half of the small intestine. With exception of a few rare conditions such as amyloidosis, 'graft versus host' effect and tropical sprue, where the mucosal pattern can be absent in a very long segment (figs. IV.167, IV.38 and IV.104), this appearance is found in every other case only in a short or limited segment. The condition is found in the proximal bowel in about 50% of celiac patients (fig. IV.43), in alcoholic duodenitis, here limited to the duodenum, in uremic enteritis and strongiloides infestation. Distally, abuse of laxatives and reflux ileitis can lead to an atrophy (figs. IV.168FH). Further, mucosal pattern can disappear, in principle, in numerous conditions affecting the entire small intestine, e.g.:

ischemia (figs. IV.169 andIV.33)
radiation enteritis (fig. IV.36A)
P.A.N. (fig. IV.35)
Henoch-Schönlein disease (fig. IV.159)
Crohn's disease (fig. IV.37)
various malignant lymphomas or Hodgkin's disease (figs. IV.109 and IV.154).

F. Translucencies in the lumen (see also chapter III.E2 and 3)

1) Bodies lying free in the lumen and those projecting into it from the mucosa or wall, both present on radiograms as translucencies in the column of contrast medium. Loose foreign bodies regularly seen in the bowel lumen include:

unidentifiable food residues (fig. III.25K)
rice grains (fig. III.27)
beans and fruit stones (figs. III.26 and III.25L)
worms (fig. IV.170)
surgical swab (fig. IV.84).

Distinction ought to be made between 'real' and 'pseudo' worms (fig. IV.170).
A surgical swab without metal thread in its weave may be difficult to distinguish from an invagination.

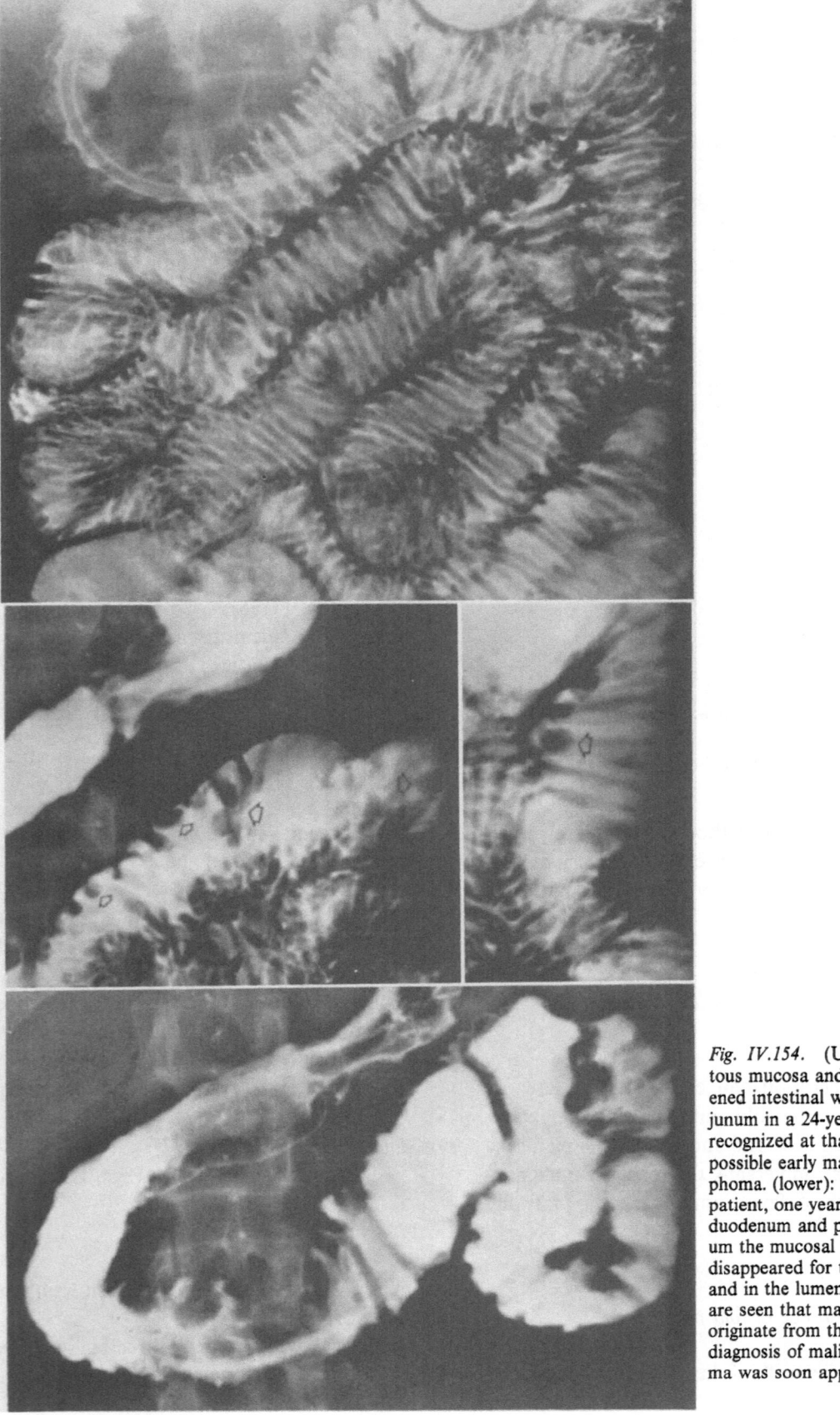

Fig. IV.154. (Upper): Edematous mucosa and slightly thickened intestinal wall of the jejunum in a 24-year-old man; not recognized at that time as a possible early malignant lymphoma. (lower): The same patient, one year later. In the duodenum and proximal jejunum the mucosal folds have disappeared for the most part and in the lumen nodular lumps are seen that may or may not originate from the folds. The diagnosis of malignant lymphoma was soon apparent.

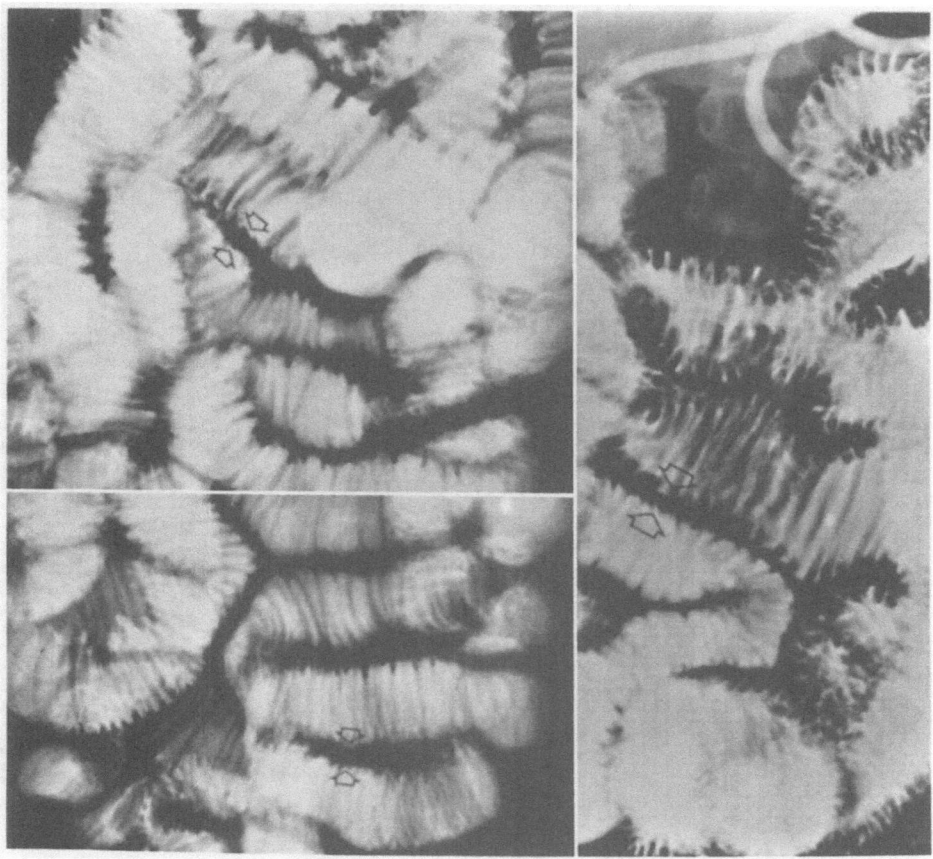

Fig. IV.155. Mesenteric arteritis of unknown origin, found during surgery, in a 10-year-old boy. The mucosal folds are moderately broadened and the wall is thickened throughout most of the intestine (arrows). The thickness of a normal bowel wall in a child can be seen at the right. Here, the mucosal folds lie so close together that they have the so-called 'stacked coin' appearance.

2) Smaller translucencies based on the mucosa are:

    lymphfollicles (figs. IV.171 and II.8)
    swollen villi in Whipple's disease (fig. IV.92)
    cobblestones in Crohn's disease (fig. IV.74).

Small gas bubbles and rice grains can deceptively resemble lymphfollicles in the distal ileum. This effect is still more pronounced in the proximal jejunum with its associated multiple overlapping projection of contractile loops rich in folds (fig. IV.172).

Gas bubbles often vary in size while that of lymphfollicles and cobblestones is more or less constant. Where insufficient anti-foaming agent is present in the contrast fluid, foam can give a very misleading impression of swollen villi but the outer edge of the contrast column still shows a sharp uninterrupted outline that is not maintained in the presence of swollen villi (fig. IV.92).

3) Larger bodies ultimately projecting from or lying within the bowel wall comprise:

    hematomata, hemangioma (fig. IV.56B)
    lipoma (fig. IV.173)
    Peutz-Jegher syndrome (fig. IV.110)
    carcinoid focus (fig. IV.174)
    melanoma metastases (fig. IV.175)
    invagination (fig. IV.85).

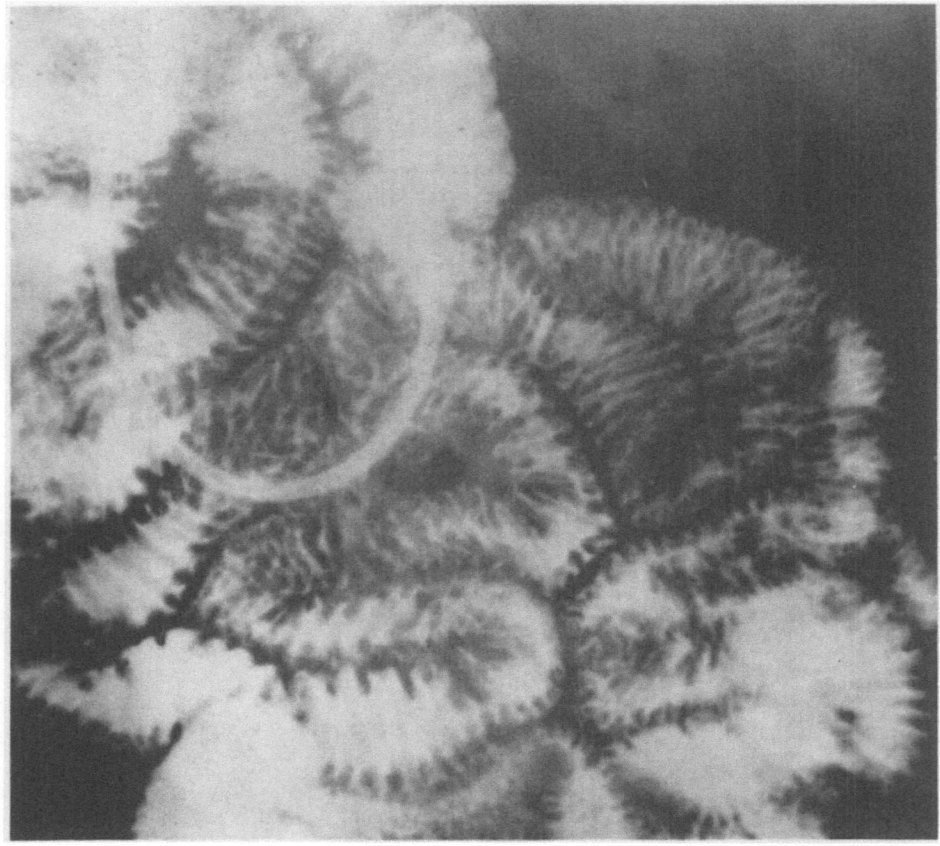

Fig. IV.156. Edematous swollen omega-shaped mucosal folds throughout the small bowel from a pronounced impairment of the venous flow as a result of liver cirrhosis. The liver is small; the spleen is greatly enlarged.

G. Disturbed motility

1. General remarks

Many markedly divergent diseases can be accompanied by changes in motility of the small bowel. Understanding and knowledge of the mechanism responsible for these motility disorders, however, can be considered as little more than rudimentary. The infusion technique has shown that motility is disturbed much more frequently than is generally assumed. On the contrary, when the contrast medium is administered orally, hypermotility is sometimes incorrectly diagnosed on the basis of an accelerated transit time. This is seen for instance in gastric aplasia or in hyperperistalsis of the stomach. In both cases there is an accelerated gastric emptying and consequent shorter transit time. The elimination of the factor – gastric

emptying time – in the enteroclysis examination has widened the possibilities of comparing transit times through the small intestine.

The greatest contribution to establishing a diagnosis of disturbed motility is that during this examination the contrast column is followed under intermittent fluoroscopy. Acute and short local changes in motility are thus as a rule no longer missed (figs. IV.63 and IV.176).

Some diseases such as the collagen diseases and diabetes mellitus are accompanied by the phenomenon of enhanced or decreased motility. Thus hypomotility is seen or a hypermotility; the latter from mild anoxia of the intestinal wall. In collagen diseases, this anoxia is due to a vasculitis, while in diabetes it is the result of an insufficiency of the peripheral circulation from arteriosclerotic changes in the walls of the arterioles. If there is diabetogenic diarrhea, then as a rule there is also

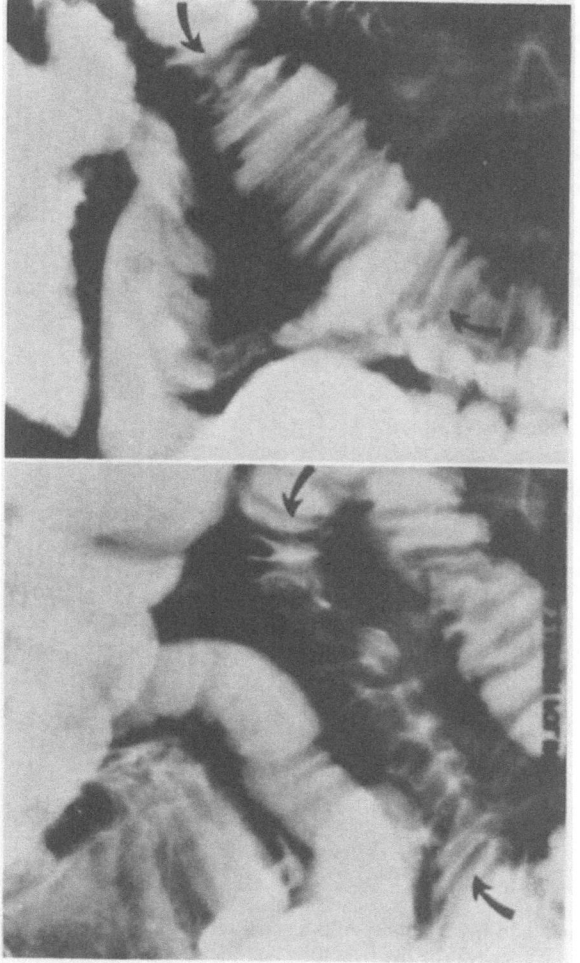

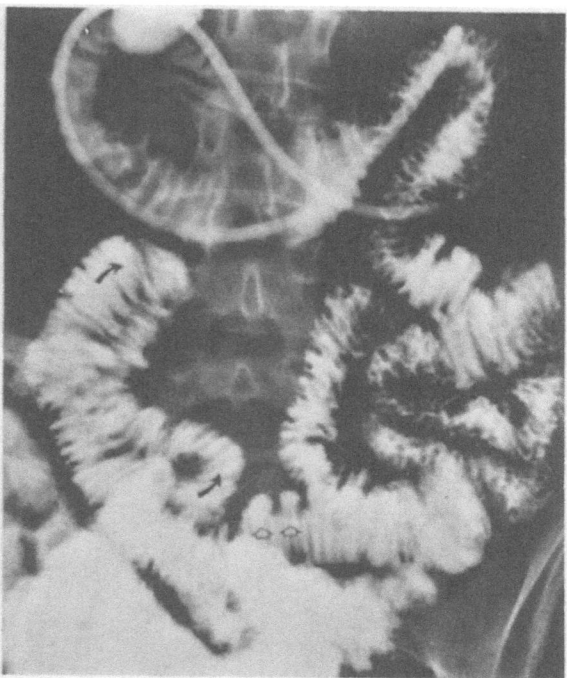

Fig. IV.157. Diffuse vascular abnormalities in the small intestine of a patient with dermatomyositis. Coarse and also irregular mucosal relief in the region of the ileojejunal junction (solid arrows). In the duodenum too the folds appear fairly coarse; the degree of filling here is, however, moderate. As in the patient with scleroderma in fig. IV.139 a number of small sacculations can also be seen (open arrows).

associated retinopathy and disturbed function of kidney and pancreas. The impaired functioning of the pancreas can be such that the resorption of diverse food substances is impaired, resulting in a pancreatogenic steatorrhea. If motility in this disease is insufficient for rapid distal transit of the contrast fluid, few intestinal loops will be seen in a state of contraction. The barium suspension then flocculates almost immediately (fig. IV.177). Statistically estimated on the number of patients and causative factors, decreased motility of the intestine is more frequently encountered than increased. Hypermotility, where seen, is more commonly an enhancement of motility throughout the entire length of the small bowel than a locally situated hyperperistalsis. Although seemingly paradoxical, most states of hypomotility alternate with periods of hypermotility. These attacks of hyperperistalsis provoke most of the subjective complaints and lead to consultation

The *causative factors of a disturbed motility* of the small intestine can be grouped in several major categories:

a) neurogenic or humoral
    increased peristalsis
        carcinoid foci
        fear and other emotions
        hyperparathyroidism
    decreased peristalsis
        medicaments
            tranquillizers
            sedatives
            antispasmodics

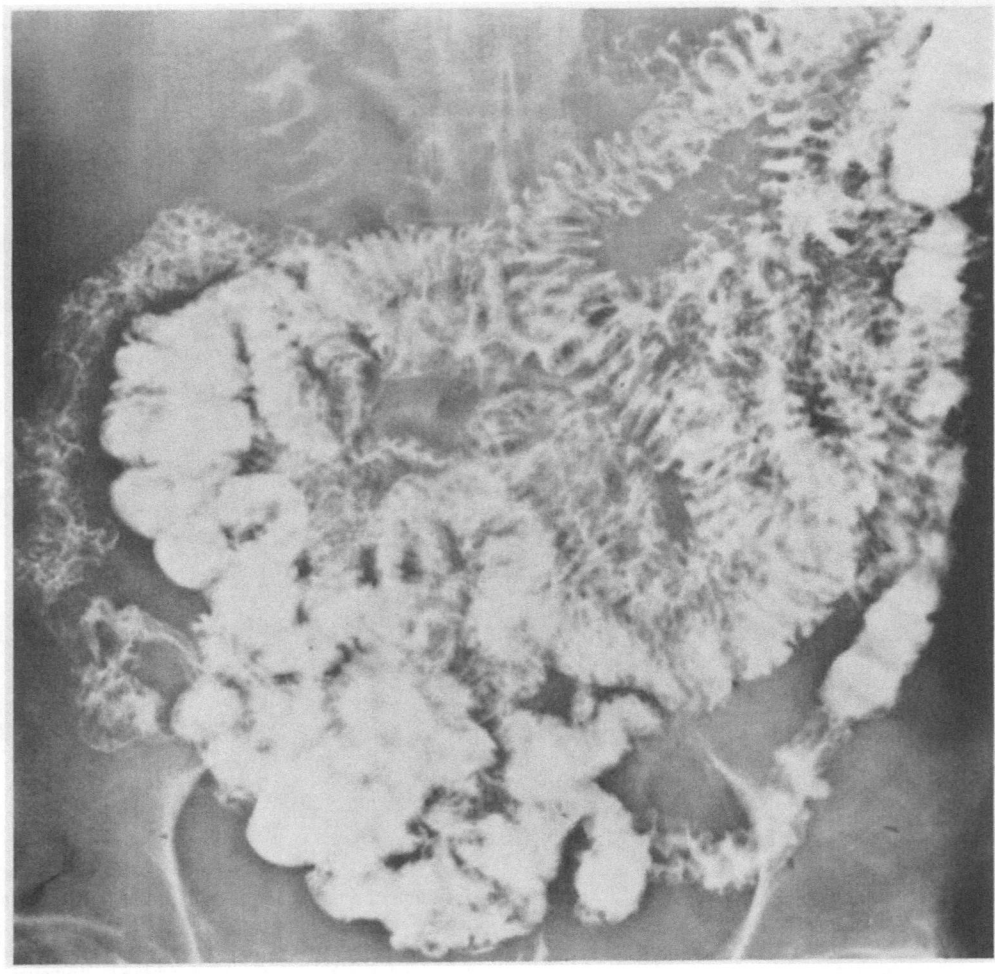

Fig. IV.158. Markedly thickened mucosal folds in the jejunum and hypermotility of the small intestine in a patient with mixed collagen disease. A marked malabsorption was apparent clinically. The hypermotility and the edema could be due to anoxia as a result of vasculitis.

heroine
systemic contraceptives
chronic use of laxatives
diabetic neuropathy
myxedema
amyotrophic lateral sclerosis
multiple sclerosis
chronic alcoholism
severe abdominal pain or abdominal
    trauma
acute inflammation
    pancreatitis
    cholecystitis
    appendicitis
    peritonitis
pregnancy

b) mechanical obstruction
Increasing dilatation towards the site of obstruction contraindicates drug-induced atony (figs. IV.178 and IV.83).
Initially there is a prestenotic hyperperistalsis. If peristalsis is still present, the obstruction is not total and a SBE examination should be considered, but obstruction in the colon must first be excluded.

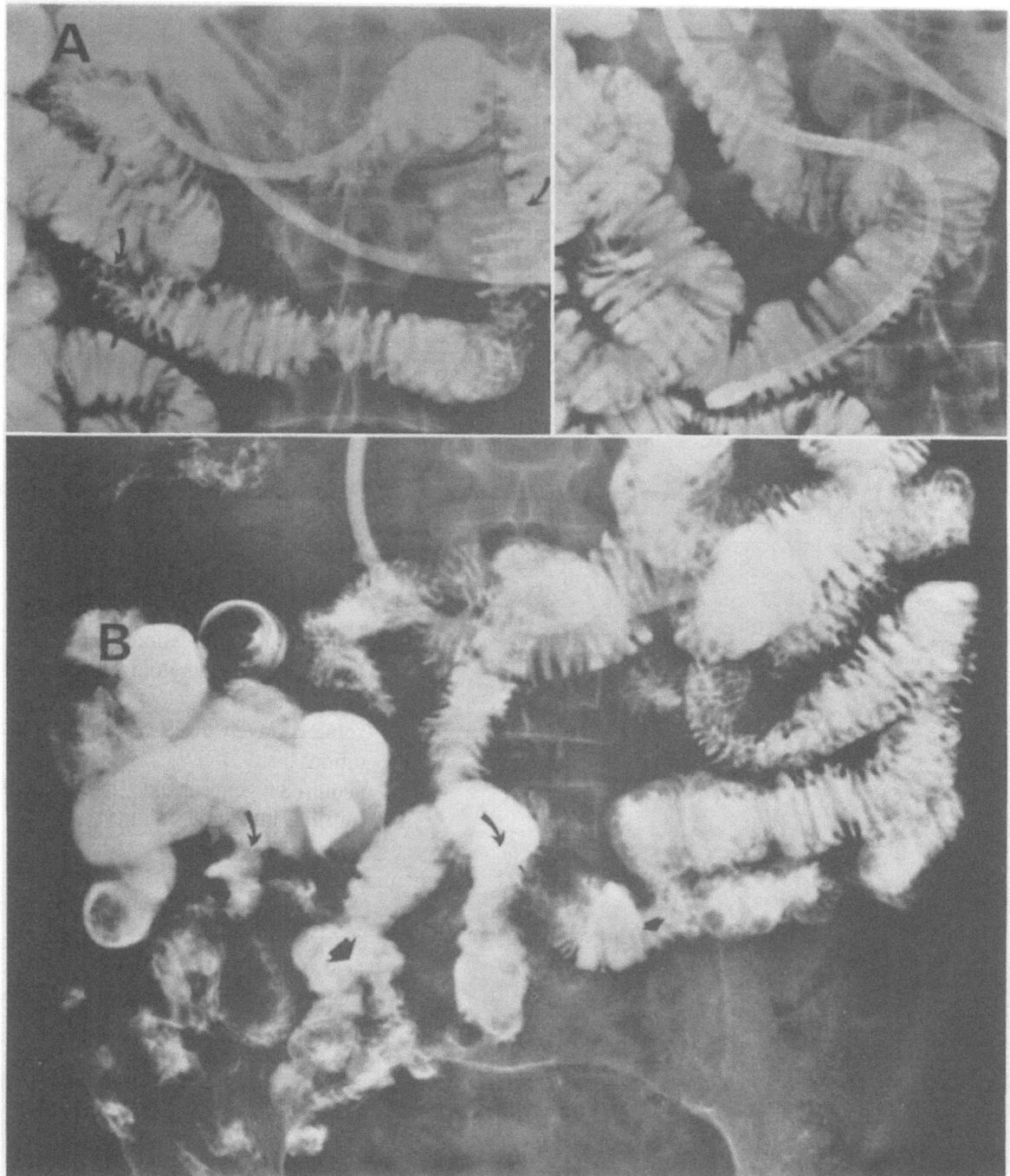

Fig. IV.159. Two patients with rectal bleeding due to Schönlein-Henoch disease. (A) Several decimetres of highly edematous swollen mucosal folds in the proximal jejunum (left), probably due to diffuse submucosal bleedings only. As so often in these patients, recovery was spontaneous and the mucosa appeared normal two weeks later (right). (B) The abnormalities can, however, also be more widespread as well as more pronounced so that complete recovery does not follow. Then the mucosal relief in several areas will be pathologically changed or completely absent. There will be an obvious hypermotility in the proximal ileum in the lower right quadrant. Similar abnormalities can be encountered in other diseases that are accompanied by arteritis – for instance dermatomyositis (see fig. IV.157).

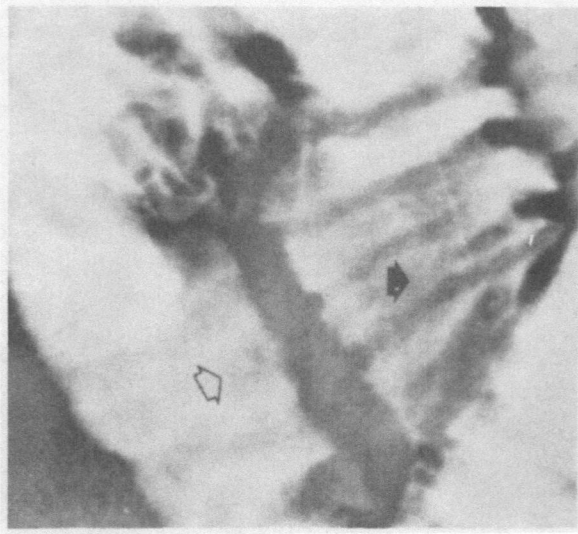

Fig. IV.160. Early stage of Crohn's disease with edematous folds and multiple aphthoid ulcerations in the distal ileum.

Fig. IV.162. Remnants of mucosal folds in Crohn's disease. No edema after healing.

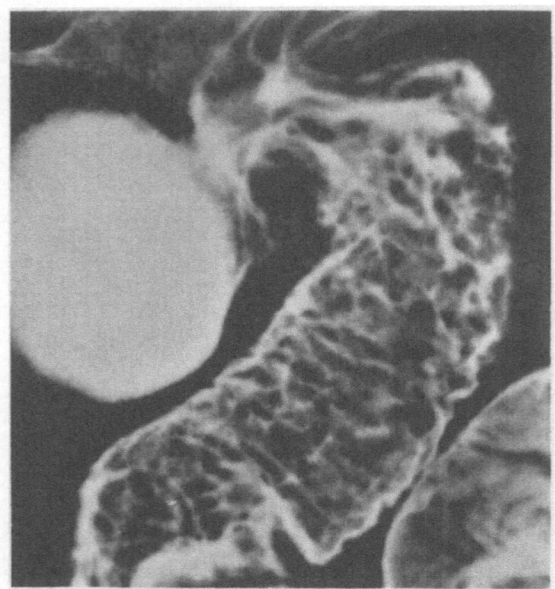

Fig. IV.161. Granular appearance of mucosal surface and very superficial, transversely directed ulcerative grooves in the distal ileum as a result of reflux ileitis in ulcerative colitis. A transverse course of ulcerations in the distal ileum is probably a result of a rather superficial edematous swelling of the mucosa. In Crohn's disease the edema is much more pronounced and necessarily leads to a predominantly longitudinal folding of the inner surface of those parts of the bowel but scarcely provided with mucosal folds (see fig. IV.150AB).

c) diseases affecting the intestinal wall
　　some cases of amyloidosis (+ local dilatations)
　　some collagen diseases (+ local dilatations)
　　acquired generalized lymphedema (normal intestinal calibre)

d) chemical enteritis
　local hyperperistalsis or spasm also possible
　　lead poisoning
　　diabetic or uremic acidosis (sometimes ulceration)
　　immunosuppressive therapy
　　gastric acid in Zollinger-Ellison's disease (hypermotility also possible)

e) allergic reactions
　violent, sometimes local hyperperistaltic movements
　　worms and parasites
　　some foods (milk)
　　Henoch-Schönlein disease

f) anoxia
　hyperperistalsis, decreased calibre of the

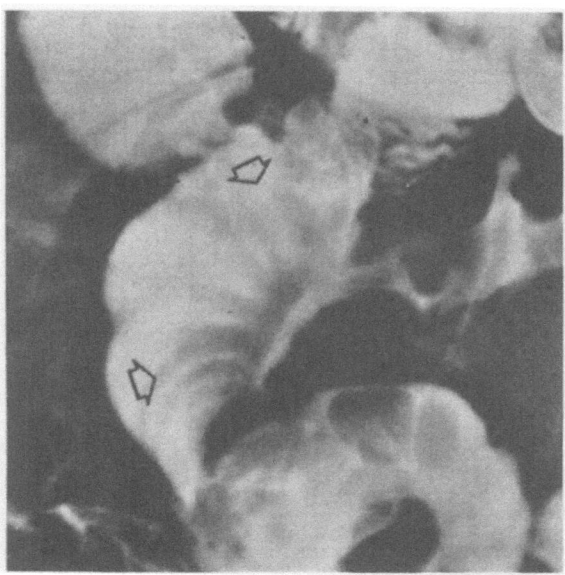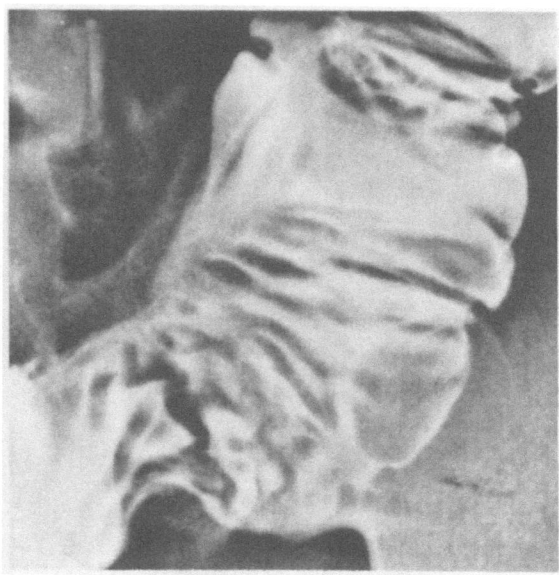

Fig. IV.163. Left: More or less concentric course of the mucosal folds directed towards the site of an ulceration in the intestinal wall. Right: In a patient with Crohn's disease, the remnants of the mucosal folds in a proximal jejunal loop radiate slightly towards the contracted mesenterial side where a healed ulcer is undoubtely present.

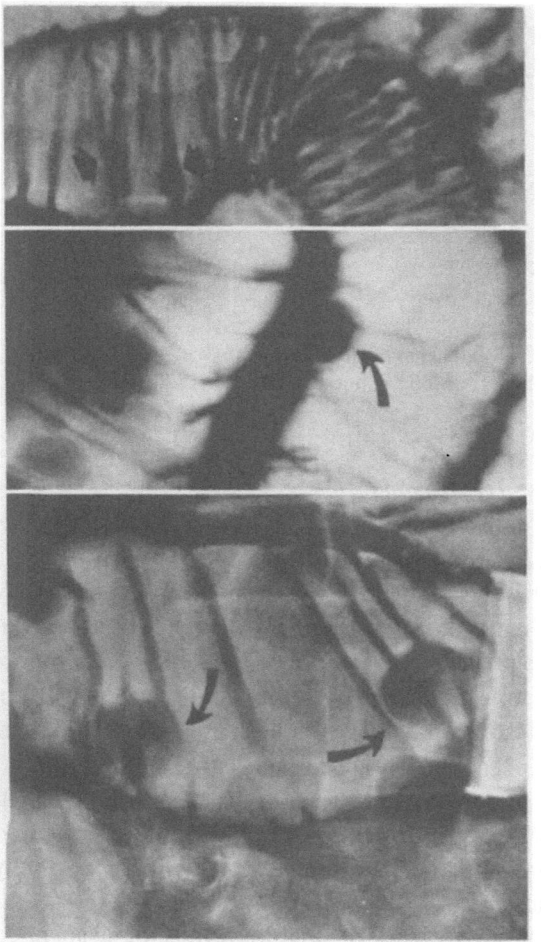

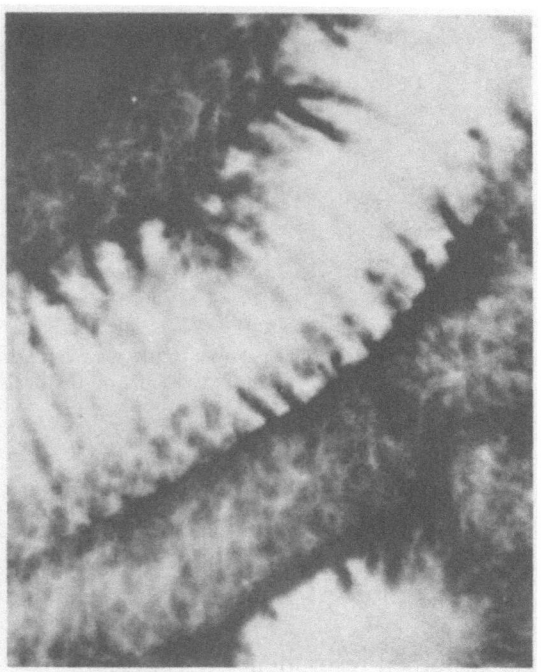

Fig. IV.165. Lymphoid nodular hyperplasia. Multiple filling defects in the contrast fluid, 1-3 mm in diameter.

Fig. IV.164. Sudden interruption of mucosal folds by metastasis of melanoma (lower) and local broadening by very small metastasis (upper).

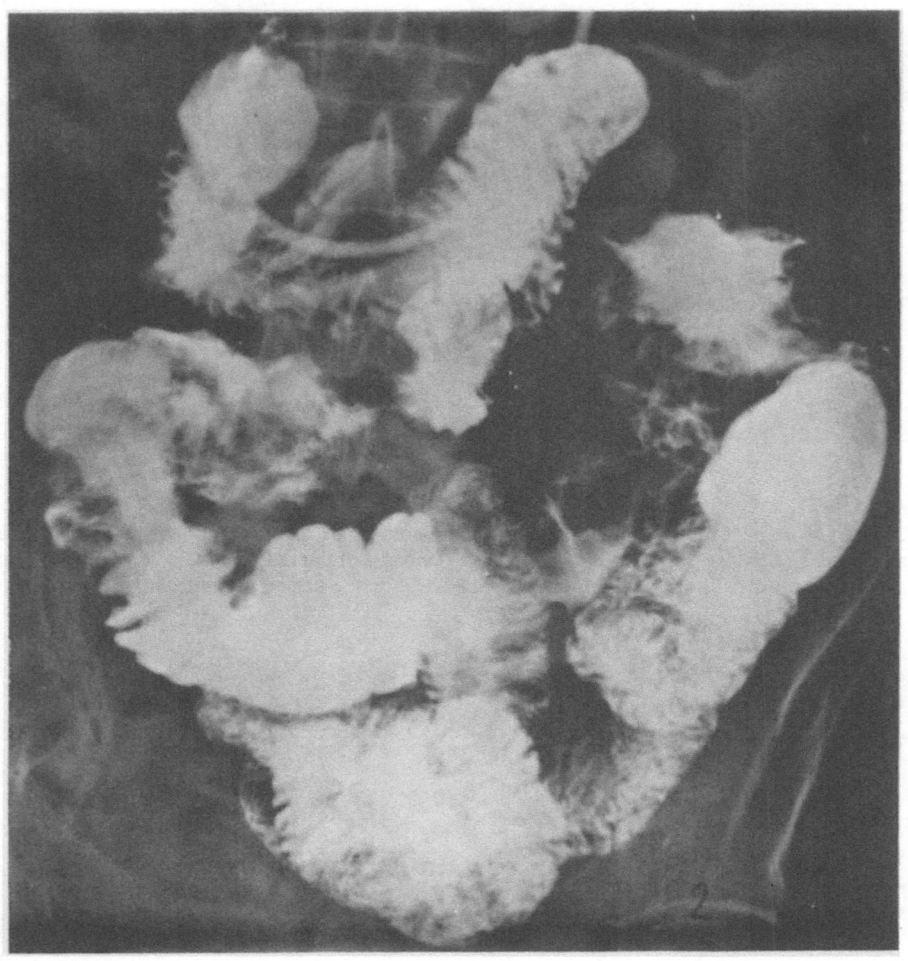

Fig. IV.166. Eosinophilic gastroenteritis with large infiltrates and extensive destruction so that differentiation from a lymphosarcoma on the basis of radiological criteria is not possible.

intestine, circular folds close together.
  vasculitis in collagen diseases
  radiation enteritis
  intestinal angina

g) disturbed resorption
  Enhancement of peristaltic movements due to an increase in the contents of the intestine because there is an impaired resorption. Strange combination of intestinal hurry and multiple dilatations.
    pancreatogenic steatorrhea
    Zollinger-Ellison's disease
    adult celiac disease

2. Hypermotility

2.1. General remarks

There is a definite suggestion of hypermotility when radiograms, taken with correct rate of infusion, show that the loops are for the half or more in contraction. Where this is associated with an intestine of narrower calibre, as is mostly the case, the cecum can be reached with 200-400 ml contrast fluid in some 3-5 min (figs. IV.67 and II.3B). In the event of dilated loops the amount required may well be in excess of the 700 ml normally indicated.

Varying degrees of dilatation may be associated with hypermotility, they are:

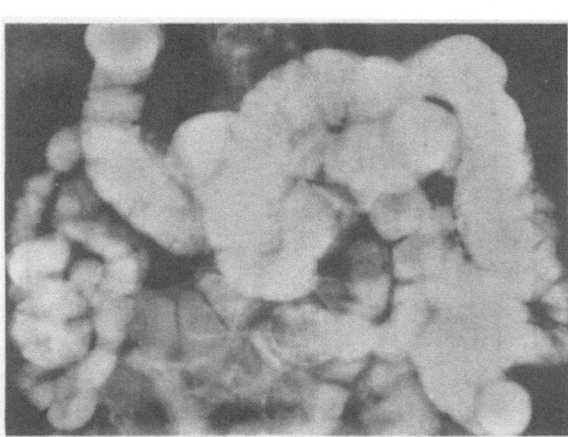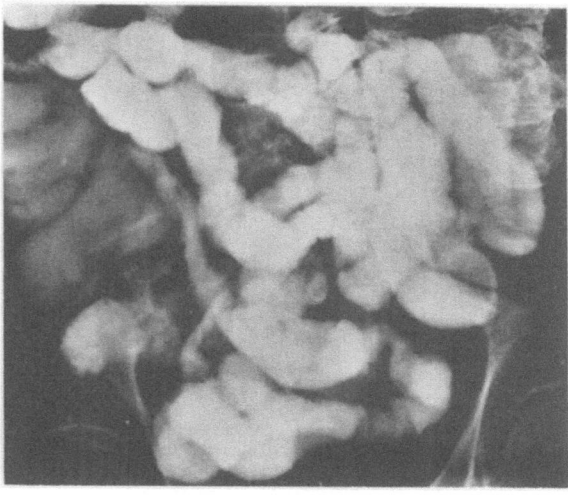

Fig. IV.167. Flat mucosal relief in the duodenum, jejunum and ileum of a patient with primary amyloidosis. In the differential diagnosis, lymphoma should also be considered. After remission of Crohn's disease and in celiac disease, the abnormalities would be less extensive and the rigidity and unequal thickening of the wall, seen here, would be absent.

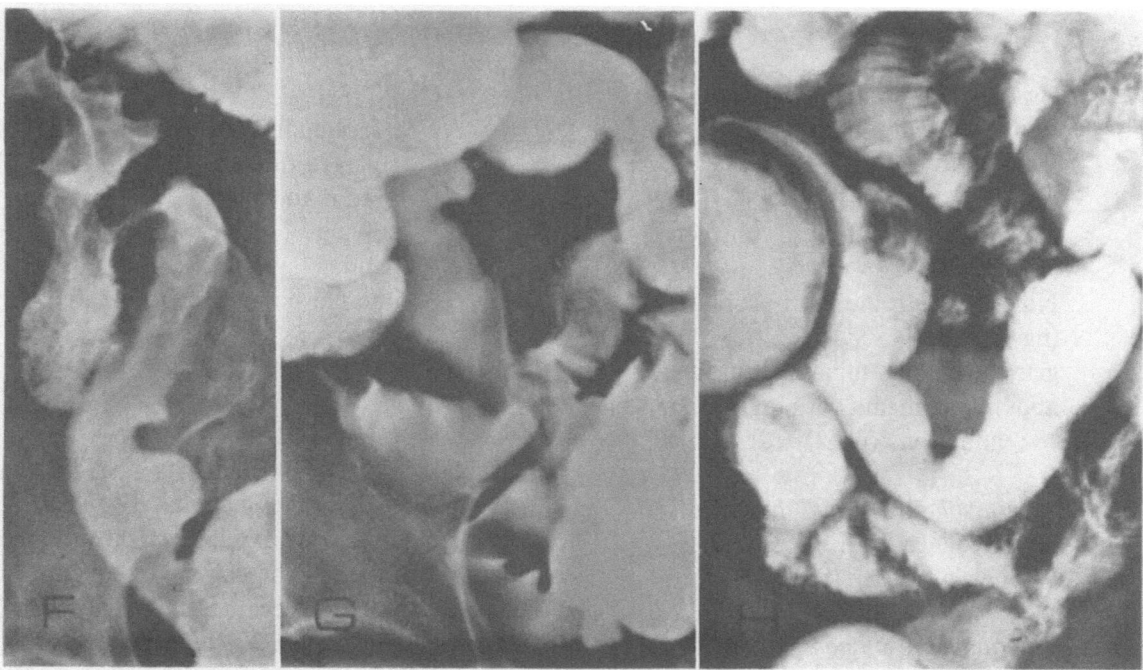

Fig. IV.168. (F) Colitis with reflux ileitis. That segment of the ileum containing the atrophied mucosa is usually only about 15 cm long. (G) Smooth mucosal surface 30 years after healing of Crohn's disease in the ileocecal region. (H) Quite pronounced atrophy of the mucosa in the ileocecal region as a result of chronic use of drugs. The marked dilatation of the cecum shown here is not found after an ileocolitis.

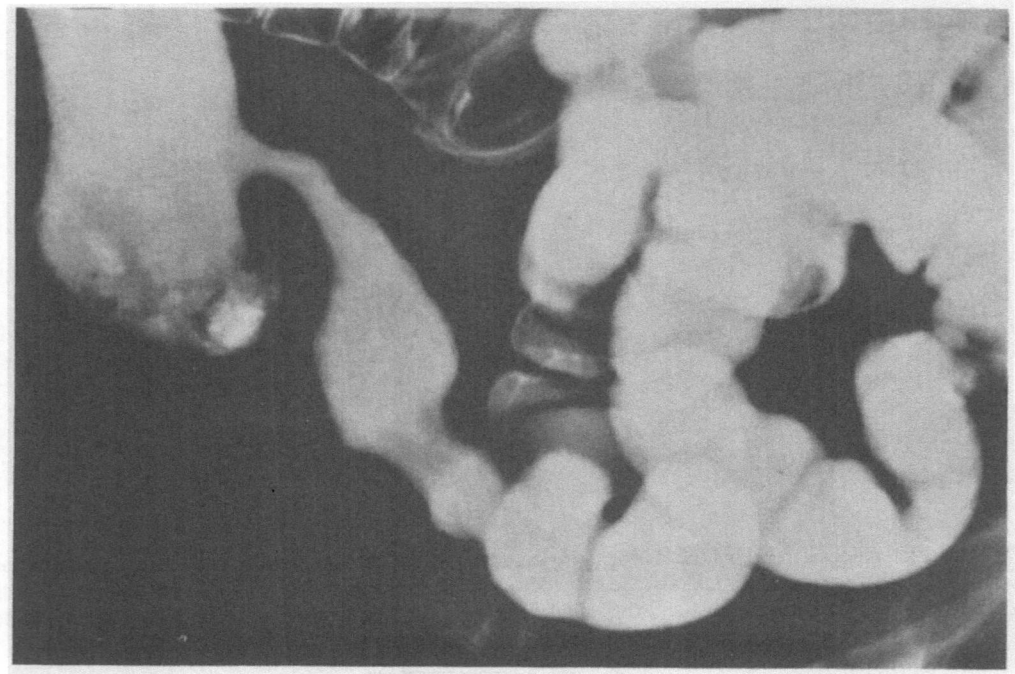

Fig. IV.169. Patient after recovery from ischemia. Smooth wall in a 50-cm segment of the cecum and distal ileum. Widely open Bauhin's valve no longer functional. In this case, differentiation from Crohn's disease on the basis of radiological examination is imposible.

2.2. Hypermotility with marked dilatation
  pancreatogenic (fig. IV.96)
  celiac syndrome (25% of cases)
  (fig. IV.180)
  Zollinger-Ellison (fewer contractions)
  (fig. IV.100)
  Naish's syndrome (non propulsive)
  (fig. IV.6)
  giardia lamblia inflammation (fig. IV.95)
  abdominal angina with massive peritoneal
    adhesions (fig. IV.70)

2.3. Hypermotility with mild dilatation
  lactase deficiency
  Whipple's disease (fig. IV.93)

2.4. Hypermotility with constriction
  fear and other emotions
  allergic (food, milk, worms and parasites)
  thyrotoxicosis
  carcinoid (eventually local hyperperistal-
    sis) (figs. IV.181 and IV.68)

anoxia: diabetic
  abdominal angina
  collagen disease (sometimes local)
  irradiation (limited segments)
  volvulus ⎫ where tran-
  bands ⎬ sient or of
  internal hernia ⎭ mild deegree

3. Hypomotility

3.1. General remarks
Reduction in motility manifests itself first and most markedly in the jejunum, the ileum can become involved only at a later stage and there it is less pronounced. The volume of contrast fluid required to reach the cecum is almost always 1200 ml (maximum dosage). A supplement of 1200 ml water (maximum dosage) is often needed. Auxilliary administration of metoclopramide via the tube is further frequently necessary. Based on extent and degree of dilatation a scala of possibilities arise with hypomotility.

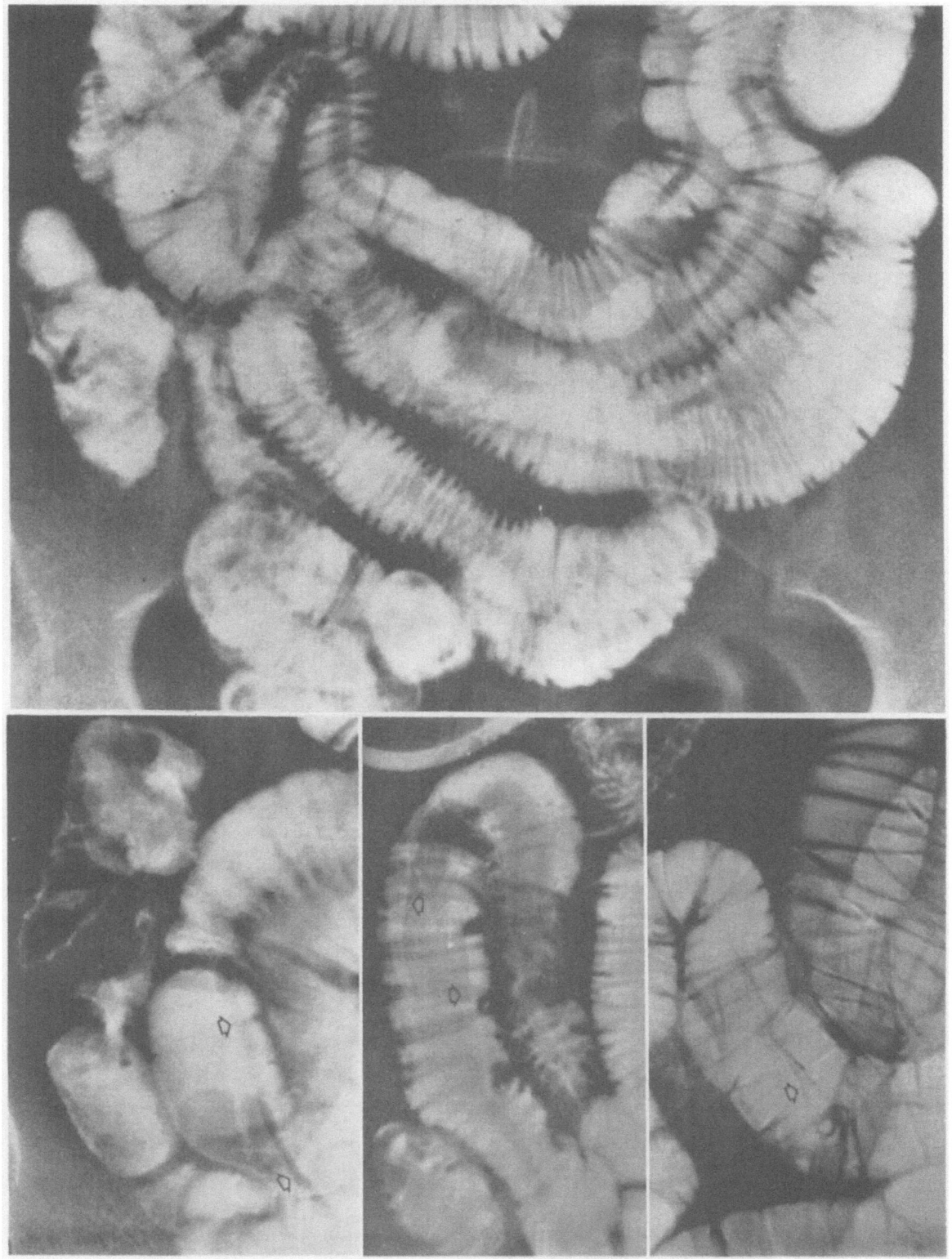

Fig. IV.170. (Upper): Ascaris or tapeworms. (Lower): Misleading pattern of worms caused by sacroiliac joint, threads of mucus and mucosal folds in other intestinal loops.

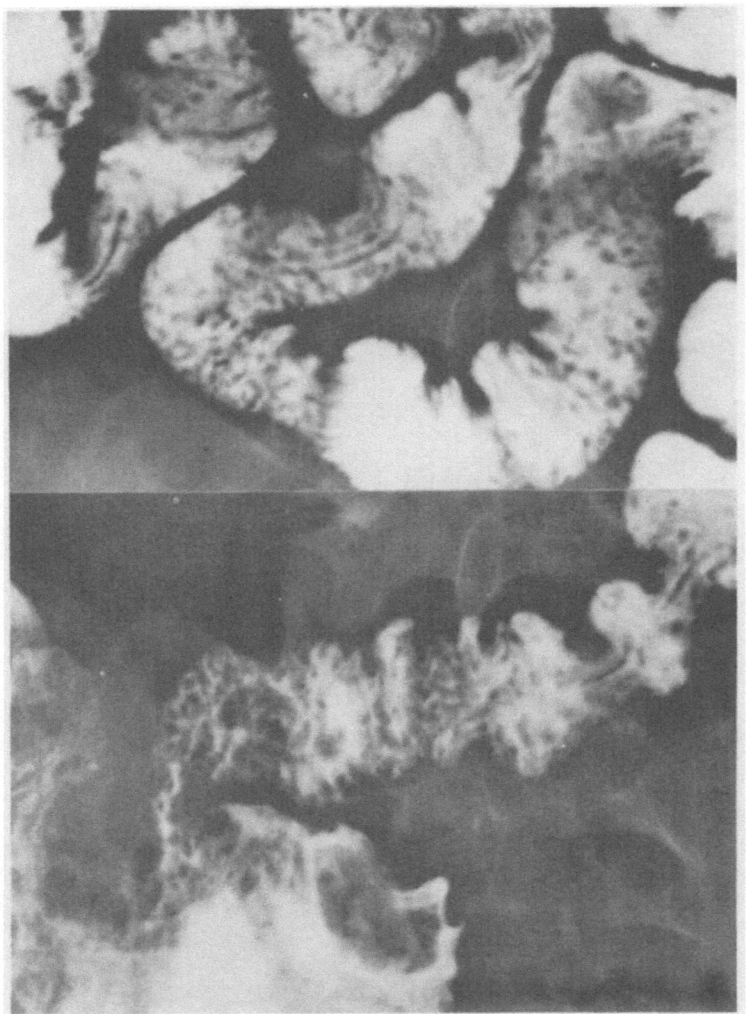

Fig. IV.171. Lymphoid nodular hyperplasia in case of immunoglobulin deficiency, involving more than 50 cm of the distal ileum (upper). During contraction, the lymph follicles can not or only with difficulty be found (lower).

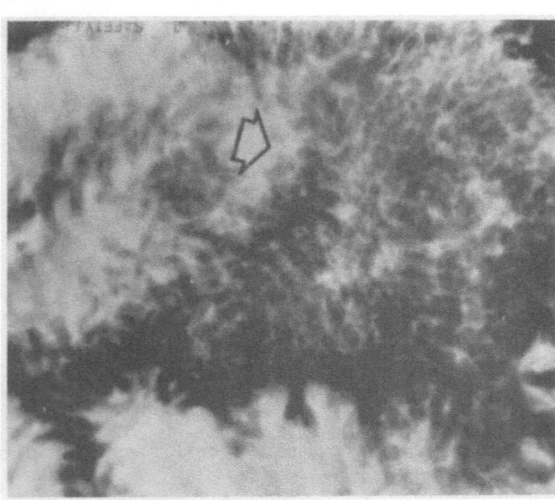

Fig. IV.172. Mucosal pattern in an irritable jejunum of a patient infected with Giardia lamblia. Rapid disintegration after 1 min although 900 ml contrast fluid was administered through the tube.

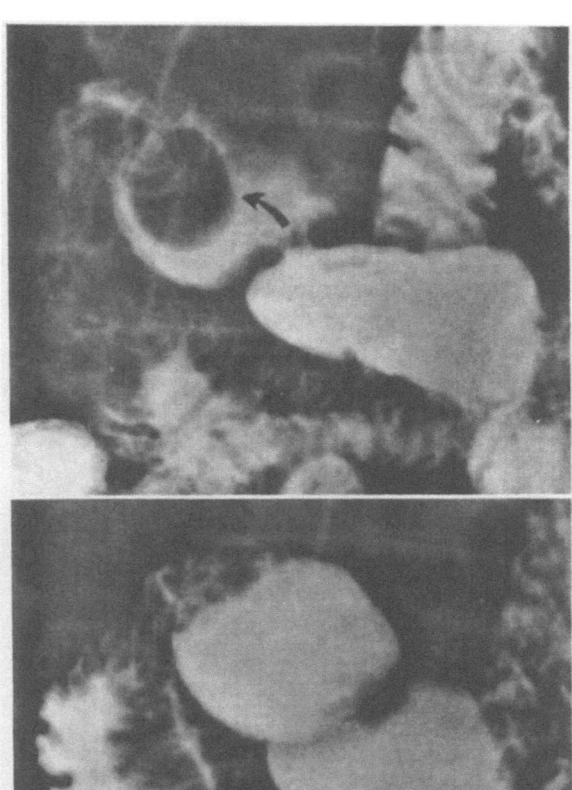

Fig. IV.173. A characteristic of lipomas is that they are easily deformed.

3.2. Generalised hypomotility with considerable dilatation

obstruction – motility initially normal

sedatives ⎫
tranquillizers ⎬ motility imme-
antispasmodics ⎭ diately disturbed (fig. IV.182)

intact fold pattern

neurogenic, alcoholism, lues
abdominal trauma
acute inflammations

scleroderma – sacculations, thin folds
amyloid disease – broad, irregular, nodular folds

3.3. Generalised hypomotility with mild dilatation

lead poisoning
immunosuppresive therapy – fold pattern lost in vascular rejection
Zollinger-Ellison – thickened folds, flocculation in jejunum, motility normal
myxedema

3.4. Partial hypomotility with mild dilatation

diabetic acidosis ⎫
uremic acidosis ⎬ jejunum

laxative abuse (fig. IV.179) ⎫ distal
ulcerative colitis ⎬ ileum

3.5. Partial hypomotility with mild constriction

celiac disease (jejunum)
lymphoretic. malig. ⎫
post vasc. acc. ⎬ entire length

3.6. Partial hypomotility with dilatation or constriction

quiescent Crohn's disease ⎫ entire
amyloid disease ⎬ length

lost musocal fold pattern

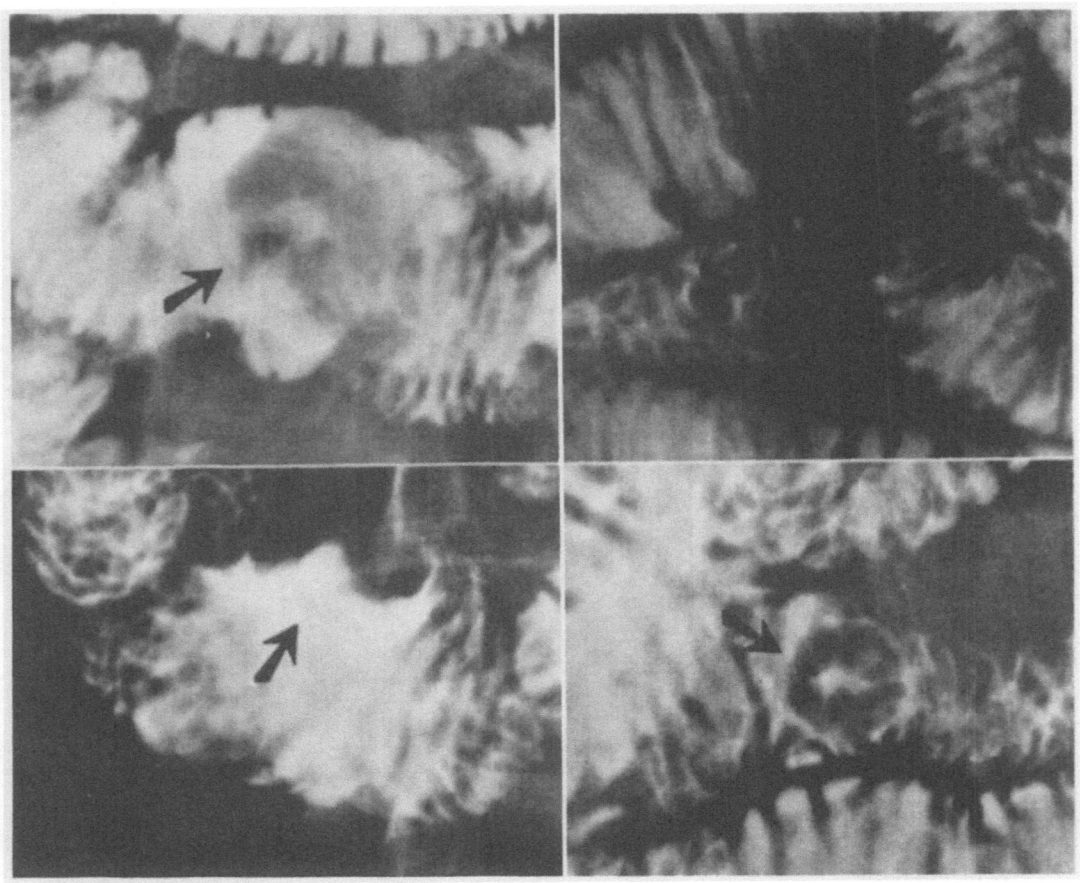

Fig. IV.175. Several examples of melanotic metastases, including one which is very small and shows central necrosis. On the left, a so-called 'bull's eye' is seen en face (upper) and in profile (lower).

Fig. IV.174. Intramural carcinoids in the distal ileum (thick arrow). Extensive fibrosis in the intestinal wall and the mesentery causes constriction of the intestinal lumen of when the intestine is well filled. These constrictions are clearly visible as deep grooves.

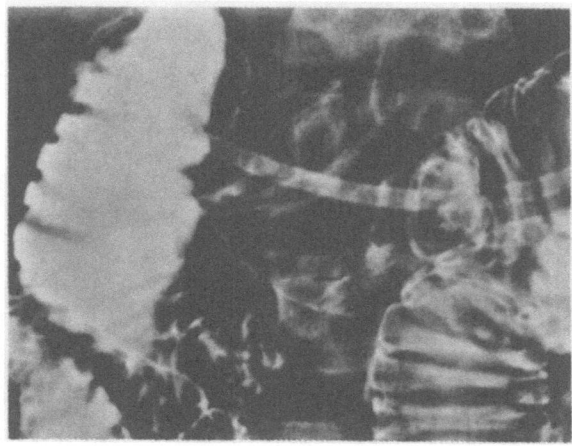

Fig. IV.176. Temporary subileus phenomenon. The examination taken after hypotonia was induced showed a stream of contrast medium ± 5 cm long in the distal duodenum that started abruptly and ended in a portio-like configuration. Since the complaints disappeared and abnormalities were no longer seen during a follow-up examination, surgical intervention was not required.

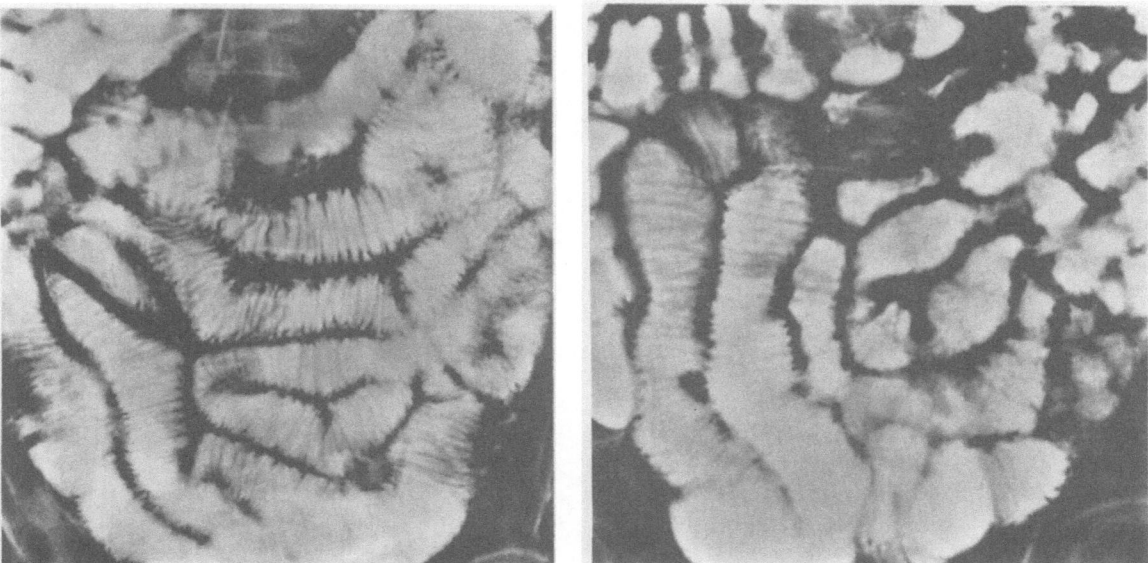

Fig. IV.177. Pancreatogenic steathorrea with some dilatation of the intestinal lumen without an increase in motility. (under the influence of drugs?). Since here the contrast fluid cannot be rapidly propelled distally, a marked flocculation develops within several minutes (right).

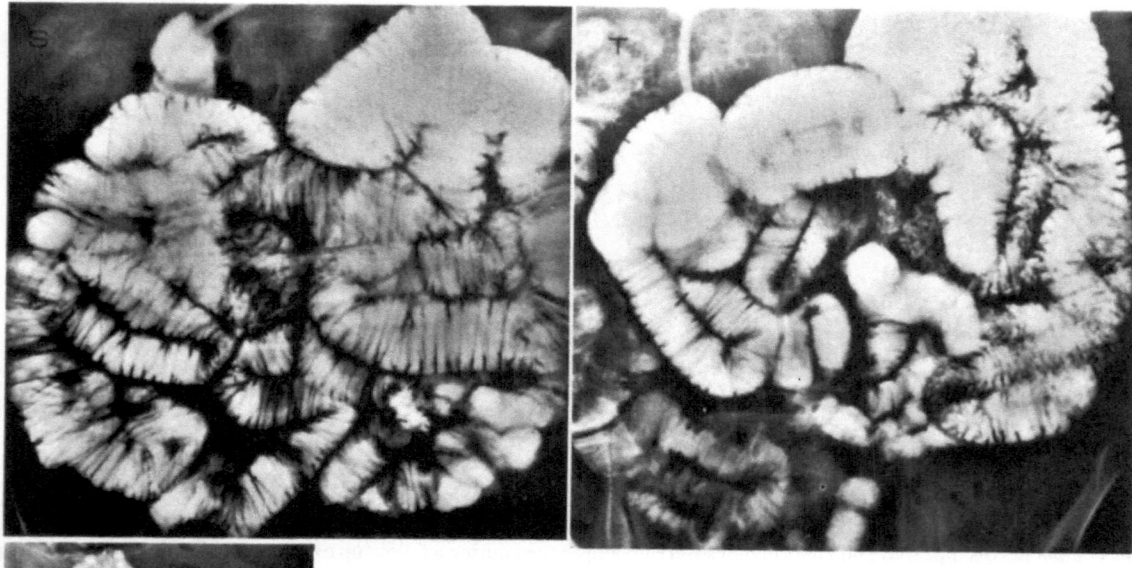

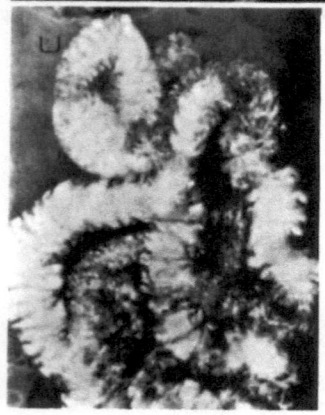

Fig. IV.178. ((s) Moderately pronounced atony of the small intestine from prolonged medication with tranquillizers. Because the patient complained of recurrent attacks of abdominal pain, antispasmodics were prescribed and the complaints *increased*. (T) All drug therapy was discontinued for three months; at the end of this period some improvement in the motility could be observed. Subjectively, however, the complaints had diminished considerably. In the first examination, 1300 ml of contrast fluid were required to reach the cecum; the subsequent examination was performed with only 900 ml. (U) 1½ years later, a follow-up examination showed that peristalsis and the calibre of the intestine had become completely normal. Experience has shown that an improvement in motility always precedes normalization of the tone of the intestine. The patient's complaints almost invariably subside before radiological improvement is noted.

Fig. IV.179. In rare cases a diminished peristalsis in the ileum can arise from chronic use of laxatives. In the classic case, atrophy of the fold relief is seen that extends to the cecum. Moreover, dilatation is not as pronounced as in patients using anti-spasmodics. In the beginning of the examination, contractions in the jejunum are completely normal; this was also the case in this patient. As soon as large quantities of contrast fluid are required to reach the cecum (here 1000 ml barium suspension followed by 1000 ml water), the loops in the jejunum also became dilated and peristalsis decreased (entero-enteral reflex mechanism).

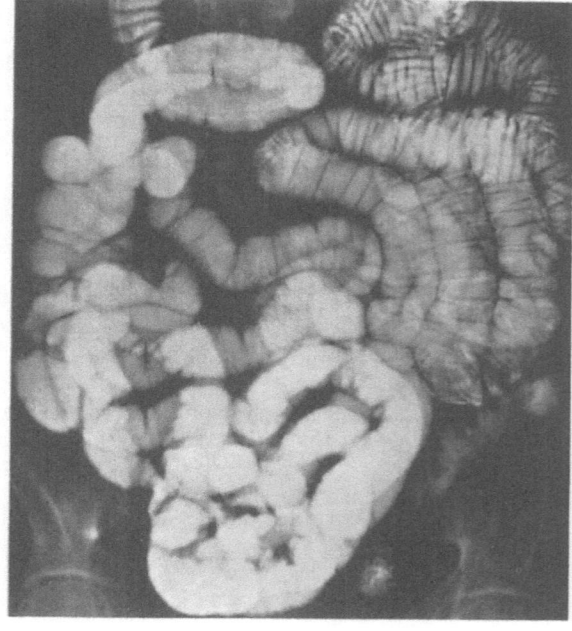

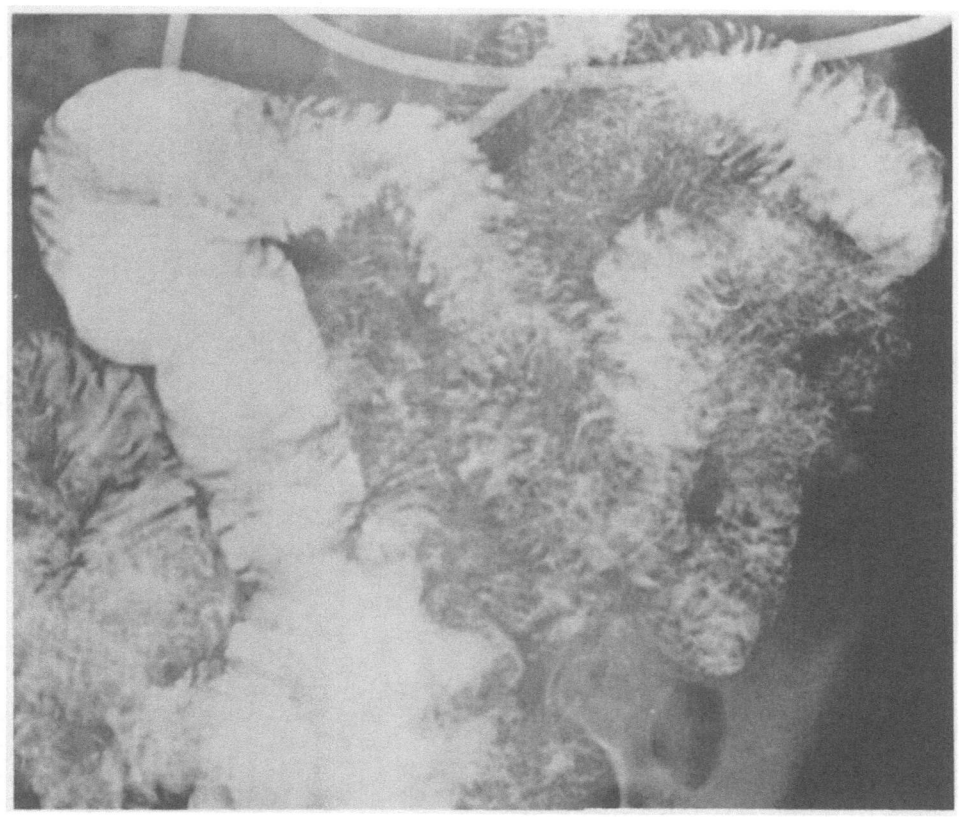

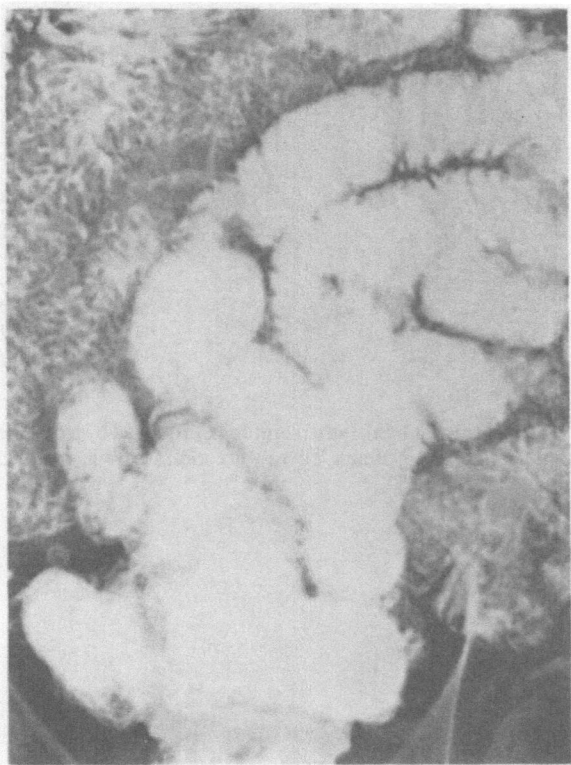

Fig. IV.180. Transplantation patient who had complained of diarrhea for two weeks. The röntgen examination showed an obvious dilatation of the jejunum and ileum together with hypermotility and a pronounced tendency to flocculation of the contrast medium. On the basis of these findings the diagnosis of celiac disease was established; this was subsequently confirmed by biopsy.

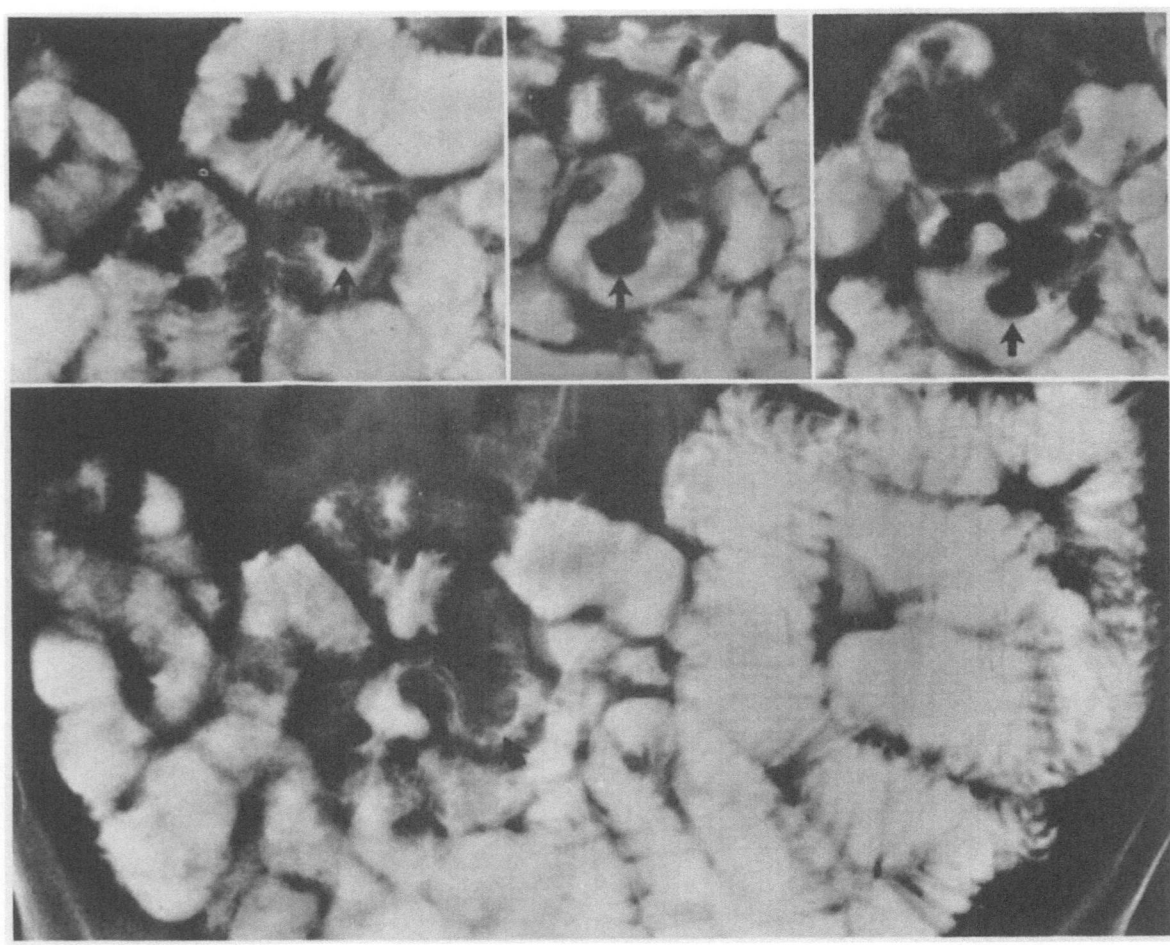

Fig. IV.181. Intestine with very local hypermotility and high tone (narrow lumen) due to serotonin, produced by a carcinoid. The marble-sized space (arrows) seen next to the lumen must be the small tumor. There were metastases in the liver.

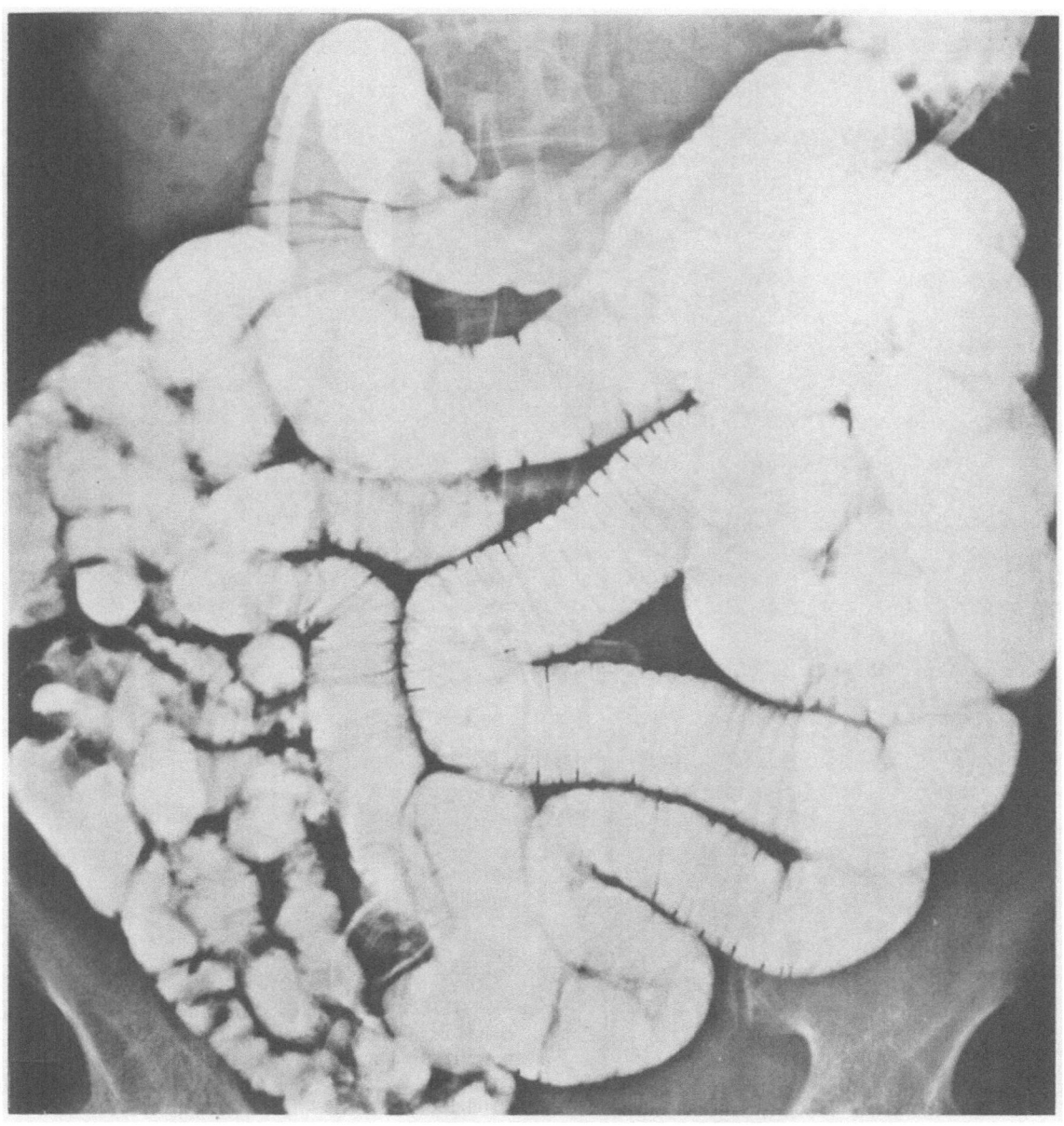

Fig. IV.182. A 57-year-old woman with invalidating 'stomach' cramps as a result of a severe drug-induced atony of the small bowel. There is pronounced dilatation with a local lack of peristalsis in the jejunum. The ileum appears practically normal. Dilatation of the ileum is seen only in the more severe cases that are called 'paralytic ileus'.

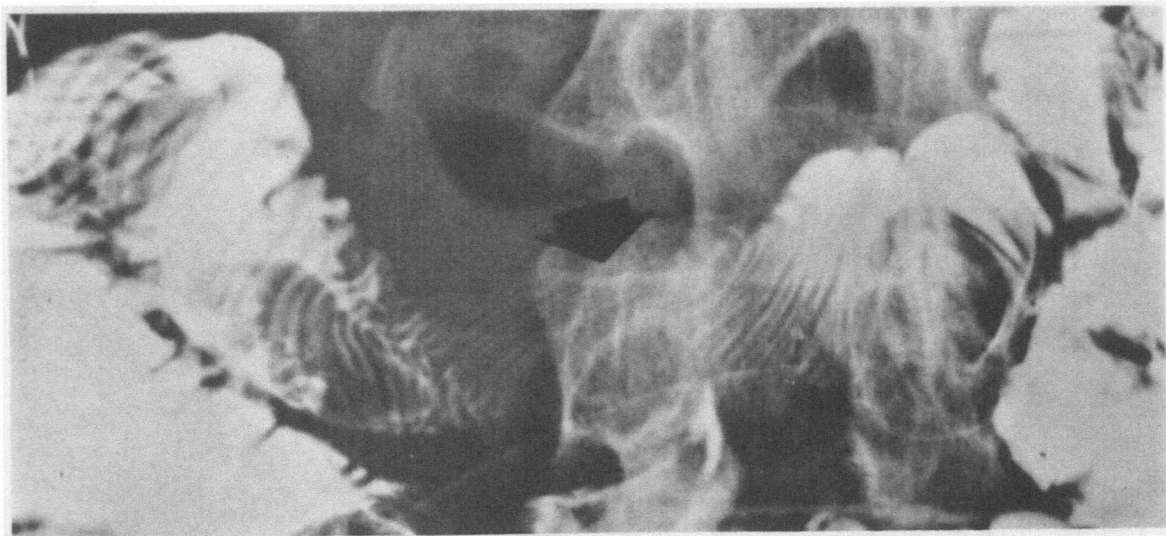

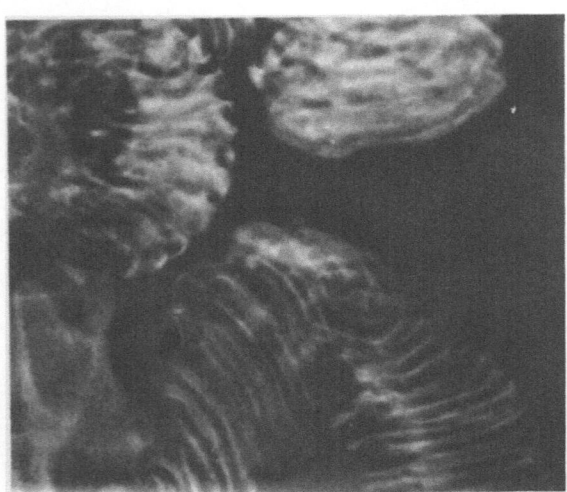

Fig. IV.183. (A): Stretched and more or less parallel mucosal folds in a rather long segment (± 10 cm) of the small bowel, caused by a leiomyosarcoma. (B): Misleading pattern resembling leiomyoma due to local compression of the intestinal loops.